Norbert Rietbrock
Barry G. Woodcock (Eds.)

Balanced Alpha/Beta Blockade of Adrenoceptors

Balancierte Blockade von Alpha- und Beta-Adrenozeptoren

Norbert Rietbrock, Barry G. Woodcock (Eds.)

Methods in Clinical Pharmacology
Number 5

Balanced Alpha/Beta Blockade of Adrenoceptors

A rational therapeutic concept in the treatment
of hypertension and coronary heart disease

Balancierte Blockade von Alpha- und Beta-Adrenozeptoren

Ein rationales Konzept zur Behandlung der
Hypertonie und der koronaren Herzerkrankungen

Springer Fachmedien Wiesbaden GmbH

The Editors

Norbert Rietbrock is Professor of Clinical Pharmacology, *Barry G. Woodcock* is Senior Lecturer in Clinical Pharmacology, University Clinic, Frankfurt am Main, Federal Republic of Germany

Set by Vieweg, Braunschweig
Produced by Lengericher Handelsdruckerei, Lengerich

ISBN 978-3-528-07922-2   ISBN 978-3-663-20205-9 (eBook)
DOI 10.1007/978-3-663-20205-9

Balanced alpha/beta blockade

Balanced alpha/beta blockade is;
Not only alpha blockade,
Not only beta blockade.
Not too little of alpha with beta
and
Not too little of beta with alpha;
but enough of each to bring out the
Therapeutic advantages of both.

The Editors

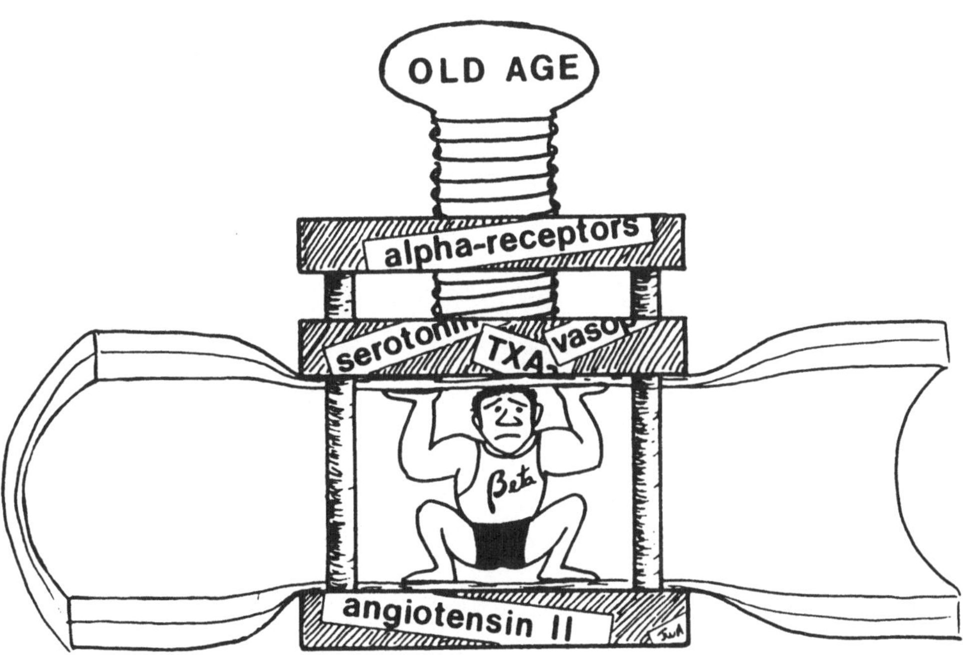

... „Perhaps it was best summed up for the arterial vascular system in a cartoon drawn by my former Lilly colleague, Dr. James Aiken (now with Upjohn Company) and reproduced on this page. In it, the worn out beta receptor system is fighting a losing battle with age to maintain vessel patency in the fact of an army of vaso-constrictors."
(Fleisch, J. H., TIPS, **2**, 337—339, 1981)

Contents / Inhaltsverzeichnis

IV Balanced Alpha/Beta Blockade in the Therapy of Coronary Heart Disease

I Clinical Pharmacology of Balanced Alpha/Beta Blockade

Das ideale Antihypertensivum – Wunschdenken und Wirklichkeit

D. Palm
Zentrum der Pharmakologie, Klinikum der Johann Wolfgang Goethe-Universität, Theodor-Stern-Kai 7, D-6000 Frankfurt/Main, FRG

Einleitung

Die Pharmakotherapie der Hypertonie hat in den vergangenen 30 Jahren geradezu atemberaubende Fortschritte gemacht. Nachdem die Risiken des hohen Blutdrucks hinsichtlich erhöhter Morbidität und Mortalität (Übersicht bei [25]) bekannt geworden waren, hat die antihypertensive Pharmakotherapie den Beweis dafür erbracht, daß eine Senkung der erhöhten Blutdruckwerte auch das Risiko, eine Sekundärerkrankung zu erleiden, trotz Weiterbestehens des Grundleidens zu senken vermag (Übersicht bei [26]).
Als anfangs der fünfziger Jahre der Ganglienblocker Hexamethonium in die Therapie der rasch zum Tode führenden malignen Hypertonie eingeführt wurde [15, 20], konnten erstmals lebensbedrohende Zustände mit hohem Blutdruck erfolgreich behandelt werden. Allerdings nahmen diese Patienten die lebensrettende therapeutische Maßnahme auf Kosten schwerer Nebenwirkungen in Kauf.
Als zwischen 1950 und 1960 Hydralazin, Reserpin und die ersten Thiadiazid-Diuretika, Anfang der 60er Jahre Methyldopa und Guanethidin Eingang in die Therapie fanden [15, 20], konnten — auf Grund der Wirksamkeit dieser Arzneimittel, aber auch auf Grund einer wesentlich höheren Nutzen/Risiko-Relation — hohe Patienten-Zahlen auch mit nicht lebensbedrohlichen Blutdruckwerten erfolgreich behandelt werden. Der Nachweis einer gesicherten Senkung von Morbidität und Mortalität (zerebrovaskuläre Ereignisse, Myokard-Insuffizienz, Niereninsuffizienz) konnte in zahlreichen kontrollierten Studien [25, 26] geführt werden.
Fraglich ist jedoch nach wie vor, ob auch die Häufigkeit der Ereignisse auf Grund einer koronaren Herzkrankheit durch eine konsequente antihypertensive Therapie gesenkt werden kann [1, 3, 17, 32]. Verbunden damit stellt sich auch die Frage: „Sollen oder dürfen" auch Patienten mit diastolischen Drücken $\leqslant$ 100 mm Hg behandelt werden, mit dem Ziel, Folgeerkrankungen zu verhindern? Das „Australian Therapeutic Trial in Mild Hypertension" [39] besagt, daß pro 1000 Patienten mit milder Hypertonie nur 2 Todesfälle verhindert werden können.
Bedeutet dies — eine scheinbare Binsenwahrheit —, daß die therapeutische Wirksamkeit zahlenmäßig geringer wird, wenn das Risiko auf Grund niedriger Blutdruckwerte geringer wird? Oder wiegen bei jahrzehntelanger Therapie der milden Hypertonie arzneimittelbedingte Risiken den Nutzen antihypertensiver Wirksamkeit auf?
In jüngster Zeit sind Zweifel laut geworden, ob bestimmte Formen der antihypertensiven Therapie bei bestimmten Patienten-Kollektiven nicht nur nichts nützen, sondern eher schaden [1, 2, 17, 32]. Zahlen der MRFT-Studie (Tabelle 1) [44] könnten so gedeutet werden, daß die Zahl der Todesfälle auf Grund einer koronaren Herzerkrankung bei

Tabelle 1: Einzelergebnisse der MRFT-Studie [44]. — Das Risiko, einen Herzinfarkt zu erleiden, scheint bei Patienten mit niedrigen diastolischen Drücken (Ausgangswerte) oder bei Patienten mit EKG-Veränderungen durch intensive antihypertensive Therapie erhöht zu werden

Multiple Risk Factor Intervention Trial (1982)		
Initial	CHD Deaths per 1000	
Blood Pressure mmHg diast	Usual Care	Special Intervention
90—94	10.2	14.7
95—99	22.5	22.9
$\geqslant 100$	29.8	20.8
Normal ECG	20.7	15.8
Abnormal ECG	17.7	29.2

Tabelle 2: Kriterien der pharmakodynamischen und pharmakokinetischen Wirkungsqualitäten eines idealen Antihypertensivums

Criteria for an Ideal Antihypertensive Drug
Decrease of Peripheral Resistance (After Oral Application: Slow Onset, Long Duration [24h], No Tolerance) No Change in Cardiac Output No Impairment of Cardiovascular Reflex Regulation No Impairment of Renal Function No Side Effects (CNS, Impairment of Ionic and Metabolic Homeostasis) No Adverse Drug-Drug Interactions No Contraindications

niedrigen Ausgangswerten der diastolischen Drücke durch aggressive Therapie erhöht werden. Auch das Risiko von Patienten mit EKG-Veränderungen scheint durch die antihypertensive Therapie anzusteigen.

Die im Thema dieses Referates gestellte Frage scheint damit — zumindest partiell — negativ beantwortet zu sein. Führen wir eine kritische Bewertung der derzeit zur Verfügung stehenden Antihypertensiva an Hand der für ein „ideales Antihypertensivum" geltenden Kriterien (Tabellen 2 und 3) durch, so müssen wir ebenfalls „summa summarum" zu einem negativen Ergebnis kommen.

Derzeit existieren weltweit etwa 500—600 blutdrucksenkende Pharmaka [32]. Nur ein geringer Bruchteil davon hat auf Grund von blutdrucksenkender Wirksamkeit und einer relativ hohen Nutzen/Risiko-Relation Eingang in die Therapie gefunden. In Abb. 1 sind die in der Bundesrepublik Deutschland für die Indikation Hypertonie zugelassenen Arzneistoffe [56] dargestellt, sowie die tatsächlichen oder vermuteten Angriffspunkte in der Herz-Kreislauf-Regulation. Entsprechend den in Tabellen 2 und 3 vorgegebenen Kriterien können die *Antisympathotonika* vom Typ der α_2-Adrenozeptor-Agonisten

Tabelle 3: Kriterien der präventiven Wirkungsqualitäten eines idealen Antihypertensivums

Criteria for an Ideal Antihypertensive Drug
High Benefit/Risk Ratio (Mild Hypertension, Pregnancy) Protection against Secondary Events: e. g. Stroke, Cardiac Failure, CHD, Renal Failure, Atherosclerosis Inhibition of Platelet Aggregation and Thrombosis Effectiveness Independent of Age

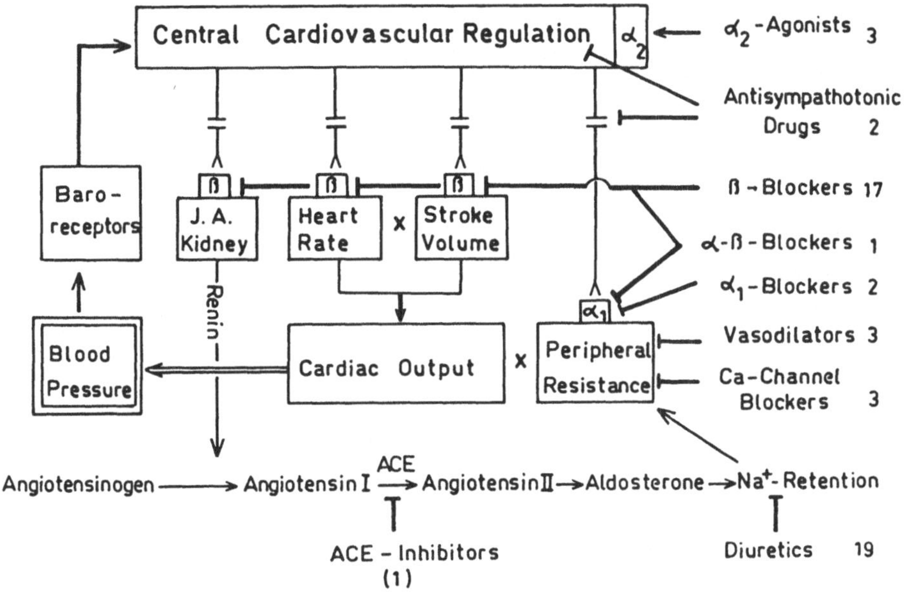

Abb. 1

Angriffspunkte von Antihypertensiva. Zahlen = Derzeitiger Stand in der BRD [56] α_2-Agonisten: Clonidin, Guanfacin, Methyldopa (bzw. α-Methylnoradrenalin). Antisympathotonika: Reserpin (zentral und peripher wirkend), Guanethidin (peripher wirkend). β-Rezeptorenblocker (relativ β_1-selektiv wirkende, solche mit partiell agonistischer Wirkung, nicht-selektiv wirkend); α-β-Rezeptorenblocker: Labetalol; α_1-Blocker: Prazosin, Urapidil; Vasodilatatoren: Hydralazin, Dihydralazin, Minoxidil; Diuretika: Thiadiazid-Derivate, Indapamid, Schleifendiuretika, K-sparende Diuretika; ACE-Inhibitoren: Captopril.

zwar auf Grund ihres Wirkungsmechanismus, nicht jedoch auf Grund ihrer zentral-nervösen unerwünschten Wirkungen, als ideale Antihypertensiva angesehen werden. Reserpin und Guanethidin scheiden ebenfalls auf Grund ihres Nebenwirkungsspektrums aus. Denn sie beeinträchtigen „Befindlichkeit" und Kreislaufregulation. Ideale Antihypertensiva sind sicherlich auch nicht die *Vasodilatatoren* vom Typ des Dihydralazin und Minoxidil, da sie auf Grund starker kardiovaskulärer Gegenregulation über den Barorezeptorenreflex zu schweren Nebenwirkungen führen. Sie können daher nur in der Kombination mit β-Rezeptorenblockern und Diuretika Verwendung finden.

Derzeit (noch?) gelten als Standard-Therapeutika der 1. Wahl, weil als „relativ ideal" angesehen, Diuretika und β-Rezeptorenblocker.

Diuretika

Diese Arzneimittel schienen bislang die Antihypertensiva mit der größten therapeutischen Breite zu sein. Ihre Anwendung beruhte auf rein empirischer Basis. Sie waren wirksam, wurden relativ gut toleriert, zeigten keine Toleranz der Wirkung und schienen oder sind unverzichtbar in der Kombinationstherapie mit anderen Antihypertensiva, die zu Na^+- und Wasserretention führen (Tabelle 4).

Tabelle 4: Erwünschte und unerwünschte Wirkungen von Diuretika (TPR = total peripheral resistance; PRA = plasma renin activity)

Diuretics	
Advantages	Disadvantages
Decrease in TPR	PRA ↑
Effective in mild hypertension (50%)	Serum-Urate ↑
	Serum-Calcium ↑
Well tolerated	Serum-Potassium ↓
No CNS-side effects	Plasma-Triglycerides ↑
Effective in combination therapy	Plasma-Cholesterol ↑
	Glucose-Tolerance ↓

⌐ ⌐ Cardiac risk factors

Den scheinbar idealen Wirkungen steht jedoch eine Reihe unerwünschter, vor allem metabolischer Wirkungen entgegen. Die Erniedrigung des Serum-Kaliums bringt die Gefahr einer erhöhten Inzidenz von u. U. tödlichem Kammerflimmern mit sich [45]. Die Morgan-Studie [43] machte wahrscheinlich, daß die Inzidenz tödlicher Herzinfarkte in einer Gruppe von nur mit hohen Dosen von Chlorothiazid behandelten Patienten deutlich höher gegenüber anderen Gruppen antihypertensiv behandelter Patienten (Abb. 2) war. Als kardiale Risikofaktoren müssen zusätzlich die Störungen des Lipid-Stoffwechsels angesehen werden (Tabelle 5), die wahrscheinlich durch alle derzeit zur Verfügung stehenden Thiazid-Diuretika ausgelöst werden [1, 2, 14, 17, 27, 30, 31, 42, 49, 57]. Ob Indapamid tatsächlich eine Ausnahmestellung einnimmt [49], bedarf weiterer Bestätigung. Die Störungen des Lipidstoffwechsels sind dosisabhängig und nehmen mit der Behandlungsdauer offensichtlich zu [49]. Wenn man akzeptiert, daß eine Erhöhung des Serumcholesterol um 10 mg/dl ein um 15 % erhöhtes kardiales Risiko mit sich bringt, so stellt sich die Frage, ob nicht die therapeutische Wirksamkeit der Thiadiazid-Diuretika durch Blutdrucksenkung bei langjähriger Therapie durch ein erhöhtes kardiales Risiko zumindest teilweise aufgehoben wird. In jüngster Zeit ist daher mehrfach die Frage aufgetaucht, ob der nur marginale Erfolg oder gar Mißerfolg zahlreicher Studien [1, 2, 31], die Folgen einer koronaren Herzkrankheit durch intensive antihypertensive Therapie zu verhindern, nicht darauf zurückzuführen ist, daß hohe (!) Dosen von Diuretika oft zur Monotherapie, fast immer in kombinierter Therapie mit anderen Antihypertensiva verwendet wurden. Zumindest scheint deutlich zu werden, daß die Progredienz der koronaren Herzkrankheit durch Diuretika weniger deutlich aufgehalten werden kann, als es

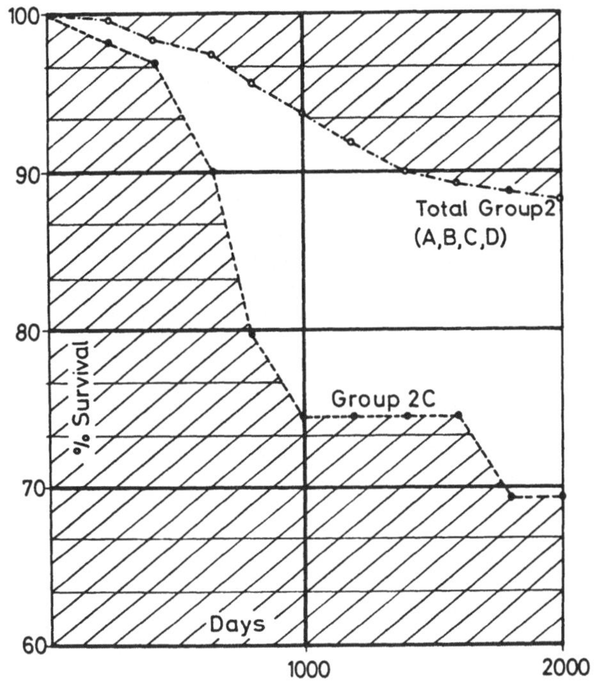

Abb. 2
Geringere Überlebensrate einer nur mit 1−2×500 mg/Tag Chlorothiazid behandelten Patientengruppe (2C) gegenüber der Gesamtgruppe (unbehandelt, mit Kochsalzrestriktion, Diuretika + Methyldopa). Daten nach [43].

Tabelle 5: Wirkungen von Diuretika auf den Lipidstoffwechsel.

Effects of Diuretics on Serum Lipids after 12 Months Treatment (Changes in mg/dl)		
	Hydrochlorothiazide	Chlorthalidone
Triglycerides	+ 39[*]	+ 36[*]
Cholesterol	+ 12[*]	+ 15[*]
HDL-Cholesterol	− 1	+ 1
Diastolic Blood Pressure (mm Hg)	− 7[*]	− 13[*]

From Ames and Hill (1982) [2]   [*] = statistisch signifikant

ihrer antihypertensiven Wirksamkeit entspricht. Es stellt sich allerdings die Frage, warum in allen bisherigen Studien Hydrochlorothiazid oder Chlortalidon in einer Tagesdosis von ≥ 50–100 mg verwendet wurden! Logisch erscheint es, daß auf Grund der „nicht-idealen" Eigenschaften der Diuretika derzeit verschiedentlich darauf hingewiesen wird, diese Antihypertensiva erst als Mittel der 2. oder 3. Wahl in der Stufentherapie der Hypertonie einzusetzen [9, 10].

β-Rezeptorenblocker

Auf Grund ihrer sicheren antihypertensiven Wirksamkeit und — bei Beachtung der Kontraindikationen — weitgehend fehlenden unerwünschten Wirkungen sind β-Rezeptorenblocker in zahlreichen Ländern die Antihypertensiva der 1. Stufe (Tabelle 6). Ein Grund hierfür ist auch die zusätzliche Wirksamkeit bei Angina pectoris und tachykarden Arrhythmien. Es ist von herausragender Bedeutung und rückt die β-Rezeptorenblocker in die Nähe idealer Antihypertensiva, daß mehrfach ihre eindeutige kardioprotektive Wirksamkeit in Bezug auf die Sekundärprävention nach Herzinfarkt nachgewiesen werden konnte [23]. Der sichere Nachweis der Primärpräventation steht zwar noch aus [4]; das Ergebnis zweier noch nicht abgeschlossener Studien muß abgewartet werden [42, 59].

Tabelle 6: Erwünschte und unerwünschte Wirkungen von β-Rezeptorenblockern

β-Adrenoceptor Blocking Drugs	
Advantages	Disadvantages
Effective in mild hypertension (~ 60%)	Contraindications
	Cardiac output $\quad\downarrow\uparrow$?
No postural hypotension	
No CNS-side effects	Peripheral resistance $\uparrow\downarrow$?
PRA $\downarrow$	Less effect in the elderly
No volume expansion	Serum triglycerides $\uparrow$
Effective in combination therapy	HDL-Serum cholesterol $\downarrow$
Antianginal and antiarrhythmic effects	Cardiac risk factors?
Primary cardioprotection?	
Secondary cardioprotection	

Ideale antihypertensive Wirkungsqualitäten sind sicherlich *nicht*:
1. der zumindest initiale Abfall des Herzzeitvolumens mit reflektorisch ansteigendem peripheren Gefäßwiderstand. Beide Veränderungen sollen zwar nach Wochen und Monaten „adaptiv" zur Norm zurückkehren [7, 40, 55]. Ob dies jedoch für alle Patienten zutrifft, muß in Zweifel gezogen werden. Lund-Johansen [37] konnte zeigen, daß trotz ausgeprägter Blutdrucksenkung nach 1- und 5-jähriger Therapie mit Atenolol der periphere Gefäßwiderstand über dem bereits erhöhten Ausgangsniveau, das Herzzeitvolumen jedoch gegenüber den Ausgangswerten gesenkt war.
2. Im Gegensatz zu anderen Antihypertensiva (z. B. Methyldopa, Reserpin, Prazosin, Labetalol) führen β-Rezeptorenblocker zu Störungen im Lipid-Stoffwechsel [2, 14, 17, 18, 30, 31, 49, 50]. Im Gegensatz zu den Thiadiazid-Diuretika nimmt zwar die Konzentration des Gesamt-Cholesterol im Serum nicht zu, wohl aber die Konzentrationen der Triglyceride und der VLDL-Fraktion bei tendenziell absinkender HDL-Fraktion (Tabelle 7). Die Abklärung, inwieweit relativ β_1-selektive β-Rezeptorenblocker (Atenolol, Metoprolol [50]), β-Rezeptorenblocker mit partiell agonistischer Wir-

Tabelle 7: Wirkungen von β-Rezeptorenblockern auf den Lipidstoffwechsel

Effects of Beta-Adrenoceptor Blocking Drugs on Serum Lipids	
Total Cholesterol	∅
Triglycerides	↑
VLDL-Fraction	↑
HDL-Fraction	↓
LDL-Fraction	∅

kung (Pindolol [35]) oder das nicht-selektive Nadolol „idealere" weil „lipid-neutralere"[14] Antihypertensiva sind und, ob die Lipidstoffwechselstörungen tatsächlich die Nutzen-Risiko-Relation dieser Pharmakon-Klasse verschlechtern [17, 30, 33], bedarf einer dringlichen Abklärung in gut kontrollierten Langzeit-Studien.

„Idealere" Anwendung von Antihypertensiva

Es ist auffallend, daß zumindest im Initialstadium ihrer Anwendung fast alle Antihypertensiva zu hoch dosiert wurden. Nach wie vor werden im ausländischen aber auch im deutschen Schrifttum für Hydrochlorothiazid oder Chlortalidon Tagesdosen von 50—100 mg empfohlen. Beide Diuretika sind schon in einer Dosis von 12,5 mg bzw. 25 mg/Tag nahezu maximal blutdrucksenkend wirksam (Abb. 3); höhere Dosen erbringen keine zusätzliche Blutdrucksenkung; sie führen hingegen zu dem Auftreten unerwünschter Wirkungen, wie Hypokaliämie u.a. (vgl. Abb. 3, rechts) [5, 11, 38, 41].
Propranolol wurde in Tagesdosen bis zu 1 g empfohlen. Von Serlin et al. [51] hingegen werden 2 × 40 − 2 × 80 mg/Tag als nahezu maximal wirkend angesehen.
Im Falle des Captopril (s. ACE-Hemmstoffe) wurden zunächst Dosen von > 600 mg/Tag verwendet; die heutigen Empfehlungen lauten auf 2 × 12,5 − 2 × 50 mg/Tag. Es ist absehbar, daß bei dieser Dosierung und ausreichender Wirksamkeit auch die Häufigkeit der schweren Nebenwirkungen dieses Antihypertensivums, die zur Einstufung von Captopril als „Antihypertensivum für sonst therapie-refraktäre Fälle" geführt hat, in den Hintergrund treten. Für Clonidin ist vor kurzem gezeigt worden, daß die zur optimalen Blutdrucksenkung notwendigen Dosen in einem Bereich (∼ 2 × 150 μg/Tag) lagen, der zu einer Konzentration im Plasma von 1−2 ng/ml führte [19]. Höhere Dosen waren von keiner stärkeren Blutdrucksenkung, wohl aber von häufiger auftretenden und stärkeren unerwünschten Wirkungen gefolgt.
Es ist eine pharmakologische Binsenwahrheit, daß die Nutzen/Risiko-Relation eines Pharmakons mit steigender Dosis abnimmt. Dies wurde in der Therapie der Hypertonie bislang nicht oder zu wenig beachtet.
Nur sehr zögernd scheint sich durchgesetzt zu haben, daß niedrigere Dosierungen bei Anwendung einer sinnvollen und nicht starren Kombination (z. B. β-Rezeptorenblocker + Diuretikum + Vasodilator = additive blutdrucksenkende Wirkung) wirksamer sind auf Grund fehlender bzw. blockierter gegenregulatorischer Prozesse. In der Vergangenheit mußten schwere Nebenwirkungen bei der Hoch-Dosis-Therapie mit Dihydralazin (> 300 mg/Tag) in Kauf genommen werden. Durch die Kombination mit β-Rezeptorenblockern erfolgt die Ausschaltung der Gegenregulation; Dihydralazin wird dadurch als

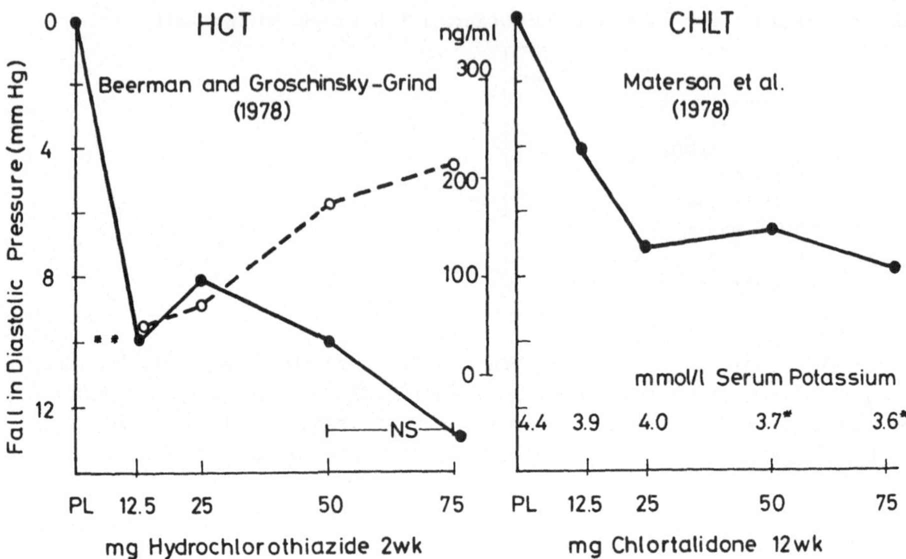

Abb. 3

Hydrochlorothiazid (HCT) bewirkt schon in einer Tagesdosis von 12,5 mg eine fast maximale Senkung des diastolischen Druckes (· —— ·). Höhere Dosen steigern zwar die Plasmakonzentrationen (o— —o); nicht aber die Drucksenkung [5]. Auch Chlortalidon erreicht schon bei 25 mg/Tag eine maximale Blutdruck senkende Wirkung. Höhere Dosen führen zu Hypokaliämie [41].

Antihypertensivum erst akzeptabel; das Diuretikum und der β-Rezeptorenblocker werden „idealer" wirkend. Ob das Prinzip der α- und β-Rezeptorenblockade + Gefäßerweiterung mit den 4 Labetalol-Isomeren ein akzeptables und idealeres Äquivalent dieser 3-fach-Kombination ist, wird die Diskussion dieses Symposiums erbringen.

Calzium-Kanal-Blocker

Ca-Kanalblocker vom Typ des Nifedipin oder Verapamil haben erst seit kurzem Eingang in die Therapie gefunden. Die endgültige Beurteilung ihres Stellenwertes ist daher noch nicht möglich. Sie werden allerdings bereits als Antihypertensiva der 1. Wahl diskutiert [8, 9, 10, 16, 22, 47]. Die Wirkungscharakteristik (Tabelle 8) im Hinblick auf die akut einsetzende und für die Therapiedauer anhaltende Senkung des peripheren Gefäßwiderstandes ohne − zumindest nach mehrwöchiger Therapie − wesentliche Gegenregulation seitens des sympatho-nervalen Systems, sowie die u. U. erwünschte antianginöse Begleitwirkung auf Grund einer Senkung des Preload, der coronaren Vasodilatation in Verbindung mit einer verbesserten Durchblutung subendocardialer Myokardschichten, scheinen sie in die Nähe der idealen Antihypertensiva zu rücken.

Ob sie tatsächlich in den vermuteten pathogenetischen Mechanismus der Hochdruckerkrankung − einer gesteigerten Konzentration freien Ca^{2+} im Intrazellulärraum − durch Hemmung des langsamen Ca^{2+}-Einstroms in die glatte Muskelzelle eingreifen [8, 9], ist m. E. bislang nur als ein Silberstreifen am Horizont zu diskutieren.

Tabelle 8: Erwünschte und unerwünschte Wirkungsqualitäten von Ca-Kanalblockern

Calcium Channel Blockers (Nifedipine, Verapamil)	
Advantages	Disadvantages
Peripheral resistance ↓ without persistent counterregulation	Short duration of action
Decrease in B.P. related to pretreatment value	Side effects:
No fluid retention	Flushing, headache, ankle oedema (N)
Antianginal action	Constipation (V)
Cardioprotection?	

Dasselbe trifft für eine mögliche, bislang jedoch nicht erwiesene kardioprotektive Wirkung zu. β-Rezeptorenblocker werden sicherlich zunächst die Antihypertensiva der 1. Stufe beim jugendlichen Hypertoniker mit einem erhöhten Herzzeitvolumen bleiben. Die Abnahme ihrer Wirksamkeit mit steigendem Lebensalter [8—10] führt jedoch zu der zunehmenden — und offensichtlich sinnvollen — Verwendung von Ca-Kanalblockern beim älteren Menschen mit einer „low-renin-hypertension". Der Vorteil des Nifedipin als oral und sicher wirkendes Antihypertensivum beim krisenhaft und lebensbedrohlich erhöhten Blutdruck darf inzwischen als gesichert gelten. Sicherlich werden uns die nächsten Jahre eine Flut neuer antihypertensiv wirkender Ca-Kanalblocker bescheren, vor allem vom Dihydro-Pyridin-Typ [6, 29]. Es bedarf jedoch m. E. genauester Abklärung, welche Ca-Kanalblocker das idealere Wirkungsspektrum haben: Die überwiegend vasodilatatorisch wirksamen (z. B. Felodipin) oder die mehr „cardiospezifischen" vom Typ des Verapamil und Diltiazem (vgl. Abb. 4). Vor allem sollte es gelingen, die 24 Stunden anhaltende Wirkung vorzugsweise durch Modifizierung der chemischen Struktur (Metabolismusresistent!) und nicht durch galenische Retardierung zu gewährleisten, die eine 1 X Tagesdosis ermöglicht.

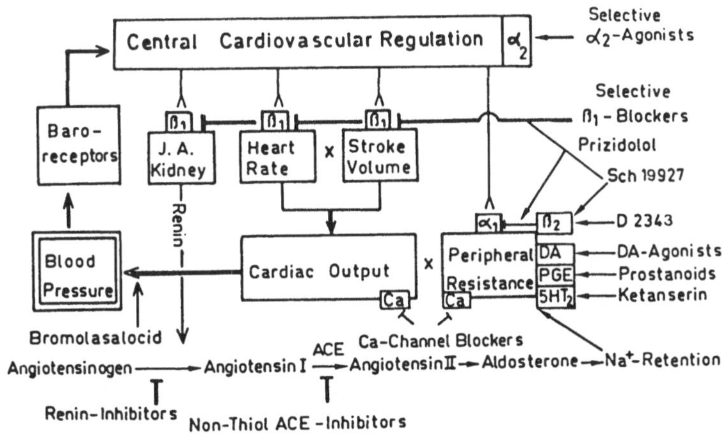

Abb. 4

Angriffspunkte neuer, noch nicht im Handel befindlicher Antihypertensiva (J. A.: Juxtaglomerulärer Apparat; DA: Dopamin-Rezeptoren). Weitere Einzelheiten siehe Text.

Angiotensin I-Converting-Enzyme(ACE)-Inhibitoren

Als jüngster Durchbruch der Pharmakotherapie der Hypertonie kann die Entwicklung der ACE-Inhibitoren bezeichnet werden [24, 53]. Es ist nicht gesichert, ob die Hemmung des Angiotensin II-bildenden Enzyms den alleinigen blutdrucksenkenden Mechanismus darstellt.

Auf Grund der in Tabelle 9 dargestellten Qualitäten der erwünschten Wirkungen — nahezu isolierte Erniedrigung des peripheren Gefäßwiderstandes — rückt auch das derzeit als einziger ACE-Inhibitor in der BRD verfügbare Captopril schon jetzt in die Nähe eines idealen Antihypertensivums [53]. Das ursprüngliche Verdikt der Gesundheitsbehörden, demzufolge Captopril nur bei der Therapie sonst therapierefraktärer Fälle indiziert sei, kann heute, nach Anwendung sehr niedriger Dosen sicherlich nicht mehr aufrecht erhalten werden [13, 53]. Es steht zu hoffen, daß die Häufigkeit des Auftretens einer Neutropenie (Häufigkeit mit 0.02 % vergleichbar derjenigen nach Behandlung mit Phenothiazinen, Phenytoin, Hydralazin u.a. [13]) mit der jetzt empfohlenen Niedrig-Dosierung weiter zurückgeht.

Patienten mit eingeschränkter Nierenfunktion sollten trotzdem noch als Risikopatienten für Captopril eingestuft werden und einer laufenden Blutbildkontrolle unterzogen werden [13].

Sollte es sich bewahrheiten, daß die neuen Non-Thiol-ACE-Inhibitoren (z. B. Enalapril [34, 54], CGS 13945, [28], RHC 3659 u.a.) (vgl. Abb. 4) die typischen unerwünschten Penicillamin-Wirkungen nicht besitzen, wäre der Schritt zum idealen Antihypertensivum nicht mehr weit.

Tabelle 9: Erwünschte und unerwünschte Wirkungsqualitäten von Angiotensin I — Converting — Enzyme (ACE)-Inhibitoren

ACE-Inhibitors (Captopril)	
Advantages	Disadvantages
Effective in all forms of hypertension	Penicillamine-like side effects
(± Diuretic)	e.g. rash, fever, disturbance of taste, leucopenia, proteinuria
TPR ↓	
Cardiac output ~ ⌀	(Presumably avoidable by using non-thiol ACE-inhibitors; e.g. Enalapril)
Aldosterone secretion ↓	
Less side effects at low dosage (< 150 mg/d)	

Ideale Antihypertensiva in der Zukunft

Wenn die Wirkungsqualitäten der bislang besprochenen Antihypertensiva an den Kriterien der Tabellen 1 und 2 gemessen werden, wird deutlich, daß „das ideale Antihypertensivum" bislang nicht existent ist. Bei den in den vergangenen Jahren eingeführten Antihypertensiva ist zwar die Nutzen/Risiko-Relation deutlich angestiegen. M. E. nähert sich schon jetzt die Entwicklung asymptotisch einem erzielbaren Optimum. Eine we-

sentliche Weiterentwicklung ist in den nächsten 10 Jahren nicht zu erwarten. Es wird eine „Entwicklung der kleinen Schritte" sein, die zum Ziel hat, nicht stark blutdrucksenkende Pharmaka, sondern zur Behandlung der Grenzwert-Hypertonie und milden Hypertonie geeignete Arzneistoffe zu schaffen [15, 21], Arzneistoffe mit dem möglichst geringen Risiko subjektiv empfundener und objektiv nachweisbarer unerwünschter Wirkungen. Neue Antihypertensiva (Abb. 4) sollten eine höhere Affinität als bislang an Rezeptoren und/oder Akzeptoren haben, wodurch eine höhere Selektivität der erwünschten Wirkungen erzielt werden könnte. Es wäre wünschenswert, wenn z.B. künftige α_2-Adrenozeptoragonisten den zentral ausgelösten blutdrucksenkenden Effekt ohne sedierende Wirkungen (und ohne periphere α_1-agonistische Wirkungen) ausüben könnten; durch β_1-Rezeptorenblocker mit höherer Selektivität und Affinität könnten die unerwünschten, durch Hemmung von β_2-Adrenozeptoren ausgelösten Wirkungen (Kontraindikation Asthma bronchiale!) vermieden werden. Es bleibt abzuwarten, inwieweit Monosubstanzen mit dualistischen Wirkungsqualitäten (Prizidolol = vasodilatierender β-Rezeptorenblocker [52]; Sch 19927-β_1-Rezeptorenblocker mit β_2-agonistischer Wirkung [3]; D 2342 — ein α_1-Rezeptorenblocker mit β_2-agonistischer Wirksamkeit [46]) von Vorteil gegenüber den seitherigen α- und β-Rezeptorenblockern sind. Ketanserin vereinigt die Wirkungsqualitäten eines 5-HT$_2$ und α_1-Rezeptorenblockers [58]. Ob gefäßerweiternde Prostanoide vom Typ stabiler PGE$_2$-Derivate [12] Vorteile gegenüber den derzeit gebräuchlichen Vasodilatatoren vom Typ des Dihydralazin oder Endralazin haben (z. B. nach percutaner Applikation) erscheint zweifelhaft. Neu ist der Versuch, mit Dopamin-Agonisten ohne α- und β-agonistische Wirkungen entweder nur die renale Strombahn oder auch das gesamte arterioläre Widerstandssystem über Dopamin$_1$-Rezeptoren zu erweitern [36]. Zentralnervöse Begleiterscheinungen werden über ihre Brauchbarkeit entscheiden. Bromlasalocid stellt den ersten Versuch dar, die noch hypothetische pathogenetische Umverteilung in Ca^{2+}-Kompartimenten der glatten Muskulatur zu beseitigen [48].
Der Wunsch nach einem idealen Arzneimittel ist so alt wie die Geschichte der Menschheit. Wir werden uns damit abfinden müssen, daß derzeit nur wenige Silberstreifen am Horizont der idealen antihypertensiven Therapie sichtbar werden.

Literatur

[1] Ames, R. P.: Negative effects of diuretic drugs on metabolic risk factors for coronary heart disease: possible alternative therapy. *Amer. Heart J.* 51, 632−638 (1983).

[2] Ames, R. P., Hill, P.: Antihypertensive therapy and the risk of coronary heart disease. *J. Cardiovasc. Pharmacol.* 4 (Suppl. 2), 206−212 (1982).

[3] Baum, T., Sybertz, E. J.: Antihypertensive actions of an isomer of labetalol and other vasodilator-β-adrenoceptor blockers. *Fed. Proc.* 42, 176−181 (1983).

[4] Berglund, G., Wilhelmsen, L., Sannerstedt, R., Hansson, L., Andersson, O., Sivertsson, R., Wedel, H., Wikstrand, J.: Coronary heart disease after treatment of hypertension. *Lancet* I, 1−5 (1978).

[5] Beermann, B., Groschinsky-Grind, M.: Antihypertensive effect of various doses of hydrochlorothiazide and its relation to the plasma level of the drug. *Europ. J. clin. Pharmacol.* 13, 195−201 (1978).

[6] Braunwald, E.: Mechanism of action of calcium-channel blocking agents. *New Engl. J. Med.* 307, 1518−1627 (1982).

[7] Breckenridge, A.: Which beta blocker? *Brit. Med. J.* 286, 1085−1088 (1983).

[8] Bühler, F. R.: Renin, renin inhibition and antihypertensive therapy. *Clin. Exp. Hypert.* — A5, 1395−1407 (1983).

[9] Bühler, F. R.: Age and cardiovascular response adaptation. Determinants of an antihypertensive treatment concept primarily based on beta-blockers and calcium entry blockers. *Hypertension* 5 (Suppl. II), 94−98 (1983).

[10] Bühler, F. R., Hulthén, L.: Calcium channel blockers: a pathophysiologically based antihypertensive treatment concept for the future. *Europ. J. Clin. Invest.* **12**, 1–3 (1982).

[11] Carney, S., Gilles, A. I., Morgan, T.: Optimal dose of a thiazide diuretic. *Med. J. Aust.* **2**, 692–693 (1976).

[12] Chan, P. S., Cervoni, P., Ronsberg, M. A., Accomando, R. C., Quirk, G. J., Scully, P. A., Lipchuk, L. M.: Antihypertensive activity of dl-15-deoxy-16-hydroxy-16(α/β)-vinyl prostaglandin E_2 methylester (Cl 115, 347), a new orally and transdermally long-acting antihypertensive agent. *J. Pharmacol. Exp. Ther.* **226**, 726–732 (1983).

[13] Cooper, R. A.: Captopril-associated neutropenia. Who is at risk? *Arch. Int. Med.* **143**, 659–660 (1983).

[14] Cutler, R.: Effect of antihypertensive agents on lipid metabolism. *Amer. J. Cardiol.* **51**, 628–631 (1983).

[15] Dollery, C. T.: A clinican looks at the future. *Brit. J. Clin. Pharmacol.* **13**, 127–132 (1982).

[16] Doyle, A. E.: Hypertension and Ca-antagonists. *Clin. Exp. Pharmacol. Physiol.*, Suppl. 6, 103–106 (1982).

[17] Editorial: Antihypertensive drugs, plasma lipids, and coronary heart disease. *Lancet* II, 19–20 (1980).

[18] Eliasson, K., Lins, L.-E., Rössner, S.: Serum lipoprotein changes during atenolol treatment of essential hypertension. *Europ. J. Clin. Pharmacol.* **20**, 335–338 (1981).

[19] Frisk-Holmberg, M.: Plasma-Konzentration und Wirkungen von Clonidin bei leichter bis mittelschwerer Hypertonie. In: Hayduk, K., Bock, K. D. eds. *Zentrale Blutdruckregulation durch α_2-Rezeptorenstimulation.* pp. 115–118. Steinkopf Verlag Darmstadt (1983).

[20] Gifford, R. W.: Three decades of antihypertensive therapy. *Clin. Pharmacol. Ther.* **28**, 1–5 (1980).

[21] Gross, F.: Can we develop new drugs for hypertension. *Brit. J. Clin. Pharmacol.* **13**, 133–136 (1982).

[22] Guazzi, M. D., Polese, A., Fiorentini, C., Bartorelli, A., Morozzi, P.: Treatment of hypertension with calcium antagonists. *Hypertension* **5** (Suppl. II), 85–90 (1983).

[23] Hampton, J. R.: Should every survivor of a heart attack be given a beta-blocker? *Brit. Med. J.* **285**, 33–36 (1982).

[24] Hodsman, G. P., Robertson, J. I. S.: Captopril; five years on. *Brit. Med. J.* **287**, 851–852 (1983).

[25] Holzgreve, H.: Die Prognose der arteriellen Hypertonie und ihre Beeinflussung durch antihypertensive Therapie. *Internist* **22**, 156–161 (1981).

[26] Holzgreve, H.: Beeinflussung der Prognose durch antihypertensive Therapie pp. 3–14. In: Distler, A., Philipp, Th. (Hrsg.): *Neuere Entwicklungen in der Hochdrucktherapie.* F. K. Schattauer Verlag Stuttgart – New York (1983).

[27] Hubbell, F. A., Weber, M. A., Winer, R. L., Rose, D. E.: Biochemical cardiac risk factors during diuretic therapy. *Arch. Int. Pharmacodyn. Ther.* **256**, 123–133 (1982).

[28] Jacot des Combes, B., Turini, G. A., Brunner, H. R., Porchet, M., Chen, D. S., Sen, S. B.: CGS 13945: A new orally active angiotensin-converting enzyme inhibitor in normal volunteers. *J. Cardiovasc. Res.* **5**, 511–516 (1983).

[29] Janis, R. A., Triggle, D. J.: New developments in Ca^{2+} channel antagonists. *J. Med. Chem.* **26**, 775–785 (1983).

[30] Johnson, B. F.: The emerging problem of plasma lipid changes during antihypertensive therapy. *J. Cardiovasc. Res.* **4** (Suppl. 2), 213–221 (1982).

[31] Kaplan, N. M.: New approaches to the therapy of mild hypertension. *Amer. J. Cardiol.* **51**, 621–627 (1983).

[32] Kaplan, H. R., Ryan, M. J., Singer, R. M., Cohen, D. M., Cygan, R. M.: Survey of new antihypertensive drugs: 1982. *Fed. Proc.* **42**, 154–156 (1983).

[33] Kaune, P.: Bei Langzeitbehandlung der Hypertonie mit Beta-Blockern kein atherogenes Risiko. *Dtsch. Med. Wschr.* **107**, 757 (19882).

[34] de Leuw, P. W., Hoogma, R. P. L. M., van Soest, G. A. W., Tchang, P. T., Birkenhäger, W. H.: Humoral and renal effects of KM-421 (enalapril) in hypertensive subjects. *J. Cardiovasc. Pharmacol.* **5**, 731–736 (1983).

[35] Leren, P., Foss, O. P., Helgeland, A., Hjermann, I., Holme, I.: Effects of pindolol and hydrochlorothiazide on blood lipids – The Oslo study. *Clinical Trials J.* **18**, 254–261 (1981).

[36] Lokhandwala, M. F., Barrett, R. J.: Dopamine receptor agonists in cardiovascular therapy. *Drug Develop. Res.* **3**, 299–310 (1983).

[37] Lund-Johansen, P.: Hemodynamic consequences of long term beta-blocker therapy. A 5-year follow-up study of atenolol. *J. Cardiovasc. Pharmacol.* **1**, 487–495 (1979).

[38] MacGregor, G. A., Banks, R. A., Markandu, N. D., Bayliss, J., Roulston, J.: Lack of effect of beta-blocker on flat dose response to thiazide in hypertension: Efficacy of low dose thiazide combined with betablocker. *Brit. Med. J.* **286**, 1535–1538 (1983).

[39] Management Committee: The Australian Therapeutic Trial in Mild Hypertension. *Lancet* **I**, 1261–1267 (1980).

[40] Man In'T Veld, A. J., Schalekamp, M. A. D. H.: How intrinsic symphomimetic activity modulates the haemodynamic responses to β-adrenoceptor antagonists. A clue to the nature of their antihypertensive mechanism. *Brit. J. Clin. Pharmacol.* **13**, 245–257 (1983).

[41] Materson, B. J., Oster, J. R., Michael, U. F., Bolton, S. M., Burton, Z. C., Stambough, J. E., Morledge, J.: Dose response of chlorthalidone in patients with mild hypertension. Efficacy of a lower dose. *Clin. Pharmacol. Ther.* **24**, 192–198 (1978).

[42] Medical Research Council Working Party. Adverse reactions to bendroflumethiazide and propranolol for the treatment of mild hypertension. *Lancet* **II**, 539–542 (1981).

[43] Morgan, T. O., Adams, W. R., Hodgson, M., Gibberd, R. W.: Failure of therapy to improve prognosis in elderly males with hypertension. *Med. J. Austr.* **2**, 27–31 (1980).

[44] Multiple Risk Factor Intervention Trial Research Group: Multiple risk factor intervention trial. *JAMA* **248**, 1465–1477 (1982).

[45] Nordrehang, J. D.: Malignant arrhythmias in relation to serum potassium values in patients with an acute myocardial infarction. *Acta Med. Scand. Suppl.* **647**, 101–107 (1980).

[46] Olsson, O. A. T., Alquist, B., Gustavsson, B.: A new β_2-adrenoceptor agonist with α_1-adrenoceptor blocking properties. *Acta Pharmacol. Toxicol.* **48**, 340–348 (1981).

[47] Opie, L. H., Jee, L. D.: Nifedipine: Expanding Indications in Hypertension. pp. 333–346. In: Opie, L. H. (ed.): *Calcium Antagonists and Cardiovascular Disease. Perspectives in Cardiovascular Research.* Vol. 9; Raven Press, New York (1984).

[48] Osborne, M. W., Kovzelove, F., Cohen, R. M., Wenger, J. J.: Bromolasalocid (Ro-20-0006) antihypertensive ionophore. *Fed. Proc.* **42**, 191–195 (1983).

[49] Perry, H. M.: Some wrong-way chemical changes during antihypertensive treatment: Comparison of indapamide and related agents. *Amer. Heart J.* **106**, 251–257 (1983).

[50] Rössner, S., Weiner, L.: Atenolol und Metoprolol: Comparison of effects on blood pressure and serum lipids, and side effects. *Europ. J. Clin. Pharmacol.* **24**, 573–577 (1983).

[51] Serlin, M. J., Orme, M. L. E., Baber, N. S., Sibeon, R. G., Laws, E., Breckenridge, A.: Propranolol in the control of blood pressure: A dose response study. *Clin. Pharmacol. Ther.* **27**, 586–592 (1980).

[52] Steiner, J. A., Chancy, A., Manghani, K. K., James, I. M.: Comparison of prizidolol hydrochloride (SK & F 92657), a new antihypertensive agent with β-adrenoceptor antagonist and vasodilator activity with propranolol and hydralazine in normal volunteers. *Brit. J. Clin. Pharmacol.* **12**, 573–578 (1981).

[53] Stumpe, K. O., Kolloch, R., Overlack, A.: Angiotensin-Converting-Enzym Hemmer. Neuer Weg in der Hypertoniebehandlung. *Herz + Gefäße* **3**, 446–459 (1983).

[54] Sweet, C. S.: Pharmacological properties of the converting enzyme inhibitor, enalapril maleate (MK-421). *Fed. Proc.* **42**, 167–170 (1983).

[55] Tarazi, R. C., Dustan, H. P.: Beta adrenergic blockade in hypertension. *Amer. J. Cardiol.* **29**, 633–640 (1972).

[56] *Transparenzliste für das Indikationsgebiet Arterielle Hypertonie.* Geschäftsstelle der Transparenzkommission beim Bundesgesundheitsamt, Berlin 1982.

[57] Tweeddale, M. G., Ogilvie, R. I., Ruedy, J.: Antihypertensive and biochemical effects of chlorthalidone. *Clin. Pharmacol. Ther.* **22**, 519–527 (1977).

[58] Vanhoutte, P. M., van Nueten, J. M., Symoens, J., Janssen, P. A. J.: Antihypertensive properties of ketanserin (R 41 468). *Fed. Proc.* **42**, 182–185 (1983).

[59] Wilhelmsen, L., Berglund, G., Elmfeldt, D., Wedel, H.: Beta-blocker versus saluretics in hypertension. *Prev. Med.* **10**, 38–49 (1981).

The Pharmacodynamics of Alpha and Beta Blockade

B. N. C. Prichard
Department of Clinical Pharmacology, School of Medicine, University College London,
5 University Street, London WC1E 6JJ, U. K.

Beta Adrenoceptor Blocking Activity

Blockade of Exogenous Stimuli

Isoprenaline given by an intravenous infusion or bolus injection exerts both $beta_1$ and $beta_2$-adrenoceptor agonist effects, and its use has become established in the identification of drugs with beta-adrenoceptor blocking properties (McDevitt 1977). Log dose response increases in heart rate and reductions in diastolic blood pressure to isoprenaline are both shifted to the right after both oral and intravenous administration of labetalol. These shifts of the heart rate response curves are similar in magnitude to those of reductions in diastolic blood pressure. This suggests that labetalol has non-selective beta-adrenoceptor blocking effects (Richards et al. 1976; Richards et al. 1977a). The comparison of the effects of labetalol and of propranolol has revealed no qualitative differences, as both inhibited the effects of isoprenaline in a similar manner, although propranolol was found to be more potent on a weight basis. Estimates of the relative potency of both $beta_1$ and $beta_2$-adrenoceptor sites fell in the range 4 to 6:1 propranolol:labetalol (Richards et al. 1978a).
The dose response curve of increase in cardiac output produced by graded doses of isoprenaline is also shifted to the right by labetalol. These responses are not influenced by the administration of phentolamine in sufficient doses to produce further alpha-adrenoceptor antagonism indicating that this is due to its beta-blocking action and that it is not influenced by the alpha-blocking activity of labetalol (Richards et al. 1978a).

Blockade of Endogenous Activity

The increase in both heart rate and systolic blood pressure from vigorous physical excercise is reduced by drugs with beta-adrenoceptor blocking properties. It has been shown with labetalol that both oral (Richards et al. 1974) and intravenous (Richards et al. 1977a) administration produce a dose related reduction in exercise heart rate and systolic blood pressure.
When labetalol and propranolol were compared similar effects were shown, but propranolol was found to be more potent by four to six-fold and similar to that shown with isoprenaline responses (Richards et al. 1977b). The tachycardia induced by tilting was inhibited by labetalol, and again propranolol was more potent. This potency difference between Plabetalol and propranolol, however, was less marked when assessing the inhibition of the tachycardia induced by Valsalva's manoeuvre (Richards et al. 1977a).

Blockade of Alpha-Adrenoceptors

Labetalol administered orally and intravenously inhibits the increases in blood pressure induced by alpha-adrenoceptor stimulation with phenylephrine, and linear log dose-response curves of these increases were shifted to the right in a parallel manner (Richards et al. 1976; Richards et al. 1977a). While exogenously infused noradrenaline in man exerts both alpha and beta-agonist effects, the predominating circulatory responses are those mediated through alpha-adrenoceptors. Hence dose-related increases in blood pressure occur which are accompanied by reflexly induced reductions in heart rate and cardiac output. It has been shown that labetalol competitively antagonizes the systolic and diastolic pressor effects induced by noradrenaline (Richards et al. 1978a) but leaves the reflex reductions in heart rate and cardiac output unaffected (Richards et al. 1979). The modification by labetalol of noradrenaline induced increases in blood pressure is similar to that observed after the administration of phentolamine (Richards et al. 1978b). By contrast, the cardioselective beta-blocking drug atenolol had no effect on the increases in blood pressure by noradrenaline. Labetalol is less pharmacologically potent at inhibiting the effects of noradrenaline compared with those of phenylephrine (Richards et al. 1978a). It appears from animal work that labetalol inhibits the cocaine sensitive uptake of noradrenaline into adrenergic neurones which would minimise the post synaptic alpha receptor blocking action of labetalol.
The systemic administration of adrenaline to man also exerts both alpha and beta-agonist effects, but its predominant effect within the circulation depends on the dose administered (Richards et al. 1979). Administration of adrenaline after previous administration of propranolol leads to marked increases in systolic and diastolic blood pressure accompanied by reductions in heart rate and probably cardiac output (Prichard and Ross 1966). Administration of high doses of adrenaline after labetalol caused increases in diastolic blood pressure but the increases in systolic blood pressure were attenuated compared with those observed before labetalol administration. At high dose levels of adrenaline after labetalol, reductions in heart rate and cardiac output occurred and this pattern of change was similar to that occurring after noradrenaline.

Blockade of Endogenous Sympathetic Acitivity

Placing a hand in ice-cold water for 60 seconds elevates blood pressure in normal man and this procedure may be used to test alpha-adrenoceptor blocking drugs (Maconochie et al. 1977). Administration of propranolol did not inhibit the cold-induced increase in blood pressure, but after a comparable beta-adrenoceptor blocking dose of labetalol there was a significant inhibitory effect on mean arterial blood pressure (Maconochie et al. 1977). In another study in which labetalol was administered intravenously, an inhibitory effect was again observed. In contrast, no similar effect occurred after administration of phentolamine and this was thought to be due to additional blocking effect of phentolamine on presynaptic alpha adrenoceptors, which in turn modified its blocking effect on post-synaptic alpha adrenoceptors. Presynaptic alpha adrenoceptor blockade does not seem to occur with labetalol (Blakeley and Summers 1977) which might explain the difference from phentolamine.
As labetalol interferes with the innervation of the alpha receptor, symptoms of postural hypotension might be expected to occur. These are uncommon with labetalol, for the possible reasons, firstly that labetalol also lowers the blood pressure because of its beta

blocking action, and secondly, as the inhibition is of the competitive type, the increased alpha sympathetic activity associated with the erect posture might be expected to at least partly overcome any partial blockade. This contrasts with the combination of the non-competitive alpha blocker phenoxybenzamine and propranolol, the additional anti-hypertensive effect is entirely postural (Beilen and Juel-Jensen 1972). Postural effects tend to occur more frequently with higher doses of labetalol (Dargie et al. 1976; Prichard and Boakes 1976), but have occurred with lower doses in series where a diuretic was used in all or most of the patients (Bolli et al. 1976; Pugsley et al. 1976). Diuretics probably produce a chronic reduction in blood volume (Prichard and Owens 1983) and this will increase sensitivity to the alpha adrenoceptor inhibition under physiological stresses such as the erect posture. Another reason for postural hypotension with lower dosages might be the abrupt administration of doses above the optimum for commence-ment of therapy, eg 400 mg and 800 mg, in double blind trials (Kane et al. 1976).

Relative Alpha and Beta Blocking Activity

Richards et al. (1976) have found that a single oral dose of 400 mg labetalol produced a shift to the right in the isoprenaline dose response curve to increases in heart rate and the fall in diastolic blood pressure. Likewise log-dose response curves to phenylephrine-induced increases in systolic blood pressure also showed a rightward parallel displacement. Comparing the shift of the curves it was found that the ratio of alpha : beta antagonism was approximately 1 : 3. When labetalol was given intravenously the ratio was 1 : 6.9 (Richards et al. 1977a).

Combined Beta and Alpha Blockade in Hypertension

Alpha receptor blocking drugs have long been demonstrated to reduce peripheral resistance and thus lower the blood pressure. The possession by labetalol, at present the only such drug generally available, of both beta and alpha receptor blocking properties, represents an additional mode of action to lower the blood pressure. While there is no controversy over the hypotensive mechanism of alpha blockade, this is not the case with beta blockade (Prichard 1982). The effect of labetalol on some of the parameters that have been suggested as relevant to the antihypertensive action of beta adrenergic blocking drugs, has been investigated. Labetalol has been found to reduce plasma renin (Weidmann et al. 1978; Lijnen et al. 1979) but this does not appear to correlate to the antihypertensive effect (Lechi et al. 1981), and others have found no consistent effect (Kornerup et al. 1979; Hauger-Klevene 1981). Some investigators have reported a fall in plasma aldosterone (Lijnen et al. 1979), others have observed a variable effect (Weidmann et al. 1978). A fall in plasma noradrenaline has been found (Kornerup et al. 1979) while others noted a rise after intravenous administration of labetalol (Lechi et al. 1981), but most have not found any effect (Weidmann et al. 1978; Lijnen et al. 1979). Agabiti-Rosei et al. (1982) observed that patients with a high basal noradrenaline responded to intravenous or oral labetalol with a fall in blood pressure greater than those with a low level; how-ever, the elevated noradrenaline also correlated with the height of blood pressure.

Acute Use

Labetalol has been reported to control the blood pressure of severely hypertensive patients (Trust et al. 1976; Brown et al. 1977; Cumming et al. 1979, 1982; McGrath et al. 1978; Pearson and Havard 1978; Pearson et al. 1979; Cumming and Davies 1979; Dal Palu et al. 1982). Labetalol has been used acutely in phaeochromocytoma (Rosei et al. 1976) and hypertensive reactions after clonidine withdrawal (Rosei et al. 1976) as well as an adjunct to produce hypotensive anaesthesia (Scott 1982). It has also been used orally to acutely control blood pressure (Ghose and Sampson 1977; Serlin et al. 1979). This immediate hypotensive action distinguishes it from beta-adrenergic blocking drugs that do not possess alpha blocking action (Prichard 1982) and is likely to have resulted predominantly from its alpha blocking component, although the beta blocking action might be expected to inhibit any tachycardia and increase cardiac output secondary to the peripheral vasodilation.

In accord with the well established anti-hypertensive effect of chronic administration of beta blocking drugs, it seems likely that with more prolonged use the beta blocking component becomes relatively more important in the antihypertensive effect of labetalol. Weidmann et al. (1978) have noted a 17% increase in blood volume with 6 weeks' oral labetalol, a finding that will reduce the hypotensive effect of the initial alpha blockade. Hunyor et al. (1980) and Rasmussen and Nielson (1980) also found labetalol increased blood volume, in contrast to propranolol. Additionally, Semplicini et al. (1983) observed an inhibition of the alpha pressor response to phenylephrine with acute labetalol, as had been previously shown (see above), which declined over 6 months of treatment, whereas the shift in the isoprenaline dose response curve was unchanged. Likewise whereas the acute administration of labetalol is associated with an inhibition of the pressor responses to noradrenaline (see above), with 4 weeks and 12 weeks' administration the response to noradrenaline is no longer inhibited and is indeed enhanced (Zschiedrich et al. 1983).

References

Agabiti-Rosei, E., Alicandri, C. L., Beschi, M., Castellano, M., Fabriello, R., Montini, E., Muiesan, M. L., Romanelli, G. and Muiesan, G., 1982: The acute and chronic hypotensive effect of labetalol and the relationship with pretreatment plasma noradrenaline levels. *British Journal of Clinical Pharmacology* 13, (Suppl. 1), 87S—92S.

Balasubramanian, V., Mann, S., Millar-Craig, M. W. and Raftery, E. B., 1979: Effect of labetalol in hypertension during exercise and postural changes. *British Journal of Clinical Pharmacology* 8 (Suppl. 2), 95S—100S.

Beilen, L. J. and Juel-Jensen, B. E., 1972: Alpha and beta adrenergic blockade in hypertension. *Lancet* 1, 979—982.

Blakeley, A. G. H. and Summers, R. J., 1977: The effects of labetalol (AH 5158) on adrenergic transmission in the cat spleen. *British Journal of Pharmacology* 59, 643—660.

Boakes, A. J., Knight, E. J. and Prichard, B. N. C., 1971: Preliminary studies of the pharmacological effects of 5-{1-hydroxy-2-[(1-methyl-3-phenylpropyl)amino]-ethyl}-salicylamide (AH 5158) in in man. *Clinical Science* 40, 18P—19P.

Bolli, P., Waal-Manning, H. J., Wood, A. J. and Simpson, F. O., 1976: Experience with labetalol in hypertension. *British Journal of Clinical Pharmacology* 3 (Suppl. 3), 765—771.

Brown, J. J., Lever, A. F., Cumming, A. M. M. and Robertson, J. I. S., 1977: Labetalol in hypertension. *Lancet* 1, 1147.

Collier, J. G., Dawnay, N. A. H., Nachev, C. H. and Robinson, B. F., 1972: Clinical investigation of an antagonist of α and β adrenoceptors — AH 5158A. *British Journal of Pharmacology* 44, 286—293.

Cumming, A. M. M. and Davies, D. L., 1979: Intravenous labetalol in hypertensive emergency. *Lancet* 1, 929—930.

Cumming, A. M. M., Brown, J. J., Lever, A. F., Mackay, A. and Robertson, J. I. S., 1979: Treatment of severe hypertension by repeated bolus injections of labetalol. *British Journal of Clinical Pharmacology* 8 (Suppl. 2), 199S–204S.

Cumming, A. M. M., Brown, J. J., Lever, A. F. and Robertson, J. I. S., 1982: Intravenous labetalol in the treatment of severe hypertension. *British Journal of Clinical Pharmacology* 13 (Suppl. 1), 93S–96S.

Dal Palu, C., Pessina, A. C., Semplicini, A., Hlede, M., Morandin, F., Palatini, P., Sperti, G. and Rossi, G. P., 1982: Intravenous labetalol in severe hypertension. *British Journal of Clinical Pharmacology* 13 (Suppl. 1), 97S–99S.

Dargie, H. J., Dollery, C. T. and Daniel, J., 1976: Labetalol in resistant hypertension. *British Journal of Clinical Pharmacology* 3 (Suppl. 3), 751–755.

Dawson, A., Smith, I. and Johnson, B. F., 1977: The transient antihypertensive effect of phentolamine in patients receiving beta-blocker treatment. *Journal International Medical Research* 5, 462–464.

Farmer, J. B., Kennedy, I., Levy, G. P. and Marshall, R. J., 1972: Pharmacology of AH 5158; a drug which blocks both α and β-adrenoceptors. *British Journal of Pharmacology* 45, 660–675.

Ghose, R. R., 1979: Acute management of severe hypertension with oral labetalol. *British Journal of Clinical Pharmacology* 8 (Suppl. 2), 189S–193S.

Ghose, R. R. and Sampson, A., 1977: Rapid onset of oral labetalol in severe hypertension. *Current Medical Research and Opinion* 5, 147–151.

Hauger-Klevene, J. H., 1981: Treatment of severe essential hypertension with labetalol: effect on active and inactive renin. *Pharmatherapeutica* 3 (1), 46–54.

Hunyor, S. N., Bauer, G. E., Ross, M. and Larkin, H., 1980: Labetalol and propranolol in mild hypertensives: Comparison of blood pressure and plasma volume effects. *Australian and New Zealand Journal of Medicine* 10, 162–166.

Kane, J., Gregg, I. and Richards, D. A., 1976: A double-blind trial of labetalol. *British Journal of Clinical Pharmacology* 3 (Suppl. 3), 737–741.

Kornerup, H. J., Pedersen, E. B., Christensen, N. J., Pedersen, A. and Pedersen, G., 1979: Effect of oral labetalol on plasma catecholamines renin and aldosterone in patients with severe arterial hypertension. *European Journal of Clinical Pharmacology* 16, 305–310.

Lechi, A., Picotti, G. B., Covi, G., Pomari, S., Pedrolli, E., Cesura, A. M., Danti, G. and Mattioli, M., 1981: Intravenous labetalol in severe hypertension: effects on blood pressure, renin activity and catecholamines. *Arzneimittel-Forschung* 33 (I), 3: 524–526.

Lijnen, P. J., Amery, A. K., Fagard, R. H., Reybrouck, T. M., Moerman, E. J. and De Schaepdryver, A. F., 1979: Effects of labetalol on plasma renin, aldosterone and catecholamines in hypertensive patients. *Journal of Cardiovascular Pharmacology* 1, 625–632.

Maconochie, J. G., Richards, D. A. and Woodings, E. P., 1977: Modification of pressor responses induced by "cold". *British Journal of Clinical Pharmacology* 4, 389P.

Majid, P. A., Meeran, M. K., Benaim, M. E., Sharma, B. and Taylor, S. H., 1974: Alpha and beta-adrenergic receptor blockade in the treatment of hypertension. *British Heart Journal* 36, 588–596.

McDevitt, D. G., 1977: The assessment of beta-adrenoceptor blocking drugs in man. *British Journal of Clinical Pharmacology* 4, 413–425.

McGrath, B. P., Matthews, P. G., Walter, N. M., Maydom, B. W. and Johnston, C. I., 1978: Emergency treatment of severe hypertension with intravenous labetalol. *The Medical Journal of Australia* 2, 410–411.

McNeil, J. J. and Louis, W. J., 1979: A double-blind crossover comparison of pindolol, metoprolol, atenolol and labetalol in mild to moderate hypertension. *British Journal of Clinical Pharmacology* 8 (Suppl. 2), 163S–166S.

Pearson, R. M. and Havard, C. W. H., 1978: Intravenous labetalol in hypertensive patients given by fast and slow injection. *British Journal of Clinical Pharmacology* 5, 401–405.

Pearson, R. M., Griffith, D. N. W., Woollard, M., James, I. M. and Havard, G. W. H., 1979: Comparison of effects on cerebral blood flow of rapid reduction in systemic arterial pressure by diazoxide and labetalol in hypertensive patients: preliminary findings. *British Journal of Clinical Pharmacology* 8 (Suppl. 2), 195S–198S.

Prichard, B. N. C., 1982: Propranolol and β-adrenergic receptor blocking drugs in the treatment of hypertension. *British Journal of Clinical Pharmacology* 13, 51–60.

Prichard, B. N. C. and Boakes, A. J., 1976: Labetalol in long-term treatment of hypertension. *British Journal of Clinical Pharmacology* 3, 743–750.

Prichard, B. N. C. and Owens, C. W. I., 1980: Mechanism of anti-hypertensive action of beta-adrenergic blocking drugs. *Cardiology* **66** (Suppl. 1), 1–11.

Prichard, B. N. C. and Owens, C. W. I., 1983: Drug Treatment of Hypertension. In: *Hypertension* (Second Edition) Eds. Genest, J., Kuchel, O., Hamet, P., Cantin, M. McGraw-Hill Book Company, New York. 1171–1210.

Prichard, B. N. C. and Ross, E. J., 1966: Use of propranolol in conjunction with alpha-receptor blocking drugs in phaeochromocytoma. *American Journal of Cardiology* **18**, 394–398.

Prichard, B. N. C. and Tuckman, J., 1977: Management and mechanisms of drug treatment of hypertension. In: *Hypertension*. Eds. Genest, J., Klow, E. and Kuchel, O. McGraw-Hill Book Company, New York. 1085–1117.

Puglsey, D. J., Armstrong, B. K., Nassim, M. A. and Beilen, L. J., 1976: Controlled comparison of labetalol and propranolol in the management of severe hypertension. *British Journal of Clinical Pharmacology* **3** (Suppl. 3), 777–782.

Rasmussen, S. and Nielsen, P. E., 1980: Blood pressure, plasma volume, and glomerular filtration rate during treatment with labetalol in essential hypertension. *Postgraduate Medical Journal* **56** (Suppl. 2), 33–36.

Richards, D. A., 1976: Pharmacological effects of labetalol in man. *British Journal of Clinical Pharmacology* **3**, 721–723.

Richards, D. A., Woodings, E. P., Stephens, M. D. B. and Maconochie, J. G., 1974: The effects of oral AH 5158, a combined α- and β-adrenoceptor antagonist, in healthy volunteers. *British Journal of Clinical Pharmacology* **1**, 505–510.

Richards, D. A., Tuckman, J. and Prichard, B. N. C., 1976: Assessment of alpha and beta-adrenoceptor blocking action of labetalol. *British Journal of Clinical Pharmacology* **3**, 849–855.

Richards, D. A., Maconochie, J. G., Bland, R. E., Hopkins, R., Woodings, E. P. and Martin, L. E., 1977a: Relationship between plasma concentrations and pharmacological effects of labetalol. *European Journal of Clinical Pharmacology* **11**, 85–90.

Richards, D. A., Woodings, E. P. and Maconochie, J. G., 1977b: Comparison of the effects of labetalol and propranolol in healthy men at rest and during exercise. *British Journal of Clinical Pharmacology* **4**, 15–21.

Richards, D. A., Prichard, B. N. C. and Dobbs, R. J., 1978a: Adrenoceptor blockade of the circulatory responses to intravenous isoproterenol. *Clinical Pharmacology and Therapeutics* **24**, 264–273.

Richards, D. A., Woodings, E. P. and Prichard, B. N. C., 1978b: Circulatory and α-adrenoceptor blocking effects of phentolamine. *British Journal of Clinical Pharmacology* **5**, 507–513.

Richards, D. A., Prichard, B. N. C. and Hernandez, R., 1979: Circulatory effects of noradrenaline and adrenaline before and after labetalol. *British Journal of Clinical Pharmacology* **7**, 371–378.

Rosei, E. A., Brown, J. J., Lever, A. F., Robertson, A. S., Robertson, J. I. S. and Trust, R. M., 1976: Treatment of phaeochromocytoma and of clonidine withdrawal hypertension with labetalol. *British Journal of Clinical Pharmacology* **3**, 809–815.

Scott, D. B., 1982: The use of labetalol in anaesthesia. *British Journal of Clinical Pharmacology* **13**, (Suppl. 1), 133S–135S.

Semplicini, A., Pessina, A. C., Rossi, G. P., Hlede, M. and Morandin, F., 1983: Alpha-adrenoceptor blockade by labetalol during long-term dosing. *Clinical Pharmacology and Therapeutics* **33** (3), 278–282.

Serlin, M. J., Orme, M. C. L'E., Maciver, M., Green, G. J., MacNee, M. and Breckenridge, A. M., 1979: Rate of onset of hypotensive effect of oral labetalol. *British Journal of Clinical Pharmacology* **7**, 165–168.

Thompson, F. D., Joekes, A. M. and Hussein, M. M., 1979: Monotherapy with labetalol for hypertensive patients with normal and impaired renal function. *British Journal of Clinical Pharmacology* **8** (Suppl. 2), 129S–133S.

Trust, P. M., Rosei, E. A., Brown, J. J., Fraser, R., Lever, A. F., Morton, J. J. and Robertson, J. I. S., 1976: Effect on blood pressure, angiotensin II and aldosterone concentrations during treatment of severe hypertension with intravenous labetalol: comparison with propranolol. *British Journal of Clinical Pharmacology* **3**, 799–803.

Weidmann, P., De Chatel, R., Ziegler, W. H., Flammer, J. and Reubi, F., 1978: Alpha and beta adrenergic blockade with orally administered labetalol in hypertension. *The American Journal of Cardiology* **41**, 570–576.

Zschiedrich, H., Neurohr, W., Lüth, J. B., Philipp, Th. and Distler, A., 1983: Sympathetic nervous activity and the pressor effect of noradrenaline under chronic α-β-adrenoceptor blockade with labetalol in hypertension. *Klinische Wochenschrift* **61**, 661–667.

Discussion

Taylor
You have talked about the possibility, during long-term-treatment, of the alpha-blocking activity of the drug being somewhat less than the beta-blocking activity. I think that it was you who showed during long-term-treatment that the effects on blood pressure were maintained for over 6 years.

Prichard
Yes. I am just a little sceptical about these curves showing the labetalol coming back because there is no shift with under 2 μg/min phenylephrine, and this is really marginal to show an effect at all acutely. I would like to see that repeated.

Taylor
It doesn't therefore really have any great clinical significance in terms of blood pressure control?

Prichard
No, we found blood pressure falls maintained for 5 or 6 years quite satisfactorily. From first principles and properties and responses of beta-blockers and alpha-blockers, I would expect that the beta-blocker component of labetalol will be making a relatively bigger contribution in time in comparison to the acute effect. I am not the least bit surprised about the blood volume compensatory changes. I expect that from any alpha-receptor blocking drug. You have for example the first dose effect with prazosin. This is mainly a blood volume effect. If you give any alpha-blocking drug you tend to get a modest compensatory increase in blood volume, as now appears to be shown with labetalol.

Taylor
That would only apply to blood pressure control and not to any ancilliary properties of alpha-blockade, such as Dr. Corr will be talking about later.

Prichard
I think it is an effect on phenylephrine. I am surprised to see it and I would like to see it repeated.

Borchard
Eine Frage zum Verhältnis der Blockade von Alpha-1- zu Alpha-2-Rezeptoren bei Labetalol. Sind dazu Untersuchungen gemacht?

Prichard
I think the alpha-2-blocking activity of labetalol is very small. Whether in animal work it can be shown to have any alpha-2-blocking activity, I don't know. I would be surprised if it had. It is practically speaking, an alpha-1-blocking drug.

N. N.
Das Verhältnis der Alpha- zur Beta-Blockade beim Labetalol ist meiner Information nach etwa 1 : 4 bis 1:6. Ist da nicht vorstellbar und möglich, daß eine Erhöhung der Dosis eigentlich nur noch eine betablockierende Wirkung zum Tragen kommen läßt?

Prichard
If you increase the dose of labetalol, the relative beta-blocking component increases faster than the alpha-blocking component as measured on phenylephrine and isoprenaline dose response curves. With the larger dose you are getting relatively more beta-blockade. The other side of the coin at first sight seems a contradiction because from the practical point of view, when one measures alpha-blockade you think in terms of a postural fall in blood pressure. The fact that you see the postural fall in blood pressure at high levels, at high dosage — that is more alpha-blockade at high dosage — is because of the following: at moderate levels of alpha-blockade, due to the innervation of the alpha-receptor in resistance vessels, there is not so much block that it prevents the compensatory vasoconstrictor impulses which occur. When we stand up we want vasoconstriction to maintain our blood pressure of course. At moderate levels of alpha-blockade, the body can produce enough vasoconstriction, so there is not a postural effect. When you get above a certain level, suddenly the physiological effects of

alpha-blockade become apparent. So, you have this contradiction as you push up the dose of labetalol. You get relatively more shift of the isoprenaline curve compared to the phenylephrine curve but at the same time as you put up the dose, physiologically you then will be going to see what is quite clearly alpha-blockade in terms of a postural effect. This effect coming in at somewhere of the order of 2 grams a day with chronic treatment.

Bahlmann

Coming back to this high dose of labetalol and the responses you have shown during exercises. I would like to know, was this after acute administration or after long-term administration? It is quite surprising that there is no fall of blood pressure during this exercise manoeuver.

Prichard

I showed the slide of exercise tachycardia with the rise in systolic pressure on exercise being inhibited with labetalol. That was acute administration and you could well show that type of effect with a straight beta-receptor-blocking drug. Of course the rise in pressure in exercise is mainly a cardiac contribution; is mainly the heart. The effect of the high dose, below and above 2 grams; here we were looking at post exercise, and as you imply perhaps, that is where you are going to see a fall in blood pressure, if you are going to see it at all. That is the most severe cardiovascular stress — looking what happens to the blood pressure immediately after exercise — and that was chronic administration. As we were discussing earlier, the main effect of acute alpha-blockade is the relaxation of blood vessels without any compensatory fluid shifts. Chronically you get, if you like, a more balanced situation as regards the alpha-blockade. You get a certain amount of compensatory fluid shifting with increase in blood volume which will tend to reduce the effects of alpha-blockade.

Zur Chronopharmakologie von Adrenozeptorenblockern

B. Lemmer
Zentrum der Pharmakologie, Klinikum der Johann Wolfgang Goethe-Universität, Theodor-Stern-Kai 7, D-6000 Frankfurt/Main, FRG

Zusammenfassung

Beim Menschen und bei Nagern lassen sich signifikante Tageszeitabhängigkeiten in den verschiedensten Funktionen des kardiovaskulären Systems nachweisen. Wirkungen und Pharmakokinetik von antihypertensiv wirkenden Pharmaka wie β-, und α- und β-Adrenozeptorenblockern sind nicht unabhängig von den Tagesrhythmen in diesen physiologischen Funktionen. Human- und tierexperimentelle chronopharmakologische Untersuchungen können somit zum besseren Verständnis der Regulationsmechanismen des kardiovaskulären Systems aber auch zur Verbesserung der Therapie der Hypertonie beitragen.

Einleitung

Fast alle bisher untersuchten physiologischen Funktionen bei Mensch und Tier weisen tageszeitabhängige Variationen auf [13]. Tagesrhythmen in kardiovaskulären Funktionen sind in der medizinischen Literatur seit fast 100 Jahren beobachtet und in der Folge detailliert nachgewiesen worden. Schon 1898 beschrieb Hill [9] den nächtlichen Blutdruckabfall beim Menschen während des Schlafens. Seine Beobachtung, daß die Höhe des Blutdrucks von der Tageszeit abhängig ist, wurde seither von zahlreichen Untersuchergruppen sowohl bei gesunden Probanden als auch bei Hypertonikern bestätigt [z. B. 1–3, 5–7, 20, 21, 25, 26]. Bei Mensch und/oder Tier werden Tagesrhythmen nicht nur im systolischen und diastolischen Blutdruck, sondern auch in Herzfrequenz, Herz-Zeit-Volumen, Meßgrößen im EKG (QRS- und QT-Intervall), Reagibilität des Gefäßsystems, Plasma-Konzentrationen an Noradrenalin, Adrenalin, cAMP, etc. nachgewiesen (Übersicht s. [13]).
Schließlich weisen verschiedene epidemiologische Studien nach, daß auch die kardiale und kardiovaskuläre Morbidität bzw. Mortalität zu verschiedenen Tageszeiten unterschiedlich hoch sind [11, 22]. Zusätzlich sind neben tageszeitabhängigen Variationen auch signifikante jahreszeitabhängige Unterschiede in Blutdruck [4] und kardiovaskulärer Mortalität [8] beschrieben worden. Alle diese Befunde weisen auf eine ausgesprochene, vor allem tageszeitliche Synchronisation kardiovaskulärer Funktionen hin. Es überrascht daher nicht, daß die Wirkungen von Arzneimitteln, die bei kardiovaskulären Erkrankungen eingesetzt werden, zu verschiedenen Tageszeiten bzw. zirkadianen Phasenlagen quantitativ unterschiedliche Wirkungen haben können.

Ergebnisse und Diskussion

In eigenen tierexperimentellen Studien an licht-dunkel-synchronisierten Nagern (Ratten, Mäuse) wurden chronopharmakodynamische und chronopharmakokinetische Effekte von β-Adrenozeptorenblockern untersucht (Übersicht s. [18]). Neben der Referenzsubstanz Propranolol wurden weitere β-Blocker in die Untersuchungen einbezogen, um vor allem die relative Bedeutung der unterschiedlichen physiko-chemischen Eigenschaft (Lipophilie) der Substanzen, für die Pharmakonwirkungen und die Pharmakokinetik zu erfassen (Tabelle 1). Dies ist deshalb von Bedeutung, da die unspezifischen Wirkungsqualitäten und das pharmakokinetische Verhalten von β-Blockern weitgehend von der physiko-chemischen Eigenschaft der jeweiligen Substanz abhängen. Bei der Bewertung der tierexperimentellen Befunde vor allem im Hinblick auf die Übertragbarkeit auf den Menschen ist ferner zu berücksichtigen, daß sich Nager und Mensch in ihren zirkadianen Aktivitätsphasen spiegelbildlich zueinander verhalten, d.h. der Mensch ist ein tagaktives, die kleinen Nager sind nachtaktive Lebewesen [13].

Tabelle 1: In chronopharmakokinetischen Studien an L-D-synchronisierten Ratten untersuchte β-Adrenozeptorenblocker [13–18].

	Rezeptor-Selektivität	Eliminationsweg (wesentlicher)	Vert. Coeff. (Okt/Puffer, pH 7)
Propranolol	$\beta_1 = \beta_2$	Leber	13.7
Metoprolol	$\beta_1 > \beta_2$	”	0.18
Sotalol	$\beta_1 = \beta_2$	Niere	0.011
Atenolol	$\beta_1 > \beta_2$	”	0.0033

Untersuchungen zur Chronotoxizität von Propranolol bei Mäusen haben entsprechende Befunde mit einer Vielzahl von anderen Substanzen in der Hinsicht bestätigt, daß schon die Toxizität eines Arzneimittels durch den Applikationszeitpunkt innerhalb von 24 Stunden beeinflußt werden kann [13]. In diesen Studien führte die sog. LD_{50}-Dosis von razemischen Propranolol (125 mg/kg, i.p.) nur um 11 Uhr morgens zu einer Mortalität von 50 % der Versuchstiere, zu anderen Tageszeiten starben jedoch bis über 90 % der Tiere auf diese Dosis [15, 28]. Während die Toxizität von Propranolol überwiegend eine unspezifische Wirkungsqualität ist, wird die Herzfrequenz durch Blockade kardialer β-Adrenozeptoren spezifisch vermindert. Entsprechende Untersuchungen an L-D-synchronisierten, wachen Ratten zeigten, daß gleiche Dosen von Propranolol zwar sowohl in der Licht- und der Dunkelphase die Herzfrequenz senkten, in der Aktivitätsperiode der Ratten jedoch im Gegensatz zur Ruheperiode eine klare Dosisabhängigkeit hinsichtlich Ausmaß und Dauer des Pharmakoneffektes nachweisbar war [15, 18, Abb. 1]. Unter Berücksichtigung der unterschiedlichen zirkadianen Aktivitätsphasen von Ratte und Mensch wurden im Prinzip gleiche Befunde mit β-Blockern beim Menschen erhalten:
Die Abb. 2 gibt repräsentativ für eine Vielzahl von Befunden, die mit verschiedenen β-Blockern von verschiedenen Untersuchergruppen erhalten wurden [1, 3, 5–7, 20, 21, 26], die Ergebnisse mit dem β-Blocker Oxprenolol bei Hypertonikern wider [6, 25]. Zunächst einmal zeigt die Abb. 2, daß auch bei Hypertonikern systolischer und diastolischer Blutdruck sowie Herzfrequenz Tagesrhythmen mit Maxima am Vormittag/Mittag

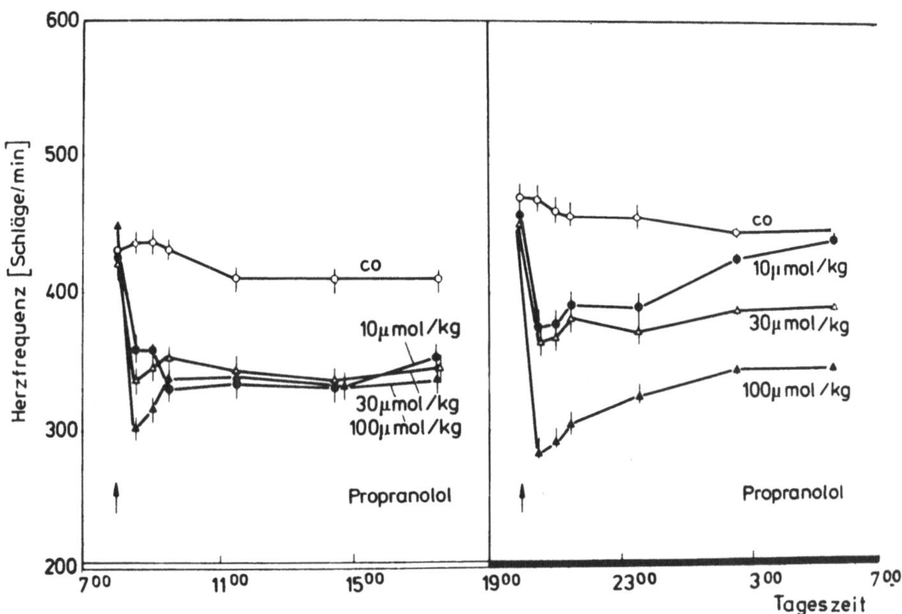

Abb. 1

Wirkungen von (±)-Propranolol (10–100 µmole/kg, s.c.) auf die Herzfrequenz wacher Ratten [13, 16, 18].

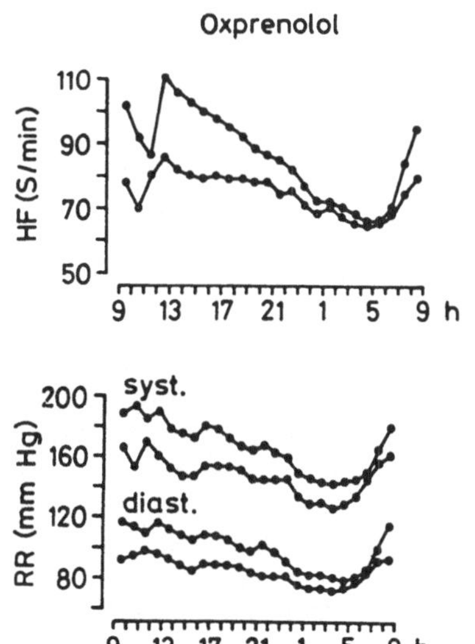

Abb. 2

Wirkung einer mehrwöchigen Behandlung mit Oxprenolol bei Hypertonikern, ●—● Kontrolle, ○—○ Oxprenolol [nach: 6, 25].

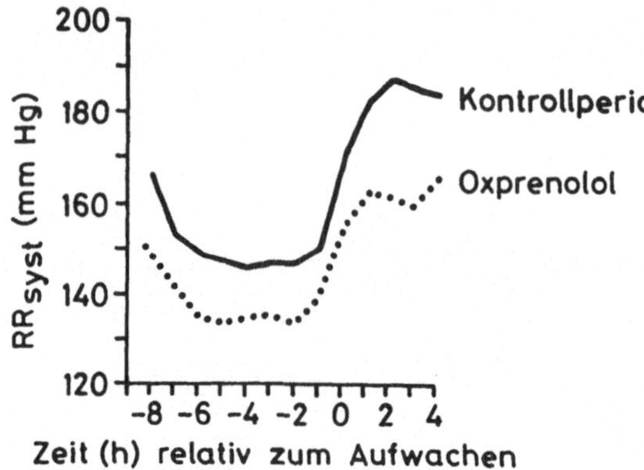

Abb. 3

Wirkung einer mehrwöchigen Behandlung mit Oxprenolol auf den Blutdruck von Hypertonikern in Bezug auf die Aufwachzeit [nach: 25].

und Minima in den Nachtstunden aufweisen. Unabhängig von den verwendeten Methoden zur Blutdruckmessung (intraarteriell, sphygmomanometrisch) sind gleiche Befunde von anderen Arbeitsgruppen erhoben worden [1, 3, 5−7, 20, 21, 25, 26], Befunde, die für Diagnostik und Therapiekontrolle von Hypertonikern − vor allem in den Praxen − noch viel zu wenig beachtet werden. Weiterhin zeigt die Abb. 2 den frühmorgendlichen Anstieg im Blutdruck, der bereits vor dem Aufwachen beginnt, dies ist zur Verdeutlichung noch einmal in Abb. 3 [25] dargestellt. β-Blocker wie Oxprenolol, Propranolol, Metoprolol, Atenolol und Mepindolol verminderten bei mehrwöchiger Gabe die tagsüber höheren Blutdruck- und Herzfrequenzwerte in dieser Periode stärker als in der Nacht, der frühmorgendliche Anstieg wurde jedoch nur wenig oder gar nicht durch diese β-Blocker beeinflußt [1, 2, 5−7, 20, 21, 25, 26].
Für die tageszeitabhängigen Unterschiede in den Wirkungen von β-Blockern bei Tier und Mensch könnten pharmakodynamische und/oder pharmakokinetische Ursachen verantwortlich sein. In tierexperimentellen Untersuchungen an Ratten konnten wir für die Razemate von Propranolol, Metoprolol, Sotalol und Atenolol in der Dunkelperiode, d. h. Aktivitätsperiode der Tiere, eine schnellere Elimination aus Plasma und Zielorganen wie Herz, Lunge, Gehirn und Muskulatur nach i.v. Gabe nachweisen [14−18]. Diese Befunde weisen darauf hin, daß [unabhängig von den Unterschieden in den spezifischen Wirkungsqualitäten der Substanzen (Rezeptorselektivität, ISA) und der relativen Lipophilie bzw. den Haupteliminationsmechanismen (s. Tabelle 1)] dieses chronopharmakokinetische Verhalten der Gruppe der β-Adrenozeptorenblocker zukommt. Nach Aufsättigung war dies chronokinetische Verhalten nur noch für das hochlipophile razemische Propranolol (Abb. 4), nicht jedoch für Metoprolol, Sotalol und Atenolol nachzuweisen [14, 17]. Entsprechende detaillierte Untersuchungen zur Tagesrhythmik in der Pharmakokinetik verschiedener β-Blocker liegen für den Menschen nicht vor. Lediglich für das lipophile Propranolol wurde nach oraler Applikation eine Tageszeitabhängigkeit in den initialen Plasmakonzentrationen nachgewiesen [23, Abb. 5], für das ähnlich wie auch für andere Pharmaka wie Diazepam [24] und Theophyllin [27] eine tageszeitlich unterschiedliche Resorption bzw. Ausmaß des first-pass-Effektes eine Rolle zu spielen scheint. Es erscheint jedenfalls unwahrscheinlich, daß die bei Nagern und Mensch nachgewiesenen tageszeitabhängigen Unterschiede in den kardiovaskulären Wirkungen von β-Blockern überwiegend oder maßgeblich durch ihr chronokinetisches Verhalten bedingt sind. Diese Annahme wird auch durch Befunde eines stereo-selektiven pharmakokinetischen Verhaltens von Propranolol gestützt [14].

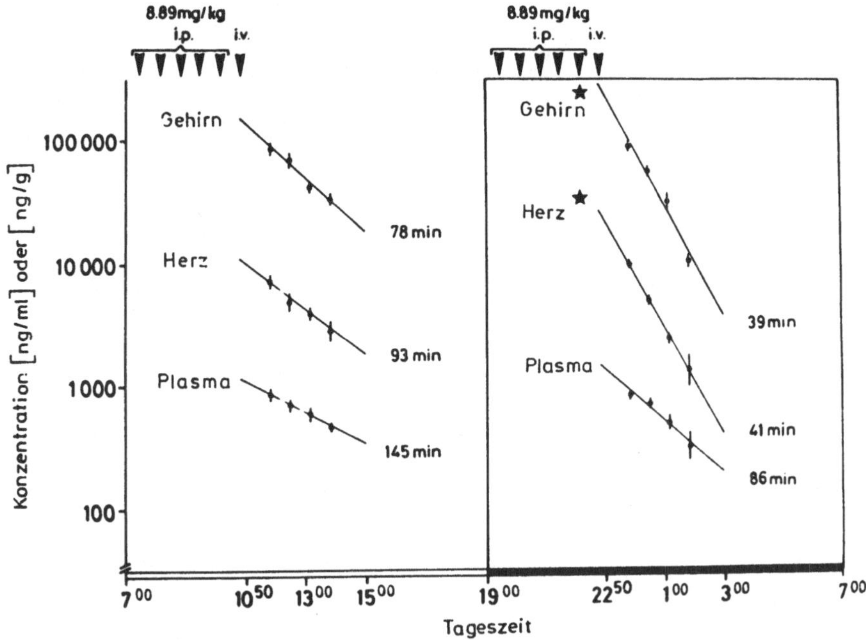

Abb. 4

Konzentrationen und Halbwertzeiten von (±)-Propranolol nach Aufsättigung in Plasma, Herz und Gehirn von L-D-synchronisierten Ratten [aus: 14, 18].

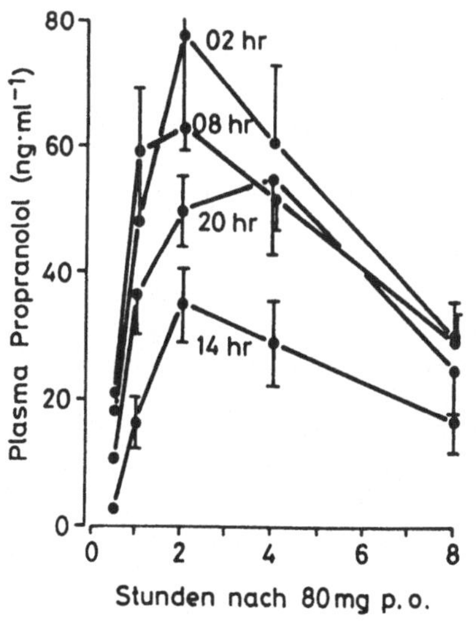

Abb. 5

Plasmakonzentration von (±)-Propranolol beim Menschen (n = 6) nach Einnahme von 80 mg p. o. zu verschiedenen Tageszeiten [nach: 23]

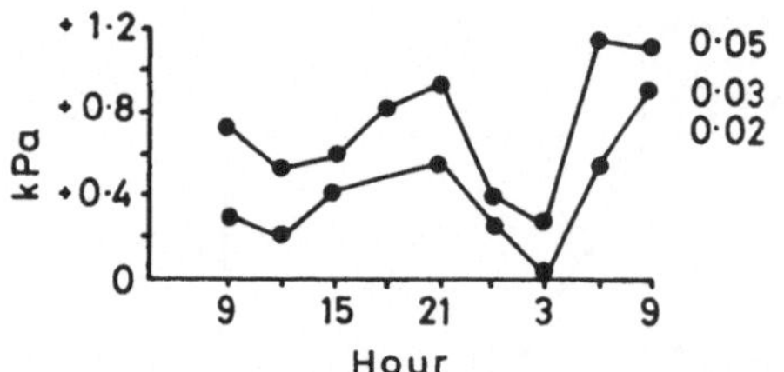

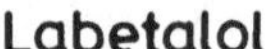

Abb. 6

Wirkung einer Noradrenalininfusion (μg/kg/min) auf den Blutdruckanstieg zu verschiedenen Tageszeiten beim Menschen [nach: 10].

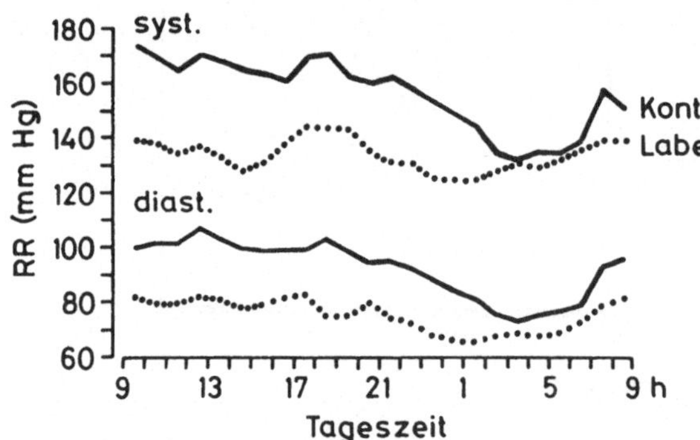

Abb. 7

Wirkung einer mehrwöchigen Behandlung mit Labetalol (3 × 100–600 mg/Tag) bei Hypertonikern [nach: 1].

Die Tagesrhythmik in den Wirkungen von β-Blockern scheint eher durch zirkadiane Variationen im dynamischen Verhalten, der Ansprechbarkeit und Reagibilität des kardiovaskulären Systems bedingt zu sein. So konnten Hossmann und Mitarbeiter [10] zeigen, daß die Infusion von Noradrenalin beim Menschen in seiner Aktivitätsperiode, d.h. am Tage, zu einer wesentlich stärkeren Blutdruckerhöhung als in der Ruheperiode führte (Abb. 6). Interessanterweise beobachteten diese Autoren ebenfalls einen frühmorgendlichen Anstieg in der Reagibilität des Gefäßsystems, wie die Abb. 5 zeigt. Diese Befunde könnten einen Hinweis dafür geben, warum die α- und β-Adrenozeptoren blockierende Substanz Labetalol nicht nur am Tage den Blutdruck bei Hypertonikern zu vermindern vermochte, sondern auch den frühmorgendlichen Blutdruckanstieg abschwächte [1, 25, Abb. 7]. Die Autoren dieser Studie stellten die Hypothese auf, daß der frühmorgendliche Blutdruckanstieg wesentlich über α-Adrenozeptoren reguliert zustande käme.

Mit niedrigeren Dosen von Labetalol (450 mg/Tag) hingegen sahen Bellamy und Mitarbeiter [2] bei Patienten mit milder Hypertonie nur einen „β-Adrenozeptoren blockierenden Effekt", d.h. die Wirkungen von Labetalol auf den Rhythmus im Blutdruck unterschieden sich nicht wesentlich von denen „reiner" β-Rezeptorenblocker. Auch wenn die Vermutung einer tageszeitlich unterschiedlichen Dominanz von α- oder β-adrenergen Mechanismen für die Blutdruckregulation noch nicht bewiesen ist, stellt sie eine interessante Arbeitshypothese dar. Daß selbst auf der Ebene des β-Adrenozeptor-Adenylatzyklase-cAMP-Phosphodiesterase-Systems signifikante tagesrhythmische Variationen nachweisbar sind, zeigten eigene Untersuchungen an Herzventrikeln von L-D-synchronisierten Ratten [12, 19].

Die eigenen Untersuchungen wurden mit Unterstützung der DFG und der Riese-Stiftung durchgeführt.

Literatur

[1] Balasubramanian, V., Mann, S., Millar-Craig, M. W., Raftery, E. B.: Effect of labetalol in hypertension during exercise and postural changes. *Brit. J. clin. Pharmacol.* 8, 955 (1979)

[2] Bellamy, G. R., Hunyor, S. N., Roffe, D., Massang, J.: Magnitude and mechanisms of the antihypertensive action of labetalol, including ambulatory assessment. *Brit. J. clin. Pharmacol.* 16, 9 (1983)

[3] Bock, K. D., Kreuzenbeck, W.: Spontaneous blood-pressure variations in hypertension; the effect of antihypertensive therapy and correlations with the incidence of complications. In: *Antihypertensive Therapy*, Edt. F. Gross, Springer-Verlag, Berlin–Heidelberg–New York 224 (1966)

[4] Brennan, P. J., Greenberg, G., Miall, W. E., Thompson, S. G.: Seasonal variation in arterial blood pressure. *Brit. Med. J.* 285, 919 (1982)

[5] Carrageta, M., Soares, R., Martins, A.: Bewertung der blutdrucksenkenden Wirkung von einmal täglich verabreichten Beta-Blockern im tagesperiodischen Verlauf. In: *Blutdruckvariabilität*, Hrsg.: D. Magometschnigg, G. Hitzenberger, Uhlen Verlagsgesellschaft Wien, 118 (1983)

[6] Craig, M. W., Mann, S., Balasubramanian, V., Raftery, E. B.: Blood pressure circadian rhythm in essential hypertension. *Clin. Sci. Mol. Med.* 55, 391 (1978)

[7] Gould, B.: Auswirkungen peripherer Vasodilatatoren auf die Blutdruckvariabilität. In: *Blutdruckvariabilität*, Hrsg. D. Magometschnigg, G. Hitzenberger, Uhlen Verlagsgesellschaft Wien, 134 (1983)

[8] Habermann, S., Capildeo, R., Rose, F. C.: The seasonal variation in mortality from cerebrovascular disease. *J. Neurol. Sci.* 52, 25 (1981)

[9] Hill, L.: On rest, sleep, and work and the consistant changes in the circulation of the blood. *Lancet* I, 282 (1898)

[10] Hossmann, V., Fitzgerald, G. A., Dollery, C. T.: Circadian rhythm of baroreflex reactivity and adrenergic vascular response. *Cardiovasc. Res.* 14, 125 (1980)

[11] Kaufmann, M. W., Gottlieb, G., Kahaner, K., Peselow, E., Stanley, M., Casadonte, P., Deutsch, S.: Circadian rhythm and myocardial infarct: a preliminary study. *IRCS Med. Sci. Biochem.* 9, 557 (1981)

[12] Lang, P.-H., Lemmer, B.: Kinetics of ^{3}H-DHA binding to rat heart membranes and circadian rhythm in sympathetic tone. *Naunyn-Schmiedeberg's Arch. Pharmacol.* 319, R68 (1982)

[13] Lemmer, B.: *Chronopharmakologie*; Wiss. Verlagsgesellschaft, Stuttgart (1983)

[14] Lemmer, B., Bathe, K.: Stereospecific and circadian-phase-dependent kinetic behavior of d,l-,l- and d-propranolol in plasma, heart and brain of light-dark-synchronized rats. *J. Cardiovasc. Pharmacol.* 4, 635 (1982)

[15] Lemmer, B., Simrock, R., Hellenbrecht, D., Smolensky, M. H.: Chronopharmacological studies with propranolol in rodents: Implications for the management of COPD patients with cardiovascular disease. In: *Recent Advances in the Chronobiology of Allergy and Immunology*, Edts.: M. H. Smolensky, J. R. Govern, A. Reinberg, Pergamon Press, Oxford–New York, 195 (1980)

[16] Lemmer, B., Bathe, K., Charrier, A., Neumann, G., Schulz, D., Winkler, H.: On the chronopharmacology of beta-adrenoceptor blocking drugs. In: *Toward chronopharmacology*, Edts.: R. Takahashi, F. Halberg, C. A. Walker, Pergamon Press, Oxford–New York, 183 (1982)

[17] Lemmer, B., Winkler, H., Fink, M.: Comparative pharmacokinetics of propranolol, metoprolol and atenolol after single and multiple dosing in the rat. *Naunyn-Schmiedeberg's Arch. Pharmacol.* 322, R33 (1983)

[18] Lemmer, B., Bathe, K., Lang, P.-H., Neumann, G., Winkler, H.: Chronopharmacology of β-adrenoceptor blocking drugs: Pharmacokinetic and pharmacodynamic studies in rats. *J. Americ. Coll. Toxicol.* 2, 347 (1983)

[19] Lemmer, B., Lang, P.-H., Bissinger, H.: Indications for circadian variations in cAMP content, adenylate cyclase and phosphodiesterase activities in rat heart ventricles. *Naunyn-Schmiedeberg's Arch. Pharmacol.* 325, R32 (1984)

[20] Magometschnigg, D., Hitzenberger, G.: Reproduzierbarkeit der Tagesblutdruckvariabilität bei Normalpersonen. In: *Blutdruckvariabilität*, Hrsg. D. Magometschnigg, G. Hitzenberger, Uhlen Verlagsgesellschaft Wien, 101 (1983)

[21] Mann, S., Millar-Craig, M. W., Balasubramanian, V., Raftery, E. B.: Propranolol LA and ambulatory blood pressure. *Brit. J. clin. Pharmacol.* 10, 443 (1980)

[22] Master, A. M.: The role of effort and occupation in coronary occlusion. *J. Amer. med. Ass.* **174**, 942 (1960)

[23] Markiewicz, A., Semenowicz, K., Korczynska, J., Boldys, H.: Temporal variations in the response of ventilatory and circulatory functions of propranolol in healthy man. In: *Recent Advances in the Chronobiology of Allergy and Immunology*, Edts.: M. H. Smolensky, J. R. Govern, A. Reinberg, Pergamon Press, Oxford—New York, 185 (1980)

[24] Nakano, S.: Time-of-day effect on psychotherapeutic drug response and kinetics in man. In: *Toward Chronopharmacology*, Edts.: R. Takahashi, F. Halberg, C. A. Walker, Pergamon Press, Oxford—New York, 51 (1982)

[25] Raftery, E. B., Millar-Craig, M. W., Mann, S., Balasubramanian, V.: Effects of treatment on circadian rhythms of blood pressure. *Biotelem. Pat. Monitor* **8**, 113 (1981)

[26] Raftery, E. B.: Klassifizierung der Beta-Blocker nach ihrer Wirkung auf Blutdruckschwankungen im tagesperiodischen Verlauf. In: *Blutdruckvariabilität*, Hrsg. D. Magometschnigg, G. Hitzenberger, Uhlen Verlagsgesellschaft Wien, 109 (1983)

[27] Scott, P. H., Tabachnik, E., Mac Loed, S., Carreia, J., Newth, C., Levison, H.: Sustained-release theophylline for childhood asthma: evidence for circadian variation of theophylline pharmacokinetics. *J. Pediat.* **99**, 476 (1981)

[28] Smolensky, M., Janovich, J. A., Kyle, G. M., Hsi, B.: Chronotoxicity in rodents challenged with propranolol HCl (Inderal[R]). In: *Chronopharmacology*, Edts.: A. Reinberg, F. Halberg, Pergamon Press, Oxford—New York, 263 (1979)

Diskussion

Borchard
Herr Lemmer, haben Sie auch einmal die Rezeptorendichte untersucht? Sie haben ja zum Schluß die Untersuchungen gezeigt über die Adenylzyklase und das cAMP.

Lemmer
Wir haben auch die Rezeptorendichte zu 2 verschiedenen Zeitpunkten untersucht. Wir sehen in Übereinstimmung damit, daß die Dichte an Beta-Adrenorezeptoren im Herzventrikel zu Beginn der Aktivitätsperiode, sprich zu Beginn der Nacht, signifikant um ca. 40 % höher ist als zu Beginn der Ruheperiode. Da haben wir allerdings nur 2 Zeitpunkte.

The Response of Plasma Catecholamines to Receptor Antagonists

R. Kirsten, K. Nelson, D. Böhmer*

Abteilung für Klinische Pharmakologie, Klinikum der Universität, Theodor-Stern-Kai 7,
* Sportärztliche Hauptberatungsstelle des Landes Hessen
D-6000 Frankfurt/Main 70, F.R.G.

Summary

1. Historical and logical reasons for linking essential hypertension to circulating catecholamines are presented. Due to lack of evidence establishing this link, the proposition is advanced that the affinity at the receptor site may be altered in essential hypertension.
2. The response of norepinephrine to various adrenoceptor blocking agents after prolonged oral therapy is reported. Propranolol, metoprolol and labetalol caused no change in norepinephrine plasma levels. Pindolol caused a decrease, and prazosin an increase in norepinephrine levels.
3. Methods for determining catecholamines are discussed, whereby it is established that fluorometric and spectrophotometric methods may account for falsely high values. The radioenzymatic determination of catecholamines is preferable.
4. The norepinephrine response to different forms of labetalol application is presented. Prolonged oral application caused no change. Intravenous and acute oral application caused increases in norepinephrine levels.
5. Feedback mechanisms accounting for the increase or no change in norepinephrine levels after acute or prolonged application, respectively, are discussed.
6. The clinical uses and implications of the various classes of adrenoceptor blocking agents are discussed.

Essential hypertension is defined as a pathological increase in blood pressure of unestablished cause. Many years of work have been invested in trying to link essential hypertension to changes in catecholamine levels. These efforts are historically and logically based on the observation of phenomena which link circulating catecholamine levels to blood pressure. In 1922 L'Abbé and his colleagues made the observation that paroxysmal crises of hypertension had occurred in a woman who at autopsy was found to have a pheochromocytoma. In 1939 such hypertensive crises were linked to marked increases in the concentration of blood epinephrine in a patient with this tumor (Strömbeck et al., 1939). Another catecholamine-blood pressure analogy is the employment of epinephrine in cases of a life threatening decrease in blood pressure. Judicious epinephrine therapy will increase blood pressure dramatically and may be life saving. These are two of the reasons why such an extensive search has been pursued for a pathological change in circulating catecholamines as a cause for essential hypertension.

Unfortunately, the proof that catecholamine levels in patients with essential hypertension are unequivocally, significantly different from those encountered in the normotensive population has remained evasive. This motivated many groups to seek another cause which they presume to have found at the catecholamine receptor site. If the catecholamine levels were not increased, perhaps the affinity at the receptor site was altered. This line of reasoning is the basis for the abundance of blocking agents which can effectively be employed in blocking the catecholamine receptor site and do indeed cause a decrease in blood pressure.

Circulating catecholamine levels are important even though no unequivocal link to essential hypertension has been established. Even a submeasurable increase in circulating catecholamine levels may cause hypertension. In the case of angiotensin II this has been adequately demonstrated by Bean et al. (1979). Low doses of angiotensin II over long periods of time caused a pronounced increase in blood pressure, even though the plasma angiotensin concentration remained within the physiological range. This is feasable in the case of catecholamines, as well. Another reason why circulating catecholamines are important is that they give clues to the modes of action of blocking agents.

Catecholamine Response to Various Oral Adrenoceptor Blocking Agents

Figure 1 shows the response of norepinephrine levels to prolonged oral treatment with various classes of receptor antagonists. Norepinephrine has been chosen since this is the catecholamine occurring in the highest concentration and is reported on by most groups.

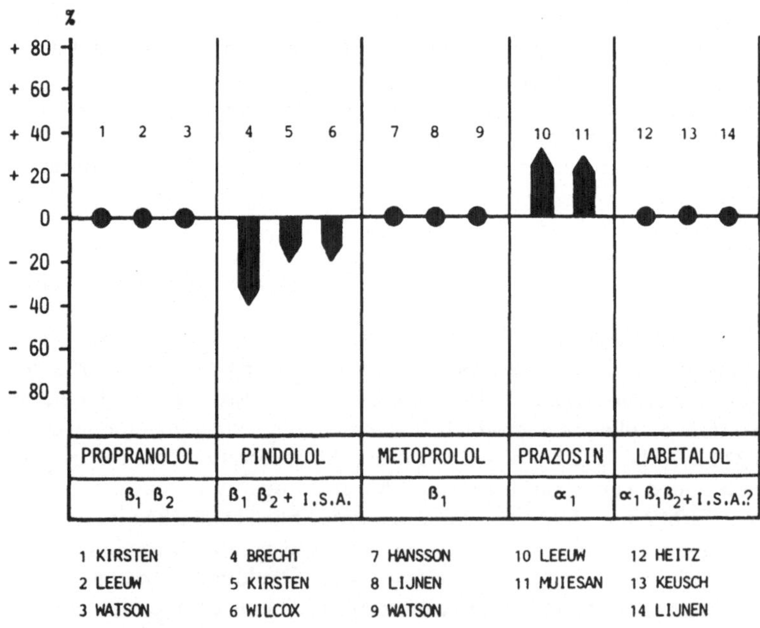

Fig. 1 Percent change in norepinephrine plasma concentration after prolonged oral treatment with receptor antagonists

The middle line represents catecholamine levels before treatment. Arrows above the line show percent increases, arrows below the line, percent decreases. A circle on the line indicates no change. Propranolol, a nonspecific beta blocker which blocks both beta 1 and 2 sites, caused no change in norepinephrine levels in three different studies, listed below the figure (Kirsten et al., 1982, de Leeuw et al., 1977, Watson et al., 1980). Pindolol, a nonspecific blocking agent which possesses intrinsic sympathomimetic activity, caused decreases of 40 and 20 percent in three different studies (Brecht et al., 1976, Kirsten et al., 1982, Wilcox et al., 1981). Metoprolol, a beta 1 blocker also caused no change in norepinephrine levels (Hannson et al., 1977, Lijnen et al., 1979, Watson et al., 1980). Prazosin, an alpha 1 blocker, caused increases in norepinephrine of about 30 percent in two different studies (de Leeuw et al., 1980, Muiesan, 1980). Labetalol, an alpha 1 blocker as well as a nonspecific beta blocker, caused no change in norepinephrine levels (Heitz et al., 1980, Keusch et al., 1980, Lijnen et al., 1979). There are conflicting reports about whether labetalol posesses intrinsic sympathomimetic activity which has been indicated by a question mark.

Discordant reports have been published about catecholamine levels after labetalol treatment. However, these discordancies are due more to difficulties in comparing studies which are not methodically alike. When the studies are separated into groups, according to methods and type of medication application, a good consensus is reached. In 1978 Weidmann et al. reported increased urinary catecholamine excretion rates after labetalol therapy, using a fluorometric method to determine catecholamines. They discounted interference with labetalol since they had incubated some samples with the drug and found no increases. Subsequent studies using the more specific radioenzymatic assay for catecholamines could not confirm these results and later comparative studies by Miano et al. (1979), Pisanti et al. (1980) and Preziosi et al. (1978) attributed the increases in catecholamine levels found by Weidmann to the presence of a metabolite of labetalol which interferes with the fluorometric and spectrophotometric methods of assay.

Catecholamine Response to Different Forms of Labetalol Application

Figure 2 shows the norepinephrine response to different forms of labetalol application. When labetalol is administered intravenously, increases of between 20 and 40 percent in the norepinephrine concentration have been reported (Carlsen et al., 1980, Lechi et al., 1981, Lin et al., 1983). As shown in figure 1, when labetalol is administered orally for prolonged periods of time, there is no increase in norepinephrine levels. After acute oral administration, Trap-Jensen (1982) reported an increase of 10 percent and Vlachakis (1979) an increase of over 100 percent. The discrepancy after acute oral administration, which is apparent here, may be attributable to different patient collectives and methods employed. Trap-Jensen's study was done after psychic stress in healthy volunteers. Norepinephrine increased only 10 percent while epinephrine increased 135 percent. Vlachakis applied labetalol to hypertensive patients and found an increase of 118 percent in norepinephrine and 64 percent in epinephrine. Even though these studies are radically different, it is evident that acute oral application does cause an increase in catecholamine levels.

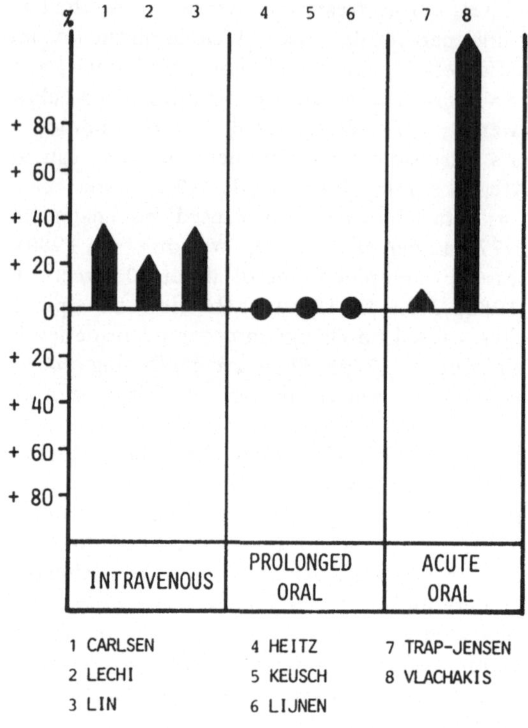

Fig. 2
Percent change in norepinephrine plasma concentration after different forms of labetalol application

Regulating Mechanisms

One reason for the increase in catecholamines after intravenous application of labetalol has been attributed to blockade of the neuronal uptake of norepinephrine (Blakeley et al., 1977, Summers and Tillman, 1977). Figure 3 shows that blockade of re-uptake would cause the plasma level to increase. Acute oral administration probably acts similarly to intravenous administration with regard to driving the norepinephrine level upwards before regulating mechanisms can come into play. During prolonged oral therapy feedback mechanisms regulating norepinephrine secretion might become effective. At slightly increased norepinephrine concentrations the extremely sensitive beta adrenoceptors facilitate an enhanced secretion of norepinephrine into the synaptic cleft. High norepinephrine levels trigger the less sensitive alpha 2 adrenoceptors which inhibit norepinephrine release, overcoming the beta adrenergic mediated positive feedback action. The result would be a normalization of the norepinephrine levels. Evidence of the alpha 2 supported negative feedback on norepinephrine release into the synaptic region has been found in studies on clonidine effects.

Clonidine, which is an alpha agonist and at first glance should cause an increase in plasma catecholamine levels, in fact, lowers catecholamines to pre-drug levels (Arndts et al., 1983). This may be attributed to the aforementioned regulating mechanism.

Another hypothesis explaining the constant levels of catecholamines during prolonged oral therapy involves cancellation of opposing effects on catecholamine levels. The alpha 1

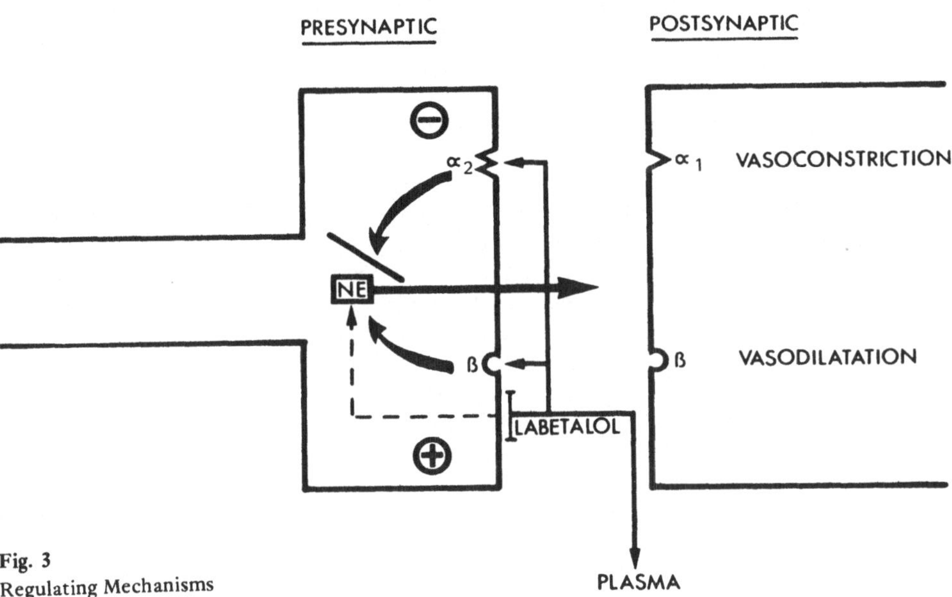

Fig. 3
Regulating Mechanisms

blocking component in labetalol alone would be expected to cause an increase in catecholamines as does prazosin (see Figure 1). The unspecific beta blocking component, which is estimated to be approximately three times stronger than the alpha component when given orally (Richards et al., 1979), would tend to have no influence on the catecholamines, like propranolol. Recent reports of Carpenter (1981) have presented evidence indicating that labetalol possesses partial agonist activity on certain beta adrenoceptor systems. Such intrinsic sympathomimetic activity would, like pindolol, influence the catecholamines, causing a downward trend. These opposing effects could cancel one another out and leave the catecholamines unchanged after longer therapy.
To summarize: it is not possible to decide at this point whether constant catecholamine concentrations during prolonged oral labetalol therapy are due to regulating mechanisms or cancellation of opposing effects of the alpha and beta blocking components of labetalol.

Clinical Implications

The clinical implications of any blocker are difficult to assess in terms of plasma catecholamine concentrations. However, if the catecholamines are raised without blockade of the alpha 1 receptors, vasoconstriction will occur which will raise the blood pressure. This occurs in the case of a norepinephrine secreting tumor. Since norepinephrine is predominantly an alpha agonist, vasoconstriction occurs, thus raising the blood pressure. Here, exclusive beta blockade is contraindicated since exposure of the alpha receptors to relatively higher catecholamine concentrations would result. In this case alpha blockade is essential. An exclusive alpha blockade in many essential hypertension patients, on the other hand, is often contraindicated. The alpha blockade leaves the beta receptors exposed to relatively high concentrations of catecholamines and orthostatic hypotension may result.

Good results have been achieved with labetolol in treating patients with pheochromocytoma (Bailey, 1979). A balanced blockade of alpha and beta receptors is theoretically advantageous since epinephrine and norepinephrine, the hormones generally secreted, possess both alpha and beta agonist activity. Labetalol also seems appropriate for treatment of high blood pressure during pregnancy (Michael, 1979). Suppression of the fetal heart rate does not occur as is often the case with exclusive beta blockade.

Alpha adrenergic blockade may alleviate the occurrence of angina pectoris and myocardial infarction by preventing alpha adrenergically mediated coronary artery vasoconstriction (Marx et al., 1979). The alpha blocking component of labetalol may be of value in treating Raynaud symptoms where cold extremities become a problem during beta blockade (Eliasson et al., 1984).

The effect of beta blockade, which is of great practical use in reducing hypertension, seems at first glance paradoxical. During beta blockade it appears logical that higher catecholamine concentrations would be available to stimulate the alpha receptors, thereby inducing vasoconstriction and an increase in blood pressure. However, epinephrine is an agonist whose beta component is greater than that of norepinephrine. This means that epinephrine would be relatively ineffectual during beta blockade. This is supported by reports of beta blocking agents being not only useful in reducing blood pressure but in controlling nervousness encountered under stress situations which is often manifested as a tremor or palpitations (Uslar et al., 1977).

The various blocking agents are of great practical use. However, at this point, it is impossible to decide which essential hypertensive patient has a disturbance in either the alpha or beta receptors or a disturbance in both systems or no disturbance at all. It is impossible to predict which patient will respond to which blocker with an acceptable blood pressure decrease and no or tolerable side effects. The state of the art is still "trial and error", with our having to say: if one blocker doesn't work, try another.

References

Arndts, D., Doevendans, J., Kirsten, R., Heintz, B.: New aspects of the pharmacokinetics and pharmacodynamics of clonidine in man. *Eur. J. Clin. Pharmacol.* **24:** 21–30 (1983.

Bailey, R. R.: Labetalol in the treatment of a patient with phaeochromocytoma: a case report. *Br. J. Clin. Pharmacol.* **8:** 141–142 (1979).

Bean, B. L., Brown, J. J., Casals-Stenzel, J., Fraser, R., Lever, A. F., Millar, J. A., Morton, J. J., Petch, B., Riegger, A. J. G., Robertson, J. I. S., Tree, M.: The relation of arterial pressure and plasma angiotensin II concentration. A change produced by prolonged infusion of angiotensin II in the conscious dog. *Cir. Res.* **44:** 452–8 (1979).

Blakeley, A. G. H., Summers, R. J.: The effects of labetalol (AH 5158) on adrenergic transmission in the cat spleen. *Br. J. Pharmacol.* **59:** 643–650 (1977).

Brecht, H. W., Banthien, F., Schoeppe, W.: Decrease in plasma noradrenaline levels following long-term treatment with prindolol in patients with essential hypertension. *Klin. Wschr.* **54:** 1095–1105 (1976).

Carlsen, J. E., Trap-Jensen, J., Svendsen, T. L., Nielsen, P. E., Rasmussen, S., Christensen, N. J.: Effect of labetalol on plasma catecholamines at rest and during increased sympathetic activity. *Postgrad. Med. J.* **56**: Suppl. 2, 43–47 (1980).

Carpenter, J. R.: Intrinsic activity of labetalol on guinea-pig isolated trachea. *J. Pharm. Pharmacol.* **33**: 806–807 (1981).

Eliasson, K. et al.: Karolinska Sjukhuset Stockholm. Kurzberichte vom Schwedischen Ärztetag "Rikstämma" vom Dec. 1983. Beim Raynaud-Phänomen nach Betablockade auf Labetalol (TRANDATE) umsetzen. Arznei-Telegramm A 4330 E p. 5, January (1984).

Hansson, B.-G., Dymling, J.-F., Manhem, P., Hökfelt, B.: Long term treatment of moderate hypertension with the beta$_1$-receptor blocking agent metoprolol. *Eur. J. Clin. Pharmacol.* **11**: 247–254 (1977).

Heitz, J., Haux, R., Gotzen, R.: Der Einfluß einer kombinierten α- und β-Rezeptoren-Blockade (Labetalol) auf die Plasmakatecholamine bei essentiellen Hypertonikern. *Therapiewoche* **30**, No. 47: 7863–64 (1980).

Keusch, G., Weidmann, P., Ziegler, W. H., de Chatel, R., Reubi, F. C.: Effects of chronic alpha and beta adrenoceptor blockade with labetalol on plasma catecholamines and renal function in hypertension *Klin. Wochenschr.* **58**: 25–29 (1980).

Kirsten, R., Heintz, B., Böhmer, D., Nelson, K., Roth, S., Welzel, D.: Relationship of plasma catecholamines to blood pressure in hypertensive patients during β-adrenoceptor blockade with and without intrinsic sympathomimetic activity. *Br. J. Clin. Pharmacol.* **13**: 397–406 (1982).

L'Abbé, M., Tinel, J., Doumer, E.: Crises solaires et hypertension paroxystique en rapport avec une tumeur surrénale. *Bull. Soc. Med. Hop.* **46**: 982–990 (1922).

Lechi, A., Picotti, G. B., Covi, G., Pomari, S., Pedrolli, E., Cesura, A. M., Danti, G., Mattioli, M.: Intravenous labetalol in severe hypertension – effects on blood pressure, plasma renin activity and catecholamines. *Arzneim.-Forsch./Drug Res.* **31** (I) Nr. 3 (1981).

de Leeuw, P. W., Falke, H. E., Kho, T. L., Vandogen, R., Wester, A., Birkenhäger, W. H.: Effects of beta-adrenergic blockade on diurnal variability of blood pressure and plasma noradrenaline levels. *Acta Med Scand* **202**: 389–392 (1977).

de Leeuw, P. W., Wester, A., Willemse, P. J., Birkenhäger, W. H.: Effects of prazosin on plasma noradrenaline and plasma renin concentrations in hypertensive subjects. *J. Cardiovasc. Pharmacol.* **2.**, (Suppl. 3): 361–372 (1980).

Lijnen, P. J., Amery, A. K., Fagard, R. H., Reybrouck, T. M.: The effects of β-adrenoceptor blockade on renin, angiotensin, aldosterone and catecholamines at rest and during exercise. *Br. J. Clin. Pharmacol.* **7**: 175–181 (1979).

Lijnen, P. J., Amery, A. K., Fagard, R. H., Reybrouck, T. M., Moerman, E. J., De Schaepdryver, A. F.: Effects of labetalol on plasma renin, aldosterone and catecholamines in hypertensive patients. *J. Cardiovasc. Pharmacol.* **1**: 625–632 (1979).

Lin, M., McNay, J. L., Shepherd, A. M. M., Keeton, T. K.: The response of plasma catecholamines to intravenous labetalol: a comparison with sodium nitroprusside. *Clin. Pharmacol. Ther.* **34**, 4: 466–473 (1983).

Marx, P. G., Reid, D. S.: Labetalol infusion in acute myocardial infarction with systemic hypertension. *Br. J. clin. Pharmacol* **8**: 233–238 (1979).

Miano, L., Kolloch, R., de Quattro, V.: Increased catecholamine excretion after labetalol therapy: a spurious effect of drug metabolites. *Clinica Chimica Acta* **95**: 211–217 (1979).

Michael, C. A.: Use of labetalol in the treatment of servere hypertension during pregnancy. *Br. J. clin. Pharmacol.* **8**: 211–215 (1979).

Muiesan, T., Discussion in: de Leeuw, P. W., Wester, A., Willemse, P. J., Birkenhäger, W. H. Effects of prazosin on plasma noradrenaline and plasma renin concentrations in hypertensive subjects. *J. Cardiovasc. Pharmacol.* **2**, (Suppl. 3): 361–372 (1980).

Pisanti, N., Vacca, M., de Natale, G., Preziosi, P.: Labetalol disposition interferes with fluorometric dosage of catecholamines: in vitro and in vivo trials with enzymatic inhibitors. *Pharmacol. Res. Commun.* **12**, No. 10: 937–44 (1980).

Preziosi, P., Pinsanti, N., Brevetti, G., Paudice, G., Moerman, E. J., de Schaepdryver, A. F.: Urinary catecholamines and labetalol. *Arch. Intern. Pharmacodyn.* **236**, No. 2: 317–19 (1978).

Richards, D. A., Prichard, B. N. C.: Clinical pharamacology of labetalol. *Br. J. clin. Pharmacol.* **8**: 89–93 (1979).

Strömbeck, J. P., Hedberg, T. P.: Tumor of the suprarenal medulla associated with paroxysmal hypertension. Report of case preoperatively diagnosed and cured by extirpation after capsular incision. *Acta. Chir. Scand.* 82: 177–189 (1939).

Summers, R. J., Tillman, J.: The effects of labetalol (AH 5158) on metabolism of ^{3}H(−) noradrenaline released from the cat spleen by nerve stimulation. *Biochem. Pharmacol.* 26: 2137–2143 (1977).

Trap-Jensen, J., Carlsen, J., Hartling, O. J., et al.: Beta-adrenoceptor blockade and psychic stress in man. A comparison of the acute effects of labetalol, metoprolol, pindolol and propranolol on plasma levels of adrenaline and noradrenaline. *Br. J. Clin. Pharmacol.* 13/Suppl. 2: 391–395 (1982).

Uslar, A., Sinn, M., Schiffter, R.: Tremorbehandlung mit dem Betarezeptorenblocker Propranolol. *Therapiewoche* 27: 490 (1977).

Vlachakis, N. D., Velasquez, M., Barr, J., Alexander, N., Maronde, R. F.: Hemodynamic and catecholamine effects of labetalol in hypertensive patients. *Clin. Res.* 27, No. 2: 546A (1979).

Watson, R. D. S., Eriksson, B.-M., Hamilton, C. A., Reid, J. L., Stallard, T. J., Littler, W. A.: Effects of chronic beta-adrenoceptor antagonism on plasma catecholamines and blood pressure in hypertension. *J. Cardiovasc. Pharmacol.* 2: 725–738 (1980).

Weidmann, P., de Chatel, R., Ziegler, W. H., Flammer, J., Reubi, F.: Alpha and beta adrenergic blockade with orally administered labetalol in hypertension — Studies on blood volume, plasma renin and aldosterone and catecholamine excretion. *The Am. J. Cardiol.* Vol. 41: 570–576 (1978).

Wilcox, C. S., Lewis, P. S., Peart, W. S., Sever, P. S., Osikowska, B. A., Suddle, S. A. J., Bluhm, M. M., Veall, N., Lancaster, R.: Renal function, body fluid volumes, renin, aldosterone and noradrenaline during treatment of hypertension with pindolol. *J. of Cardiovasc. Pharmac.* 3: 598–611 (1981).

Discussion

Borchard
Herr Prichard teilte uns heute morgen mit, daß vorwiegend die Alpha-1-Rezeptoren geblockt werden. Sie nehmen an, daß die Beta-Rezeptoren deutlich stärker gehemmt werden. Dann frage ich mich, ob überhaupt der präsynaptischen Modulation der Alpha-2-Rezeptoren eine wesentliche Rolle zukommt.

Kirsten
Für Labetalol trifft das zu. Die Effekte von Labetalol unter Ruhebedingungen lassen sich durch postsynaptische Alpha-1-Blockade und durch präsynaptische Betablockade erklären. Es handelt sich hierbei jedoch um eine Interpretation. Hinzuzufügen ist, daß die Empfindlichkeitsunterschiede zwischen Alpha-1-/Alpha-2-Rezeptoren für einzelne Pharmaka verschieden ist. Außerdem gibt es Empfindlichkeitsunterschiede zwischen Arterien, Venen und Herz.

Borchard
Haben Sie die Veränderungen der Katecholamine auch unter dynamischer Belastung gemessen?

Kirsten
Unter Belastungsbedingungen habe ich nur Propranolol, Pindolol, Clonidin und Co-Dergocrinmesylat untersucht. Weidmann hat unter Labetalol die Plasmakatecholamine bestimmt und gefunden, daß bei Belastung die präsynaptische Feedbackkontrolle der Katecholaminausschüttung unbeeinflußt bleibt.

N. N.
Die von Ihnen zitierten Literaturbefunde stimmen gut überein, wobei Sie allerdings die Veränderungen prozentual angeben. Gilt dies auch bei einem Vergleich der absoluten Werte?

Kirsten
Bedingt durch die beträchtlichen Unterschiede der benutzten analytischen Bestimmungsmethoden für die Katecholamine lassen sich die absoluten Werte nur bedingt vergleichen. Allerdings wird mit der zunehmenden Anwendung radioenzymatischer Methoden die Übereinstimmung immer besser.

N. N.
Wie erklären Sie die im Gegensatz zu Propranolol fehlende fötale Herzfrequenzbeeinflussung von Labetalol und Pindolol?

Kirsten
Propranolol hat einen größeren Verteilungsraum infolge größerer Lipidlöslichkeit und ist leichter membrangängig.

N. N.
Die Plasmakatecholaminveränderungen ließen sich erklären durch unterschiedliche Beeinflussung der
Clearance durch die verschiedenen Betablocker, bedingt durch Effekte auf die Herzdynamik.

Kirsten
Sowohl Propranolol als auch Pindolol erniedrigen die Katecholaminclearance (veröffentlicht in: Die
Beta-Rezeptorblockade aus pathophysiologischer Sicht, Hrsg. H. Roskamm & H. Holzgreve, Schattauer
Stuttgart, 1982). Das unterschiedliche Verhalten der Plasmakatecholamine ist auf präsynaptische Effekte zurückzuführen. Viel eher spiegeln die Plasmaveränderungen synaptisch beeinflußte Änderungen
des peripheren Gefäßwiderstandes wider.

II Extra-Cardiovascular Effects and Adverse Reactions

The Clinical Profiles of Long Term Labetalol Therapy

P. Feldschreiber

Glaxo Pharmaceuticals Ltd., 891/995 Greenford Road, Greenford, Middlesex UB6 0HE, England

Summary

Labetalol is an effective antihypertensive agent that has a good record of safety, as indicated by the Adverse Reation Data Base collated over the past seven years. The principal side effects are scalp tingling, acute retention of urine, postural hypotension, bronchospasm, and gastric disturbance. These did not occur with a higher incidence than those encountered with other antihypertensives, and were dose related.

Labetalol is a unique drug entity that acts as a competitive antagonist at both alpha and beta-adrenoceptors [1]. The structure is shown in Figure 1. The drug was first synthesised by Glaxo Group Research Ltd. in the UK and was developed as an antihypertensive agent in man during the period 1973–1976. The drug acts acutely by reducing peripheral vascular resistance via post-synaptic alpha blockade and the resultant reflex tachycardia is suppressed by labetalol's beta-blocking activity [2]. Long term use of the drug will reduce systemic arterial pressure by beta-blocking activity and a consistent alpha-blockade induces reduction in vascular resistance. This paper will describe the safety and efficacy of the drug used in its indication for all grades of hypertensive disease since it became available on the United Kingdom prescribing list in 1976.

Results

Database

The figures presented in the following sections are based on:

(a) UK multicentre studies performed.
(b) Monitored release study performed from 1976 to 1978. This study was requested by the UK committee on Safety of Medicines.

Fig. 1
Labetalol

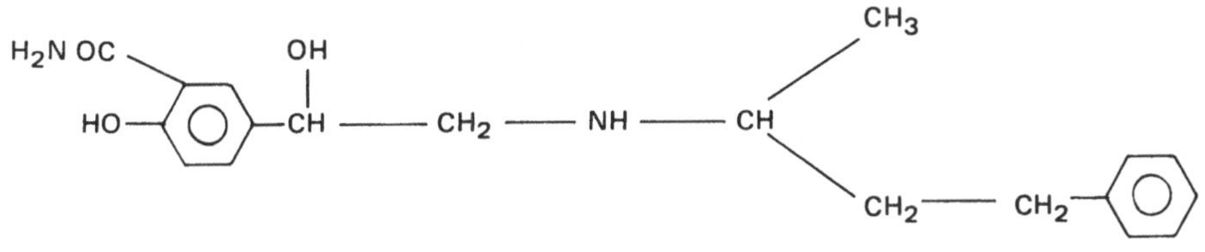

"""

These data reflect usage which is estimated to be 16,647 patient years worldwide.
In 1976, the UK CSM requested clinical data on 3000 patients treated with labetalol for a year. Glaxo complied with this request by setting up a 'monitored release survey'. 6000 patients were recruited in the first year, of which 3000 were followed up for two years.
Patients were checked for antihypertensive response and adverse events at 2 and 4 weeks, 3, 6, 9, 12, and 24 months. The final recruitment figures are shown in Figure 2.

Fig. 2
Monitored Release Survey

Patients	
Initial recruitment	6,785
Available at one year	4,345
Available at two years	3,253
Demography	
Essential hypertension	97 %
Other hypertensive disorders (e.g. renal, diabetic)	3 %

Scalp tingling (2.8 %) and acute retention of urine (0.15 %), were the important positive findings in this survey.
Figure 3 shows the absolute number of patients withdrawn from the study.

Fig. 3
Monitored Release Survey

	Number of Patients	
	Recorded	*Withdrew*
Acute retention of urine	10	5
Ejaculatory failure	14	2
Dreams/nightmares	48	10
Dry eyes	7	2

Fig. 4
Labetalol Safety

Proven Side-Effects
Postural hypotension
Scalp tingling
Bronchospasm
Lichenform skin rash
Acute retention of urine
Systemic lupus erythematosus (2 cases)
Toxic myopathy (1 case)
Drug interactions with cimetidine, tricyclic antidepressants, and urinary catecholamine estimations

Worldwide adverse events reporting: these figures include those reported in multicentre USA studies [3]. Proven side effects (Fig. 4, 5, 6) included postural hypotension, scalp

Fig. 5

Other Proven Side Effects

Postural hypotension	4.2 %
Bronchospasm	1.8 %
Lichenform skin rash	8 cases Worldwide
Systemic lupus	2 cases

Fig. 6

Proven and Unique Side Effects

Scalp tingling	2.8 %
Acute retention of urine	0.15 %
Toxic myopathy	1 case

Fig. 7

Liver Problems

Spontaneous Reports (N = 23)*	jaundiced	not jaundiced
Resolved on drug	4	5
Resolved off drug	5	4
Total	9	9
*5 reports were partly documented		

tingling, bronchospasm, lichenform skin rash, urine retention, SLE (2 cases), toxic myopathy (1 case), and interactions with cimetidine, tricyclic antidepressants, and urinary catecholamine estimations.

In addition to these proven side effects (Fig. 7), 23 cases of hepatic dysfunction have been reported from worldwide sources. These included patients with raised transaminases and 9 patients with frank jaundice. Professor Sheila Sherlock reviewed clinical details of these cases and came to the conclusion that 15 cases did have a hepatitic reaction to labetalol, and therefore the suspicion arose that the drug may induce disturbance in liver function leading rarely to cholestatic jaundice. Our advice is that the drug should be stopped immediately if jaundice is noted.

Minor Events

As with all drugs there was a definite incidence of non-serious adverse reactions. The notable event in this list is headache (9.1 %) (Figure 8). Other problems included peripheral vascular symptoms (claudication 1.7 %), chest pain (not associated with myocardial ischaemia), palpitations and tremor.

Muscular aches	2.8 %
Bowel disturbances	4.4 %
Dreams	0.7 %
Headache	9.1 %

A comparative view is shown by the side effects encountered in the pivotal registration study carried out in the United States, and presented to the Food and Drugs Administration. This was a double blind placebo controlled study comparing labetalol 200 mg — 1600 mg daily and propranolol 80 mg — 160 mg daily. Of particular note is the increased description of fatigue encountered with propranolol (12 %) and bradycardia (5 %). Labetalol treatment caused a higher incidence of gastrointestinal upset than propranolol.

Discussion

The incidence and frequency of adverse events reported with labetalol from this data show the drug to be comparable in safety to other antihypertensives, particularly beta-blocking drugs.

Kane et al. [4] have compared the side effect profiles of methyldopa, propranolol, slow release oxprenolol, and labetalol (Figure 9), and this confirms the data quoted above.

Fig. 9

Side effect profile of labetalol in comparison with methyldopa, propranolol and slow-release oxprenolol (Kane and Gregg [4]).

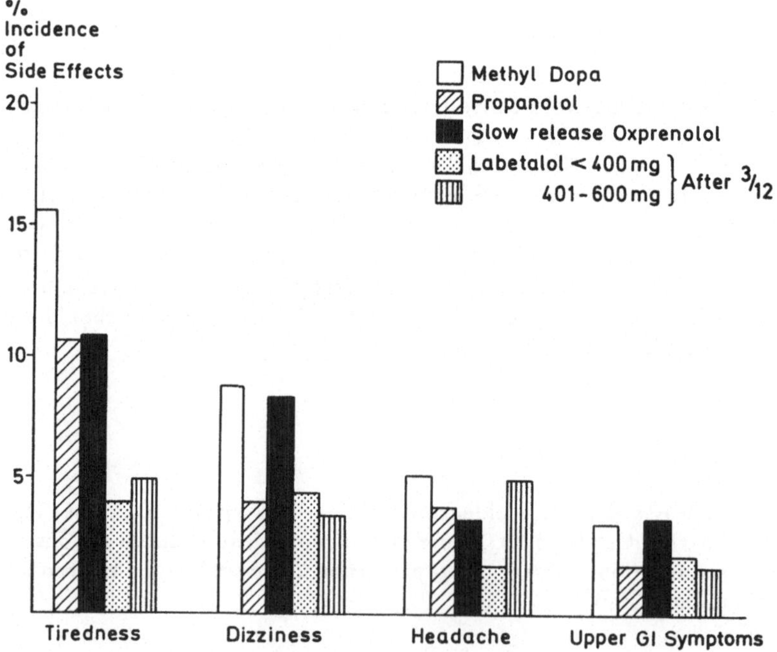

48

These workers also showed that the withdrawals of patients due to tiredness and dizziness in the Monitored Release Study progressively decreased with time. This probably indicates a 'first dose' effect of the drug.

A recent study from the MRC Blood Pressure Unit in Glasgow [5] confirmed that labetalol's side effect profile was dose dependent. The drug should be introduced at a low dose when replacing full doses of a previously administered beta-blocker.

Conclusion

Labetalol is an effective antihypertensive agent that has a good record of safety, as indicated by the Adverse Reaction Data Base collated over the past seven years. The principal side effects are scalp tingling, acute retention of urine, postural hypotension, bronchospasm, and gastric disturbance. These did not occur with a higher incidence than those encountered with other antihypertensives, and were dose related.

References

[1]   Brittain, R. T., and Levy, G. P. (1976). *Br. J. Clin. Pharmacol.* **3**, 681–694.

[2]   Richards, D. A., and Prichard, B. N. C. (1979). *European Society of Cardiology Symposium on Labetalol.* Florence, pp. 16–19.

[3]   Michaelson, E. L. et al. (1983). Multicenter clinical evaluation of long term efficacy and safety of labetalol in the treatment of hypertension. *American Journal of Medicine*, Dallas Symposium Oct. 17th 1982, pp. 68–80.

[4]   Kane, J., Gregg, I., and Stephens, M. D. B., (1979). Long term study of labetalol in general practice. *Br. J. Clin. Pharmacol.* **8**, Suppl. 2, 167.

[5]   McAreavey, D. et al. (1984). "Third Drug" Trial: comparative study of antihypertensive agents added to the treatment when BP remains uncontrolled by beta-blockers plus thiazide diuretic. *B. M. J.* **288**, 106–110.

Discussion

O'Malley
You showed the dose levels used starting at 2 weeks going up to 9 months, and the gradual shift to higher doses. Was it titration or tolerance?

Feldschreiber
It was titration. This is an important question, which I'm sure will be addressed later on in this symposium. This is a titratable drug, and it has to be used as such. You have to titrate the dose of the drug carefully using blood pressure as a response.

Schulz
Wie erklären Sie die Harnretentionen und die trockenen Augen als unerwünschte Wirkung?

Feldschreiber
Dry eyes; I don't think we have any adequate pharmacological answer. There were only two cases recorded in the 6000 patients. We have been following these patients for several years now, and we have not found a significant incidence of this side effect. So, I really cannot explain that on pharmacological grounds but I think that it is a clinically insignificant problem. Urine retention may be related to alpha-blockade, but again the incidence of that from the worldwide literature was only 0.15 %, and we have not seen this as a clinically significant problem.

Hain

Your first comment is, I think, a bit misleading because it is not only one molecule. Labetalol is actually a racemate. That is, you are treating your patients with a fixed combination of an alpha-1, and a bit alpha-2-adrenoceptor-blocking drug, with a beta-1- and beta-2-blocking drug and may be with a drug with some other effect which also is enhancing activity. How is it possible for you to ascribe to one or other molecule, or enantiomer, some special side effects which are special for labetalol, i.e., in contrast to propranolol?

Feldschreiber

Yes. This is a very interesting question. I certainly didn't mean to be misleading, and I did use the word entity rather than molecule. As you say, the drug is a mixture, a racemic mixture of 4 enantiomers. We have not yet adequately defined the different beta-blocking or alpha-blocking components of these four enantiomers. Detailed investigation, however, has now concentrated on one of the enantiomers, that is the R,R-isomer of the drug, and there we do find, as an example to answer your question, that this particular enantiomer when looked at individually, does have a far greater ratio of beta-blocking to alpha-blocking activities; It has 10 times the beta-blocking activity to that found with the racemic mixture as opposed to the 25 % alpha-blocking component of the racemic mixture. However, this particular isomer still does have significant activity in reducing peripheral vascular resistence. We are not sure whether that is due to intrinsic beta-2-agonist activity, or whether it has direct vasodilating properties. I don't think that we have adequately defined the pharmacology of these individual components, and you are quite right. I think, from this database it would be impossible to give you firm answers on which particular enantiomer is responsible for which particular side effect. One interesting thing that we do know on a positive note, about the R,R-isomer, is that when the R,R-isomer is tested in patients with obstructive airways disease the drug induced reduction in FEV is far less than with the racemic mixture. So, that may be evidence of beta-2-agonist activity, but we are certainly not sure of that. You are quite right, we have not properly delineated that.

Beta-Blocker Induced Changes in the Cholesterol: HDL-Cholesterol Ratio and Risk of Coronary Heart Disease

B. G. Woodcock, N. Rietbrock

Department of Clinical Pharmacology, University Clinic Frankfurt, Theodor-Stern-Kai 7, D-6000 Frankfurt, FRG.

Summary

The lowering of blood pressure with β-blocking drugs has had a low impact on coronary heart disease mortality and the question has been raised whether adverse changes in plasma lipoproteins offset the benefits of blood pressure reduction.

Comparison of plasma lipoprotein concentrations in hypertensive patients treated with commonly used β-blockers with lipoprotein concentrations in patients with coronary heart disease shows that these drugs can cause clinically important shifts in the cholesterol ratio (Total cholesterol: HDL-cholesterol) and reductions in the atheroprotective lipoprotein HDL-cholesterol. The magnitude of these changes is sufficient to increase the risk of heart attack 2 to 4 fold depending on the initial cholesterol ratio and the duration of treatment.

Only β-blockers with marked intrinsic sympathomimetic agonist activity (Pindolol) or combined alpha/beta blocking properties (Labetalol) appear free of adverse effects on plasma lipoproteins and triglycerides. Chronic treatment with other β-blockers should be accompanied by cholesterol and HDL-cholesterol measurements at the beginning of therapy. Plasma lipoprotein measurements at 3–6 month intervals seem mandatory in patients with cholesterol values greater than 6 mmol/l (230 mg/dl) and total cholesterol: HDL-cholesterol ratios above 5 at the start of treatment. The risk of a coronary event must be regarded as unacceptable when the cholesterol ratio exceeds a critical value of about 6.

Further controlled studies are needed to evaluate the effects of β-blockers in hypertension when administered for periods of up to a year or more. More information is required on the behaviour of lipoprotein sub-species and apo-proteins. Since the changes in lipoproteins reported in studies referred to in this review may have been submaximal the risks and the benefits from β-blocker therapy must be carefully considered.

The lowering of blood pressure with drugs has had a low impact on coronary heart disease mortality and the question has been recently raised [1] whether metabolic side effects of antihypertensive agents offset the potential benefits. There have been many reports on the effect of β-blockers on lipoprotein metabolism in patients with hypertension. Where the treatment period has been long enough and the patient group large enough, β_1-selective and non-selective β-blockers usually increased the atherogenic lipoprotein species (cholesterol, low-density lipoprotein-cholesterol (LDL-C), very low-density lipoprotein triglycerides (VLDL-TG) and decreased the so-called atheroprotective species high-density lipoprotein-cholesterol (HDL-C)) [2–10]. These observations raise two important questions: —

Are such changes in plasma lipoproteins clinically relevant?

Are there important differences between β-blockers in the extent to which they show these potentially adverse reactions?

Answers to these questions are difficult to obtain from a superficial inspection of the published results. There are, for example, more than 12 different lipoproteins and at least three types of HDL-C, together with their respective apo-proteins all of which may change during drug treatment. Not all of these fractions have been sufficiently well investigated for their possible role in coronary heart disease (CHD) and arteriosclerosis, however most investigators have measured total triglycerides, VLDL-TG, LDL-C, HDL-C and cholesterol.

The Risk Factor "Cholesterol Ratio" and Coronary Heart Disease

Raised plasma cholesterol levels have long been recognised as a risk for the development of ischemic heart disease [11–13]. The plasma concentration of HDL-C in contrast shows an inverse relationship, an observation confirmed in a number of recent epidemiological and clinical studies [11–17] and there is angiographic evidence that the severity of coronary artery disease is related to a decreasing HDL-C concentration [15].

In the Framingham Study [13] HDL-C was the best discriminator in separating patients with arteriosclerotic heart disease from healthy subjects in the group aged 50 years and over and the plasma concentration of this lipoprotein could be used to help identify even asymptomatic persons who were at greater risk of having coronary heart disease [12]. Miller et al. [18] reported that dependence of the risk of coronary heart disease on HDL-C was 300% greater than on LDL-C and found that of the 8 variables measured, HDL-C made the most important independent contribution to the 'prediction' of future coronary heart disease in young men.

In the aged, where arteriosclerosis is also present, there is evidence that the cholesterol ratio is a better predictor of underlying cardiac disease [11]. Carew at al. [19] have shown that when porcine smooth muscle cells are incubated in lipoprotein rich media LDL alone causes an increase in the cholesterol content of the cells whilst LDL + HDL results in no net increase in cholesterol content. If cholesterol is taken into the cell by way of LDL, and HDL is involved with its removal or reduction of uptake, then the ratio should be a better index of risk than the level of cholesterol or HDL-C alone and particulary so if the HDL_2 subfraction is also measured.

Measurement of HDL_2 requires ultra-centrifugation techniques however and LDL is often omitted from lipoprotein results reported [15, 20]. For these reasons the cholesterol ratio based on total cholesterol (TC), although not a simple risk factor since it includes the HDL-C, has more practical value. This ratio, (TC/HDL-C), was applied in estimates of coronary risk by Uhl et al. [12] in a coronary angiographic study of 128 asymptomatic pilots, mean age 40 years, undergoing cardiac work-up. The TC: HDL-C ratio was strongly correlated with the presence of arteriosclerosis regardless of age, evidence that it was a reliable index of risk. The equation Age × (TC/HDL-C) = 230 divided normals from patients with definite coronary artery disease with surprising sharpness.

In the following retrospective examination of lipids in coronary heart disease and of β-blocker effects on plasma lipids the cholesterol ratio TC/HDL-C has been taken as the most convenient index of risk. By plotting this ratio against the HDL-C plasma levels we should be able to separate patients with CHD or with a high risk of CHD from those without. Fig. 1a is a plot of TC/HDL-C ratio against HDL-C for patient groups with coronary heart disease published in 10 authoritative studies from 1980 or later, together with corresponding data on low risk groups (students, japanese joggers etc.) and non-cardiac patients including some groups in whom the absence of coronary lesions has been confirmed angiographically eg airline pilots and patients with valvular dysfunction (see Key to Fig. 1a). The patient groups cover a wide range of plasma cholesterol concentrations and thus the curve is similar to that given by the results of the Framingham Study which showed a near exponential change in the probability of a coronary event within 4 years after a myocardial infarction when this parameter was plotted against the plasma HDL-C concentration [21, 22].

The division between coronary heart disease and low risk groups shows a critical value for cholesterol ratio of about 5 and this is an agreement with the observations on patients over 50 years of age examined angiographically [12] and the data of Kladetzky et al. [28], (not shown in the figure) who reported cholesterol ratios for normal subjects (4.48), subjects with coronary vascular disease, 1 vessel, less than 50% stenosis (5.42), 1 vessel disease, more than 50% stenosis (6.27) and 2 or more vessel disease (5.88). In the study of Uhl et al. [12] a critical value of 6 was exceeded by only 2 of 93 subjects above 35 years and without significant coronary artery disease but was exceeded by 16 of 18 in whom the disease was present. This comparison is based on mean values. For the individual asymptomatic subject undergoing cardiac catheterisation the calculated probability of having significant coronary heart disease with a cholesterol ratio less than 6 was only 2%.

Fig. 1a also shows that in these diverse groups of subjects a decrease in HDL-C is not associated with a corresponding decrease in plasma cholesterol, but more probably an increase. The observation that the 'healthier' the subjects (the lower the risk) the higher is the HDL-C and the lower the cholesterol ratio shows that the original premiss, to use the cholesterol ratio TC/HDL-C as an index of risk, is valid.

Cholesterol Ratio Shifts Induced by β-Blockers

If there is a relationship between the cholesterol ratio and coronary heart disease then we should be able to assess the negative effect of antihypertensive therapy on metabolism by the change it induces in the plasma HDL-C and cholesterol ratio. In Fig. 1a a shift in a plotted point upwards and to the left means an increase in the risk of coronary heart disease. Conversely, a movement downwards and to the right means a reduction in the risk or an increased cardioprotective effect.

Fig. 1b is a curve analogous to Fig. 1a for patients with hypertension or CHD who have been treated with antihypertensive drugs. The results have been taken from 10 β-blocker studies listed in Table 1, where the duration of treatment was at least 3 months. The arrows show how the cholesterol ratio and HDL-C plasma levels changed during the treatment period. Even though differences were present in the dosage used, in the under-lying severity of disease and in the previous and concomitant drug therapy, all β-blockers examined, with the exception of pindolol and labetalol, increased the TC/HDL-C ratio

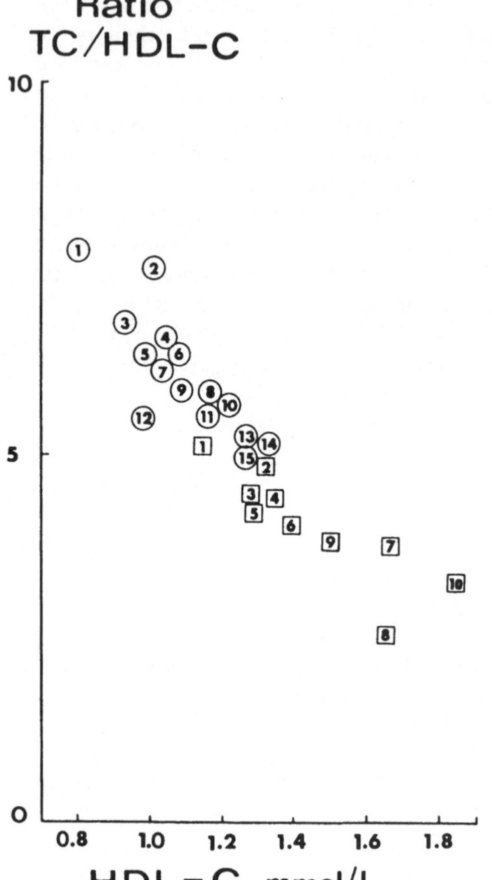

Figure 1a

Relationship between plasma HDL-C and the cholesterol ratio TC/HDL-C for groups of male patients with coronary heart disease or in a high risk category (circles) and groups of male subjects with no coronary heart disease and in a low risk category (squares). Each point is the mean for each of the groups detailed in the Key to Figure 1a.

Key to Fig. 1a

circles		Reference
1	Hyperlipidaemia with hypertension/angina, n = 5.	[2]
2	Pilots with coronary artery disease (angiographic), n = 16.	[12]
3	Post myocardial infarction-sedentary patients, n = 45.	[23]
4	Myocardial infarction/CHD, n = 11.	[8]
5	Coronary heart disease —Framingham study, n = 38.	[13]
6	Cardiac insufficiency with 3 vessel coronary lesions, n = 66.	[11]
7	Coronary heart disease with peripheral vascular disease, n = 10.	[1]
8	Coronary heart disease (category severe), n = 104.	[24]
9	Bypass patients (pre-surgical), n = 19.	[25]
10	Coronary lesions (category moderate severe), n = 68.	[24]
11	Hyperlipidaemia with hypertension/angina, n = 8.	[2]
12	Coronary heart disease, n = 7.	[1]
13	Post myocardial infarction (3 months), n = 19.	[26]
14	Post myocardial infarction, n = 23.	[26]
15	Coronary lesions (category moderate), n = 33.	[24]

squares		
1	No coronary heart disease-Framingham study, n = 1274.	[13]
2	Cardiac catheter-no coronary lesions, some valvular dysfunction, n = 21.	[24]
3	Pilots-no coronary lesions (angiographic), n = 102.	[12]
4	"Low risk" subjects, n = 440.	[12]
5	Non-cardiac hospitalised patients, n = 37.	[25]
6	Cardiac insufficiency-no stenosis (Catheter), n = 32.	[11]
7	"Employees"-random selection, n = 24.	[25]
8	Students, n = 11.	[25]
9	Healthy Japanese, n = 20.	[27]
10	Japanese joggers, n = 20.	[27]

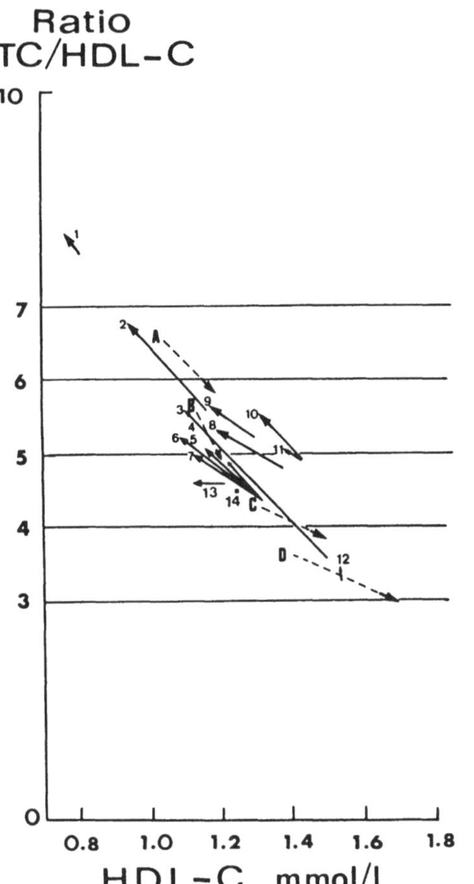

Key to Fig. 1b

		Reference
1	Metoprolol	[2]
2	Propranolol	[2]
3	Sotalol	[9]
4	Atenolol	[4]
5	Oxprenolol	[4]
6	Propranolol	[4]
7	Metoprolol	[4]
8	Metoprolol	[5]
9	Atenolol	[5]
10	Metoprolol	[6]
11	Atenolol	[6]
12	Metoprolol	[7]
13	Metoprolol	[41]
14	Labetalol	[41]
A	Pindolol	[8]
B	Pindolol	[3]
C	Prazosin	[10]
D	Pindolol	[7]

Figure 1b

Relationship between the cholesterol ratio and plasma HDL-C concentration during prolonged (3 months or longer) treatment with antihypertensive drugs, mainly β-blockers, in patients with essential hypertension and coronary heart disease (Details of each investigation are shown in Table 1). When cholesterol ratio data for individual patients were not available the ratio has been determined using mean lipid/lipoprotein values for the group. The arrows indicate the direction of change produced during the drug therapy. Numbers 1 to 12 are increases in cholesterol ratio and letters A to D decreases in cholesterol ratio for drugs detailed in Key to Figure 1b.

and decreased plasma HDL-C. Pindolol, the drug with the highest intrinsic sympathomimetic activity (ISA), was the only β-blocker of those shown here which decreased the cholesterol ratio and this occured in all 3 studies in which pindolol was included. In one study prazosin was included and like pindolol, prazosin too decreased the cholesterol ratio. The largest change was seen with sotalol, but the sotalol study lasted for 12 months,

Table 1: Clinical details and authors of long-term treatment studies with antihypertensive drugs used to obtain figures 1b and 2

Ref.	Author	Previous anti-hypertensive treatment	n=*	Treatment period	Diagnosis	Comments
[2]	Beilmann et al. (1982)	Yes	5 or 8	12 weeks	Hyperlipid-aemia/ Hypert. Angina	
[3]	Lehtonen et al. (1982)	No	20	6 months	Hyper-tension	
[4]	Day et al. (1982)	No	53	13 weeks	Hyper-tension	
[5]	England et al. (1980)	Yes	34	13 weeks	Hypert./ CHD	males or females?
[6]	Rössner et al. (1983)	Yes	50	12 weeks	Hyper-tension	non-random, low doses? Triglyceride concentra-tions unusually low
[7]	Passoti et al. (1982)	Yes	16	12 weeks	Hyper-tension	
[8]	Karmakoski et al. (1983)	Yes	11	4–6 months	CHD/Myo-cardial infarction	Patients also on prazosin etc.
[9]	Lehtonen et al. (1979)	?	12	1 year	Hyper-tension	Longest study
[10]	Kokubu et al. (1982)	Yes	14	12 weeks	Hyper-tension	
[41]	Frishman et al. (1983)	Yes	⩽44	12 weeks	Hyper-tension	includes 1 month dose titration – 20% on diuretics

* Most studies have approximately equal numbers of males and females.

at least twice as long as the other studies. Since most treatment periods covered only 3 months and since in 2 studies the increase in cholesterol ratio was greater than 1 unit it can be concluded that β-blockers used in these studies, with the exception of labetalol and pindolol, increase the risk of coronary heart disease and that the magnitude of this change may have clinical importance. An assessment of risk in this way is not new. La Porte et al. [29] determined the risk of heart attack across a spectrum of physical activity using the Framingham results based on HDL-C concentrations [30]. There was a gradient in HDL-C concentrations ranging from a mean of 0.9 mmol/l in patients with spinal cord injuries to 1.57 mmol/l in marathon runners. These values were considered to mean a 350% greater likelihood of a heart attack in the paraplegics than in the runners. Fig. 1b shows that changes approaching this magnitude can occur during β-blockers therapy. They are large enough to suggest an answer to the question posed by Leren and co-workers [31] on the MRFIT study which was 'Why had antihypertensive drug treatment (propranolol/diuretics) a possible adverse effect when hypertension was associated with a high cholesterol level'.

β_1-Selectivity and Combined Alpha/Beta Blockade

It has been claimed that the changes in HDL-C caused by β_1-selective adrenergic blocking agents are less marked than with non-selective drugs. The evidence for this is limited (Fig. 2). Only the study of Day et al. [4] with propranolol and oxprenolol (non-selective plus weak ISA) provides suitable results and no investigation is available where the drugs have been administered in the same study for longer than 3 months*. The only other study in which selective and nonselective drugs have been compared with oneanother over a sufficiently long period was carried out in patients with lipoprotein metabolism disorders where there were large differences between the baseline values for the propranolol and

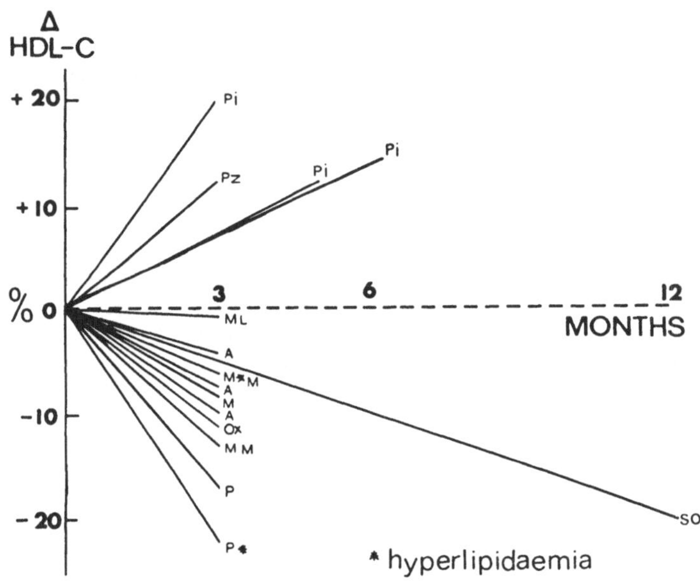

Figure 2 Percentage change in HDL-cholesterol for long-term studies (listed in Table 1) with β-blockers and prazosin where the treatment period is 3 months or longer. Key to symbols: A — atenolol; M — metoprolol; L — labetalol; Ox — oxprenolol; P — propranolol; Pi — pindolol; Pz — prazosin; So — sotalol.

* Note added in press: Evidence for a decrease in HDL-cholesterol during long-term treatment with nadolol but not atenolol has recently been reported by Franz, I. W., Lohmann, F. W., and Röcker, L. *Herz/Kreislauf* **3**, 115—122 (1984).

metoprolol (selective) groups [2]. Metoprolol in the study of Day et al. produced a greater increase in the cholesterol ratio than oxprenolol, and in the study of England et al. [5] the increase in the cholesterol ratio and decrease in HDL-C for atenolol (selective) were equal to those for oxprenolol in the study of Day et al. In the 3 studies in which metoprolol and atenolol have been compared with oneanother within the same study [4–6], it is noteworthy that atenolol produced smaller changes in the cholesterol ratio but differences were sometimes small, the treatment did not last longer than 3 months and the β-blocking potency of the doses used may not have been equivalent. Whilst the ability of β_1-selectivity 'per se' to cause a moderation of the changes in lipoproteins is still equivocal, clinical [10, 32] and experimental [33] investigations show convincingly that selective alpha$_1$-blockade produces effects analogous to intrinsic sympathomimetic activity i.e. like pindolol. Indeed, in clinical studies in hypertensive patients when β-blockade is combined with alpha-blockade using a propranolol-prazosin combination or labetalol mono-substance, the increases in triglycerides and decreases in HDL-C seen with β-blocking agents are less marked or absent [34–37, 41].

Observations for β-blockers with and without β_1-selectivity, with and without combined alpha-beta-blockade are summarised in Table 2 for VLDL-TG, LDL-C (low density lipoprotein) and HDL-C. Only changes significant at or greater than the 5% level are included. The effect of combining β-blockade, even when this is non-selective, with alpha blockade is impressive. In some instances there is evidence that alpha blockade may not only leave the lipids unchanged but also produce beneficial changes eg in VLDL-TG [10]. The precise reason why combined alpha/beta blockade should produce an opposite effect on these lipid parameters is not known. One possible explanation [4] is that a lowering in the HDL-C concentration by β-blockers occurs through an inhibition of lipoprotein lipase due to unopposed alpha stimulation by endogenous agonists. The effect of this on lipoproteins is not incompatible with a secodary Type IV/V hyperlipidaemia [42]. Prazosin, a selective alpha$_1$-adrenergic antagonist, like labetalol, lowers plasma triglycerides by inhibiting the secretion of VLDL-TG by the liver possibly by lowering the levels of circulating free-fatty acids [33]. When the mechanism of lipid changes induced by adrenergic drugs is better understood we should be better able to assess the clinical importance of the lipid changes produced by β-blockers. Until then β-blocker therapy and lipid changes in coronary heart disease must be kept under surveillance and the potential risks avoided.

Table 2: Effects of alpha- and beta-blockade ($>$ 35 days oral drug application) on plasma triglycerides and lipoproteins

Type of blockade	Drug (s)	Total triglycerides	VLDL-TG	HDL-C
alpha-blockade	Prazosin	− 16 [34] NC [10[NC [38]	NC [38]	NC [34] + 12 [10] NC [38]
	Prazosin + Propranolol	NC [34]		− 7 [34]
alpha-beta blockade	Labetalol	NC [39] NC [41] NC [36] NC [37] NC [35]	− 27 [39]	NC [35]c NC [41]
beta-blockade (mainly selective β_1)	Metoprolol	+ 14 [4] NC [41]d NC [2] + 10 [5] + 25 [6]	+ 36 [4] NC [2] NC [6]a	− 13 [4] NC [41] NC [2] − 13 [5] − 8 [6]
	Atenolol	+ 36 [4] + 27 [36] NC [34] NC [6]	+ 48 [4] NC [6] + 25 [40]b	− 7 [4] NC [34] − 10 [5] NC [6]
beta-blockade (non-selective, $\beta_1 + \beta_2$)	Oxprenolol	+ 27 [4] + 22 [34]	+ 53 [4]	− 11 [4] NC [34]
	Propranolol	+ 51 [4] + 31 [38] + 24 [34] + 26 [35]	+ 71 [4] + 32 [38]	NC [35] − 17 [4] − 22 [2] − 13 [34] NC [38]
	Sotalol	+ 66 [9]	+ 32* [9]	− 26 [9]
	Propranolol/ Hydrochlorthiazide	+ 44 [34]		− 18 [34]

VLDL-TG = Very low density lipoprotein triglycerides
HDL-C = High density lipoprotein cholesterol
NC = no change
All percentage changes shown are significant at the 5 % level or less (versus baseline or pre-treatment).
* LDL-C + VDL-C
a = + 34 % (P $>$ 0.05)
b = P value unknown
c = N.B also no change in HDL-C with Propranolol.
d = + 12 % (p $>$ 0.05)
[ ] References to literature

References

[1] Kaliman, J., Widhalm, K., Strobl, W.: Serum lipoproteins in patients with clinical signs of atherosclerosis, peripheral vascular and coronary heart disease. *Artery* **8**, 547–552 (1980).

[2] Beilmann, P., Brun, D., Gagné, C., Moorjani, S., Jéquier, J.-C., Bertrand, M., Lupien, P.-J.: Beta blockers and their effects on lipoproteins, phospholipids, apoproteins A and A_1 in whole plasma and the different fractions. *Int. J. clin. Ther. Toxicol.* **20**, 259–264 (1982).

[3] Lehtonen, A., Hietanen, E., Marniemi, J., Peltonen, P., Niskanen, J.: Effect of pindolol on serum lipids and lipid metabolising enzymes. *Br. J. clin. Pharmac.* **13**, 445S–448S (1982).

[4] Day, J. L., Metcalfe, J., Simpson, C. N.: Adrenergic mechanisms in control of plasma lipid concentrations. *Br. Med. J.* **284**, 1145–1148 (1982).

[5] England, J. D. F., Simons, L. A., Gibson, J. C., Carlton, M.: The effect of metoprolol and atenolol on plasma high density lipoprotein levels in man. *Clin. Exp. Pharm. Physiol.* **7**, 329–333 (1980).

[6] Rössner, S., Weiner, L.: Atenolol and metoprolol: Comparison of effects on blood pressure and serum lipoproteins, and side effects. *Eur. J. clin. Pharmac.* **24**, 573–577 (1983).

[7] Passoti, C., Capra, A., Fiorella, G., Vibelli, C., Chierichetti, S. M.: Effects of pindolol and metoprolol on plasma lipids and lipoproteins. *Br. J. clin. Pharmac.* **13**, 435S–439S (1982).

[8] Karmakoski, J., Viikari, J. Rönnemaa, T.: Effect of pindolol on serum lipoproteins in patients with coronary heart disease. *Int. J. clin. Pharm. Ther. Toxicol.* **21**, 189–191 (1983).

[9] Lehtonen, A., Viikari, J.: Long-term effect of sotalol on plasma lipids. *Clin. Sci.* **57**, 405S–407S (1979).

[10] Kobuku, T., Itoh, I., Kurita, H., Ochi, T., Murata, K., Yuba, I.: Effect of prazosin on serum lipids. *J. Cardiovasc. Pharmacol.* **4** (Suppl. 2): 228S–232S (1982).

[11] Swanson, J. O., Pierpont, G., Adicoff, A.: Serum high density lipoprotein cholesterol correlates with presence but not severity of coronary artery disease. *Am. J. Med.* **71**, 235–239 (1981).

[12] Uhl, G. S., Troxler, R. G., Hickman, J. R., Clark, D.: Relation between high density lipoprotein cholesterol and coronary artery disease in asymptomatic men. *Am. J. Cardiol.* **48**, 903–910 (1981).

[13] Wilson, P. W., Garrison, R. J., Castelli, W. P., Feinleib, M., McNamara, P. M., Kannel, W. B.: Prevelance of coronary heart disease in the Framingham offspring study: Role of lipoprotein cholesterols. *Am. J. Cardiol.* **46**, 649–654 (1980).

[14] Franzén, J., Fex, G.: High density lipoprotein composition versus heredity for acute myocardial infarction in middle-aged men. *Acta. Med. Scand.* **211**, 121–124 (1982).

[15] Miller, N. E., Hammett, F., Saltissi, S., Rao, S., van Zeller, H., Coltart, J., Lewis, B.: Relation of angiographically defined coronary artery disease to plasma lipoprotein subfractions and apolipoproteins. *Br. Med. J.* **282**, 1741–1744 (1981).

[16] Castelli, W. P., Doyle, J. T., Gordon, T., et al.: HDL-cholesterol and other lipids in coronary heart disease. The Cooperative lipoprotein phenotyping study. *Circulation* **55**, 767–772 (1977).

[17] Rhoads, G. G., Gulbrandsen, C. L., Kagan, A.: Serum lipoproteins and coronary heart disease in a population study of Hawaiian Japanese men. *New. Engl. J. Med.* **294**, 293–298 (1976).

[18] Miller, N. E., Førde, O. H., Thelle, D. S., Mjøs, O. D.: The Tromso heartstudy, high density lipoprotein and coronary heart disease: A prospective case-control study. *Lancet* **1**, 965–968 (1977).

[19] Carew, T. E., Koschinsky, T. Hayes, S. B., Steinberg, D.: A mechanism by which high-density lipoproteins may slow the atherogenic process. *Lancet* **1**, 1315–1317 (1976).

[20] Buckley, B. M., Bold, A. M.: Managing hyperlipidaemias. *Br. Med. J.* **285**, 1293–1294 (1982).

[21] Rouffy, J., Chanu, B., Bakir, R., Goy-Loeper, J., Miro, I.: Lipides, lipoprotéines, apoprotéines et manifestations clinique artériopathiques. *Path. Biol.* **31**, 261–270 (1983).

[22] Castelli, W. P., Doyle, J. T., Gordon, T., Hames, C., Hulley, S. B., Kagan, A., McGee, D., Vicic, W. J., Zukel, W. J.: High density lipoprotein cholesterol levels (HDLC) in coronary heart disease (CHD): A cooperative lipoprotein phenotyping study. *Circulation* **52** (Suppl. 2): 11 (Abs. 378) (1975).

[23] Berg, A., Keul, J. Ringwald, G. Stipping, J., Deus, B.: Serumlipoprotein cholesterol in sedentary and trained male patients with coronary heart disease. *Clin. Cardiol.* **4**, 233–237 (1981).

[24] Naito, H. K., Greenstreet, R. L., David, J. A., Sheldon, W. L., Shirey, E. K. Lewis, R. C. Proudfit, W. L., Gerrity, R. G.: HDL-cholesterol concentration and severity of coronary atherosclerosis determined by cine-angiography. *Artery* **8**, 101–112 (1980).

[25] Leszczynski, D. E., Cleveland, J., C. Kummerow, F. A.: Plasma lipoprotein patterns in patients hospitalised for coronary artery bypass. *Clin. Cardiol.* 3, 252–259 (1980).

[26] Ballantyne, F. C., Clark, R. S., Simpson, H. S., Ballantyne, D.: The effect of moderate physical exercise on the plasma lipoprotein subfractions of male survivors of myocardial infarction. *Circulation* 65, 913–918 (1982).

[27] Nakamura, N., Uzawa, H., Maeda, H., Inomoto, T.: Physical Fitness: Its contribution to serum high density lipoprotein. *Atherosclerosis* 48, 173–183 (1983).

[28] Kladetzky, R. G., Assmann, G., Walgenbach, S., Tauchert, P., Helb, H.-D.: Lipoprotein and apoprotein values in coronary angiography patients. *Artery* 7, 191–205 (1980).

[29] La Porte, R. E., Brenes, G., Dearwater, S., Murphy, M. A., Cauley, J. A. Dietrick, R., Robertson, R.: HDL cholesterol across a spectrum of physical activity from quadriplegia to marathon running. *Lancet* 1, 1212–1213 (1983).

[30] Kannel, W. B., Gordon, T., Castelli, W. P.: Role of lipids and lipoprotein fractions in atherogenesis. The Framingham Study. *Prog. Lipid Res.* 720, 339–348 (1981).

[31] Leren, P., Helgeland, A., Hjermann, I., Holme, I.: MRFIT and the Oslo study. *J. Amer. Med. Ass.* 249, 893–894 (1983).

[32] Leren, P., Helgeland, A., Holme, I., Foss, P. O., Hjermann, I., Lund-Larsen, P. G.: Effect of propranolol and prazosin on blood lipids: The Oslo Study. *Lancet* 2, 4–6 (1980).

[33] Dall'Aglio, E., Chang, H., Reaven, G.: Disparate effects of prazosin and propranolol on lipid metabolism in a rat model. *Metabolism* 32, 510–513 (1983).

[34] Leren, P., Eide, I., Foss, O. P., Helgeland, A., Hjermann, I., Holme, I., Kjeldsen, S. E., Lund-Larsen, P. G.: Antihypertensive drugs and blood lipids: The Oslo Study. *J. Cardiovasc. Pharmacol.* 4 (Suppl. 2): S222–S224 (1982).

[35] Ponti, G. B., Carnovali, M., Banderali, G., Missaglia, A.: Effects of labetalol on the lipid metabolism in hypertensive patients. *Curr. Ther. Res.* 33, 466–471 (1983).

[36] Thulin, T., Henningsen, N. C., Karlberg, B. E., Nilsson, O. R.: Clinical and metabolic effects of labetalol compared with atenolol in primary hypertension. *Curr. Ther. Res.* 30, 194–204 (1981).

[37] McGonigle, R. J. S., Williams, L., Murphy, M. J., Parsons, V.: Labetalol and lipids. *Lancet* 1, 163 (1981).

[38] Gemma, G., Montanari, G., Suppa, G., Paralovo, A., Franceschini, G., Mantero, O., Sirtori, C. R.: Plasma lipid and lipoprotein changes in hypertensive patients treated with propranolol and prazosin. *J. Cardiovasc. Pharmacol.* (Suppl. 2): S233–S237 (1982).

[39] Pagnan, A., Pessina, A. C., Hlede, M., Zanetti, G., Dal Palu, C.: Effects of labetalol on lipid and carbohydrate metabolism. *Pharmacol. Res. Commun.* 11, 227–236 (1979).

[40] Eliasson, K., Lins, L.-E., Rössner, S.: Serum lipoprotein changes during atenolol treatment of essential hypertension. *Eur. J. Clin. Pharmacol.* 20, 335–338 (1981).

[41] Frishman, W. H., Michelson, E. L., Johnson, B. F., Poland, M. P.: Multi-Clinic comparison of labetalol to metoprolol in treatment of mild to moderate systemic hypertension. *Am. J. Med.* (Suppl. – Hypertension and Hemodynamics) p. 54–67 (1983).

[42] Fredrickson, D. S., Levy, R. I., Lees, R. S.: Fat transport in lipoproteins: An integrated approach to mechanism and disorders. *N. Engl. J. Med.* 276, 34, 94, 148, 215, 273 (1967).

Lipid-Stoffwechsel unter Beta-Rezeptoren-Blockade – klinische Konsequenzen

F. W. Lohmann
I. Innere Abteilung des Krankenhauses Neukölln, Rudower Str. 56, 1000 Berlin 47

Zusammenfassung

Unter Beta-Rezeptoren-Blockade kann es zu Veränderungen der Lipoproteine kommen. Dabei können die „very low density"-Lipoproteine (VLDL) entsprechend einer Erhöhung der Plasmatriglyceride ansteigen und es kann zu einer Abnahme der „high density"-Lipoproteine (HDL) kommen. Derartige Veränderungen der Lipoproteine finden sich aufgrund eines komplexen biochemischen Mechanismus unter gleichzeitiger Beta-1- und Beta-2-Rezeptoren-Blockade häufiger und ausgeprägter als unter alleiniger beta-1-selektiver Rezeptoren-Blockade. Die klinische Dignität derartiger biochemischer Befunde unter Beta-Rezeptoren-Blockade ist schwer abzuschätzen. Die klinischen Erfahrungen sprechen jedoch dafür, daß der therapeutische Nutzen der Beta-Rezeptoren-Blocker bei der jeweiligen kardiovasculären Zielindikation einen eventuellen atherogenen Effekt deutlich überwiegt. Im Einzelfall ist jedoch, bei pathologischen Ausgangswerten, eine klinisch relevante Veränderung der Lipoproteine nicht auszuschließen. Daher sollte vor und unter Beta-Rezeptoren-Blockade eine Kontrolle des Lipidstatus erfolgen (Triglyceride und Gesamtcholesterin; bei pathologischem Ausfall eines dieser Werte auch Bestimmung der HDL-Fraktion und daraus abgeleitet des LDL-Cholesterins). Da beta-1-selektive Rezeptoren-Blocker selbst bei Patienten mit einer primären Hyperlipoproteinämie geringere, und zudem nur passagere Auswirkungen auf die Lipoproteine haben, ist ihnen auch unter diesem Aspekt der Vorzug zu geben. Bei Feststellung bzw. Auftreten pathologischer Werte ist neben diätetischen Maßnahmen besonders auf die Reduktion von Übergewicht, eine ausreichende körperliche Aktivität und die Einhaltung einer Nikotinabstinenz zu achten. Da es unter Alpha-Rezeptoren-Blockade zu einer Abnahme der Triglyceride bei gleichbleibenden bzw. sogar ansteigenden HDL-Lipoproteinen kommen kann, ist hierdurch die Möglichkeit einer eventuellen Zusatz- oder Alternativtherapie gegeben.

Seit einigen Jahren ist bekannt, daß auch die Beta-Rezeptoren-Blocker den Fettstoffwechsel und die Serumlipide verändern können [41–46, 63, 66]. In diesem Zusammenhang wurde eine Erhöhung der Triglyceride bzw. der „very low density Liporoteine" (VLDL) und eine Verminderung der „high density Lipoproteine" (HDL) beschrieben. Diese möglichen Veränderungen der Lipoproteine unter Beta-Rezeptoren-Blockade sind in den letzten Jahren zunehmend in den Vordergrund der Diskussion getreten, da eine

Erhöhung der VLDL bei Abnahme der HDL nach heutigem Verständnis eine potentielle Erhöhung des Risikos für arteriosklerotisch ausgelöste kardiovaskuläre Komplikationen, insbesondere der koronaren Herzkrankheit, bedeutet [2, 7, 47, 51, 62, 72]. Daher wird auch immer wieder die Frage diskutiert, ob die unter Beta-Rezeptoren-Blockade möglichen Veränderungen der Serumlipide den therapeutischen Nutzen der Beta-Rezeptoren-Blocker ggf. einschränken können. In dieser Verallgemeinerung ist diese Frage eindeutig zu verneinen; denn es gibt keine Studie, welche eine klinisch faßbare Bedeutung dieser biochemischen Befunde aufzeigt. Allerdings erscheint zur Beantwortung der in diesem Zusammenhang gestellten Fragen eine differenziertere Analyse erforderlich.

Zum Verständnis der Beeinflussung der Lipolyse und der Lipoproteine durch Beta-Rezeptoren-Blocker ist es erforderlich, einige Anmerkungen zur Steuerung der Lipolyse unter akuter und chronischer Beta-Rezeptoren-Blockade zu machen. Bei der Regulation der Lipolyse ist zwischen einer katecholamin-induzierten Lipolyse und einer katecholamin-unabhängigen Lipolyse durch andere Hormone zu unterscheiden [18, 20, 21, 35, 42, 43]. Im menschlichen Fettgewebe finden sich mehr Beta-1-Rezeptoren als Beta-2-Rezeptoren. Daher führt eine akute gemischte Beta-Rezeptoren-Blockade, welche gleichstark die Beta-1- und Beta-2-Rezeptoren blockiert, zu einer stärkeren Unterdrückung der Lipolyse als eine akute beta-1-selektive Rezeptoren-Blockade, da eben unter gemischter Beta-Rezeptoren-Blockade die katecholamin-induzierte Lipolyse stärker unterdrückt wird [1, 9, 12, 24, 34, 37, 42, 43, 56, 59, 64, 65]. Bei der in der Regel notwendigen Langzeit-Therapie mit Beta-Rezeptoren-Blockern dominiert nun bei entsprechend eingeschränkter katecholamin-abhängiger Lipolyse die reaktive und kompensatorisch gesteigerte katecholamin-unabhängige Lipolyse. Unter chronischer Beta-Rezeptoren-Blockade ist nun die katecholamin-unabhängige Lipolyse um so stärker aktiviert, je stärker die über Beta-Rezeptoren vermittelte Lipolyse blockiert ist. Das bedeutet, daß unter gemischter Beta-Rezeptoren-Blockade die reaktive Gegenregulation stärker ausfällt als unter beta-1-selectiver Rezeptoren-Blockade (Abb. 1). Dabei kann die auf diese Weise gesteigerte Lipolyse unter ge-

Lipolyse	Beta-Rezeptoren-Blockade			
	Akut		Chronisch	
	β_1	β_1, β_2	β_1	β_1, β_2
Katechol-amin-induziert	↓	↓	↓	↓
Katechol-amin-unabhängig	↑	↑	↑	↑
Bilanz	–	–	± bis +	+ bis + +

↓ Hemmung   ↑ Aktivierung

Abb. 1
Beeinflussung der Katecholamin-abhängigen und -unabhängigen Lipolyse durch akute und chronische Gabe von Beta-Rezeptorenblockern

mischter Beta-Rezeptoren-Blockade sogar den aktuellen Bedarf überschreiten. Dementsprechend fanden Tanaka et al. [69] nach 8-wöchiger Propranolol-Therapie auch einen höheren Spiegel freier Fettsäuren als vor dieser Behandlung. Aus den Veränderungen des Lipidstoffwechsels bei der Akut- bzw. Kurzzeitanwendung eines Beta-Rezeptoren-Blockers kann somit nicht auf die endgültigen Veränderungen unter chronischer Behandlung geschlossen werden [18, 20, 21].

Die durch die Aktivierung der katecholamin-unabhängigen Lipolyse im Rahmen einer Langzeit-Therapie mit Beta-Rezeptorenblockern unter Umständen vermehrt gebildeten freien Fettsäuren werden nun in der Leber zu Triglyceriden resynthetisiert. Auf diese Weise können die Befunde erhöhter Plasmatriglyceride bzw. „very low density"-Lipoproteine (VLDL) unter chronischer Beta-Rezeptoren-Blockade eine Erklärung finden [3, 5, 6, 10, 11, 15, 30, 31, 39, 40, 53, 60, 61, 69, 71]. Die gleichzeitig vermindert gefundenen „high density"-Lipoproteine (HDL) sind durch eine unter Beta-Rezeptoren-Blockade gleichzeitig nachgewiesene Hemmung der Lipoproteinlipase und dadurch bedingter Änderung der Konversion innerhalb der Lipoproteinfraktionen erklärbar [14, 69, 70]. Ein gegensätzliches Verhalten der Lipoproteine findet sich unter Alpha-Rezeptoren-Blockade [46]. Dabei ist eine Abnahme der Triglyceride bei gleichbleibender bzw. sogar ansteigender HDL-Konzentration gefunden worden. Eine mögliche Erklärung für dieses Verhalten der Lipoproteine liegt darin, daß unter Alpha-Rezeptoren-Blockade das Wachstumshormon und damit die katecholamin-unabhängige Lipolyse supprimiert ist und gleichzeitig eine Aktivierung der Lipoproteinlipase vorliegt [10, 11, 33, 46]. Durch diese beiden Mechanismen ist das zur Beta-Rezeptoren-Blockade unterschiedliche Verhalten der Lipoproteine bei Blockade der Alpha-Rezeptoren (z.B. durch Prazosin) erklärbar. So wurde weiterhin auch unter Labetalol [23, 52, 58], also der kombinierten Blockade von Beta- und Alpha-Rezeptoren keine signifikante Veränderung der Lipoproteine gefunden.

Entsprechend der unter gemischter Beta-Rezeptoren-Blockade stärker aktivierten katecholamin-unabhängigen Lipolyse können die Veränderungen der Lipoproteine unter gemischter Beta-Rezeptoren-Blockade häufiger und ausgeprägter als unter beta-1-selektiver Rezeptoren-Blockade vorkommen [23, 42—44, 46, 53, 61]. Die Sichtung der hierzu vorliegenden Literatur bestätigt bei aller Schwierigkeit des unmittelbaren Vergleichs in der Tendenz diese Aussage. Auch bei Patienten mit einer primären Fett-Stoffwechselstörung kam es unter einer gemischten Beta-Rezeptoren-Blockade zu ungünstigeren Veränderungen als unter beta-1-selektiver Rezeptoren-Blockade [5, 6]. Welche Bedeutung in diesem Zusammenhang gerade die Blockade der Beta-2-Rezeptoren hat, konnte in umgekehrter Weise demonstriert werden [32]: unter der beta-2-mimetischen Behandlung mit Terbutalin kam es für die Dauer dieser Therapie zu einem Anstieg der HDL-Konzentration, welche nach Absetzen des Terbutalins wieder auf den Ausgangswert abfiel. Da weiterhin bekannt ist, daß es unter beta-2-mimetischer Behandlung zu einer Abnahme der STH-Konzentration kommt [25, 32], können diese Befunde als Folge der Abschwächung der katecholamin-unabhängigen Lipolyse gewertet werden. Interessant ist in diesem Zusammenhang auch die Mitteilung [49], daß eine Lipidspeichermyopathie sich nach 12-jährigem Verlauf mit Beginn einer Propranolol-Behandlung klinisch, laborchemisch und bioptisch besserte. Möglicherweise ist dieser Befund auf die unter gemischter Beta-Rezeptoren-Blockade mit Propranolol besonders aktivierte katecholamin-unabhängige Lipolyse zurückzuführen [48]. Weiterhin ist es verständlich, daß die Veränderungen der Lipoproteine unter gemischten Beta-Rezeptoren-Blockern mit sympathischer Eigenaktivität (ISA) geringer in Erscheinung treten (Abb. 2), da die „ISA" den beschriebenen reaktiven Ver-

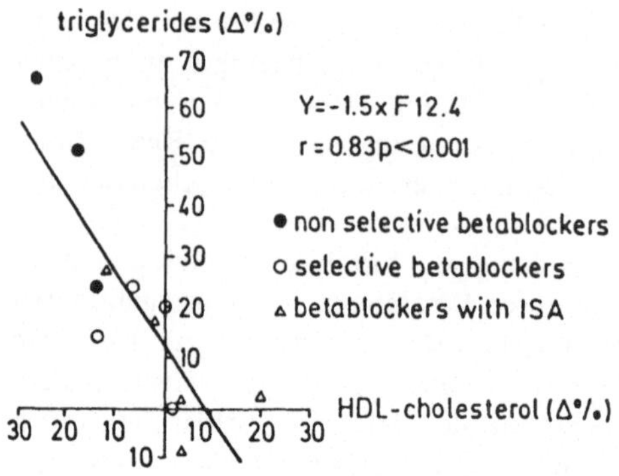

Abb. 2

Korrelation zwischen den mittleren prozentualen Veränderungen des HDL-Cholesterols und der Plasmatriglyceride (aus 8)

Tabelle 1: Veränderungen der Lipoproteine unter pharmakologischer Beeinflussung des sympathischen Nervensystems

	VLDL	HDL
α_1-Blockade	↓	↑
β_1-Blockade	(↑)	(↓)
β_1, β_2-Blockade	↑	↓
β_2-Stimulation		↑

änderungen der Lipoproteine teilweise entgegenwirkt [8, 50, 57]. Die Tabelle 1 faßt die unter pharmakologischer Beeinflussung des sympathischen Nervensystems möglichen Veränderungen der Lipoproteine noch einmal schematisch zusammen.
Dementsprechend sind die stärksten Veränderungen der Lipoproteine unter einem gemischten Beta-Rezeptoren-Blocker ohne sympathische Eigenaktivität mit zudem noch langer Halbwertzeit zu erwarten, da in diesem Fall die reaktive Aktivierung der Lipolyse am stärksten ausfallen wird. So fanden wir bei stoffwechselgesunden Hypertonie-Patienten [22] im Überkreuzversuch unter chronischer Behandlung mit dem beta-1-selektiven Rezeptoren-Blocker Atenolol und dem gemischten Beta-Rezeptoren-Blocker Nadolol bei gleich starker Blutdrucksenkung in Ruhe und unter Belastung ein unterschiedliches Verhalten der Lipoproteine. Beide Beta-Rezeptoren-Blocker führten zu keiner Beeinflussung des Gesamtcholesterins und des LDL-Cholesterins. Dagegen kam es unter beta-1-selektiver Rezeptoren-Blockade zu einer nicht signifikanten, unter gemischter Beta-Rezeptoren-Blockade jedoch zu einer signifikanten Abnahme des HDL-Cholesterins nach jeweils 4-wöchiger Behandlung. Auffallend war nun, daß es nach 16-monatiger Behandlungsdauer unter beta-1-selektiver Rezeptoren-Blockade zu einem Wiederanstieg der HDL-Konzentration kam. Dagegen blieb nach 16-monatiger Behandlung mit dem gemischten Beta-Rezeptoren-Blocker die HDL-Konzentration gleich stark abgesenkt, stieg jedoch bei diesen Patienten nach Umsetzen auf den beta-1-selektiven Rezeptoren-Blocker und weiterer 6-monatiger Behandlung wieder deutlich an (Abb. 3). Die Triglyceride stiegen nach 4-wöchiger Behandlung sowohl unter beta-1-selektiver als auch unter gemischter Beta-Rezeptoren-Blockade an, jedoch deutlich stärker unter gemischter Beta-Rezeptoren-Blockade. Nach 16-monatiger Behandlung hatten sich die Triglyceride unter beta-1-

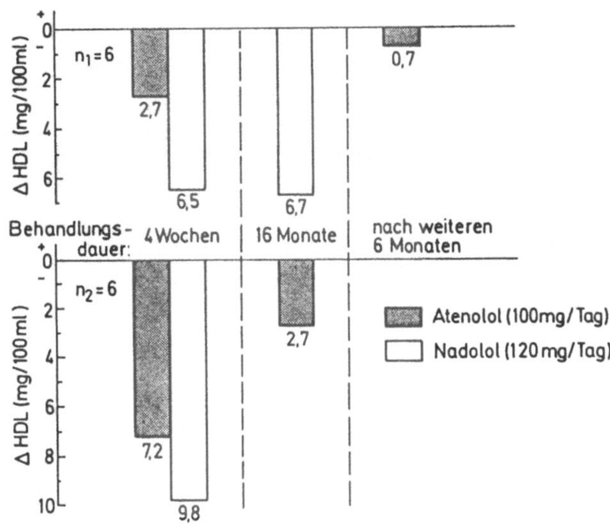

Abb. 3

HDL unter chronischer β_1-selektiver und β_1-β_2-Rezeptorenblockade

selektiver Rezeptoren-Blockade normalisiert, während sie unter gemischter Beta-Rezeptoren-Blockade nach wie vor deutlich erhöht waren. Diese Untersuchungen bestätigen, daß es unter gemischter Beta-Rezeptoren-Blockade zu deutlichen und anhaltenden Veränderungen der Lipoproteine kommen kann. Dagegen war unter beta-1-selektiver Rezeptoren-Blockade eine geringere und nur vorübergehende Abweichung der Lipoproteine von den Ausgangswerten nachweisbar. Das bedeutet, daß für die Langzeit-Therapie mit beta-1-selektiven Rezeptoren-Blockern nicht mit nennenswerten potentiell ungünstigen Veränderungen der Lipoproteine zu rechnen ist.

Die bisher vorliegenden umfangreichen klinischen Erfahrungen und Studien sprechen nun eindeutig dafür, daß der therapeutische Nutzen der Beta-Rezeptoren-Blocker allgemein bei der jeweiligen kardiovasculären Zielindikation einen eventuellen atherogenen Effekt deutlich überwiegt. Andernfalls hätte es nicht zur Prägung des Begriffes von der kardioprotektiven Wirkung der Beta-Rezeptoren-Blocker kommen können. Es sei in diesem Zusammenhang auf die Postinfarktstudien sowie auf die Göteborg-Studie bei Hypertonie-Patienten hingewiesen [45], in denen einheitlich eine kardioprotektive Wirkung der Beta-Rezeptoren-Blocker demonstriert werden konnte. Es bleibt daher zu bezweifeln, ob selbst in langfristigen prospektiven Studien [38] je die klinische Dignität der unter chronischer Beta-Rezeptoren-Blockade beobachteten Veränderungen der Lipoproteine quantifizierbar sein wird. Aufgrund epidemiologischer Analogieschlüsse kann jedoch für Patienten, die bereits vor einer notwendigen Therapie mit Beta-Rezeptoren-Blockern pathologische Ausgangswerte ihrer Serumlipide aufweisen (insbesondere eine Erhöhung des risikoträchtigen LDL-Cholesterins), nicht ausgeschlossen werden, daß es therapiebedingt nicht doch zu ungünstigen Veränderungen der Lipoproteine kommt. Aber auch für Patienten mit einer vorbestehenden Hyperlipoproteinämie konnte ja gezeigt werden [5, 6], daß bei derartigen Patienten der beta-1-selektive Rezeptoren-Blocker vergleichsweise von Vorteil ist. Hieraus ist jedoch die Konsequenz abzuleiten, daß vor und während einer Langzeit-Therapie auch mit beta-1-selektiven Rezeptoren-Blockern eine Kontrolle des Lipidstatus erforderlich ist (Triglyceride und Gesamtcholesterin, sowie bei pathologischem Ausfall eines dieser Parameter zusätzliche Bestimmung des antiatherogen wirksamen HDL-Choesterins und des LDL-Cholesterins). Weiterhin konnte in wenigen bereits vorliegenden Langzeitstudien mit einem Verlauf bis zu über 6 Jahren hinsichtlich des Verhaltens der Serumlipide unter Beta-Rezeptoren-Blocker-Therapie gezeigt werden [4, 36, 54], daß es dabei unter bestimmten Voraussetzungen überhaupt nicht zu relevanten Veränderungen der Lipoproteine kommen muß. Die günstigen Voraussetzungen bestanden in diesen Studien vor allem in einer Abnahme des Körpergewichtes im Rahmen einer begleitenden Patientenbetreuung. Mit diesen Befunden scheint in derartigen diätetischen Maßnahmen zugleich eine Möglichkeit aufgezeigt zu werden, ungünstige Veränderungen der Lipoproteine unter Beta-Rezeptoren-Blockade zu vermeiden bzw. zu behandeln. Darüber hinaus ist bekannt, daß körperliche Aktivität [13, 26, 28, 67] sowie Nikotinabstinenz [68] pathologischen Veränderungen der Lipoproteine entgegen wirken. Selbst ein mäßiger Alkoholkonsum (etwa 30 g/Tag) ist in diesem Zusammenhang nicht abträglich [16, 27, 55].

Hinsichtlich der Beeinflussung des Lipidstoffwechsels durch Beta-Rezeptoren-Blocker ergeben sich somit folgende Schlußfolgerungen:

1. Da beta-1-selektive Rezeptoren-Blocker selbst bei Patienten mit einer vorbestehenden Hyperlipoproteinämie die geringsten potentiell ungünstigen Auswirkungen auf die Lipoproteine haben, ist ihnen auch unter diesem Aspekt der Vorzug zu geben.

2. Vor und während einer Langzeit-Therapie auch mit beta-1-selektiven Rezeptoren-Blockern ist eine Kontrolle des Lipidstatus erforderlich (Triglyceride und Gesamtcholesterin, sowie bei pathologischem Ausfall eines dieser Parameter zusätzlich Bestimmung des HDL-Cholesterins und daraus Errechnung des LDL-Cholesterins). Bei Feststellung bzw. Auftreten pathologischer Werte ist neben diätetischen Maßnahmen besonders auf die Reduktion von Übergewicht, eine ausreichend körperliche Aktivität (dynamischer Bewegungssport) und die Einhaltung einer Nikotinabstinenz zu achten. Nur äußerst selten dürfte im Einzelfall aus den hier zur Diskussion stehenden Gründen eine andere Zusatz- oder Alternativtherapie notwendig sein.

3. Nach den bisher vorliegenden Befunden ist die kardioprotektive Wirkung der Beta-Rezeptoren-Blocker generell und eindeutig größer als ein potentielles atherogenes Risiko einer derartigen Therapie. Unter Beachtung und Einhaltung der zuvor erwähnten Kontrolluntersuchungen und eventuellen Maßnahmen erfährt daher die Anwendung der beta-1-selektiven Rezeptoren-Blocker bei gegebener Indikation auch in diesem Zusammenhang keine Einschränkung. Dieses gilt auch für die Kombinationstherapie mit einem Saluretikum, da die durch Saluretika verursachten Veränderungen der Lipoproteine durch Beta-Rezeptoren-Blockade weitgehend rückgängig gemacht werden [46].

Abschließend ist somit festzustellen, daß bei der Behandlung der arteriellen Hypertonie sowie von Herz-Kreislauf-Erkrankungen mit Beta-Rezeptoren-Blockern ein beta-1-selektiver Rezeptoren-Blocker vorzuziehen ist, um nachteilige metabolische Auswirkungen einer derartigen Therapie zu vermeiden. Dieses gilt nicht nur bezüglich der Beeinflussung des Fettstoffwechsels durch Beta-Rezeptoren-Blockade, sondern vor allem auch für den Kohlenhydratstoffwechsel: Im Gegensatz zu den gemischten Beta-Rezeptoren-Blockern kommt es unter beta-1-selektiver Rezeptoren-Blockade zu keiner Beeinträchtigung der Insulinreserve und zu keiner Beeinträchtigung der Glykogenolyse der Skelettmuskulatur; so kommt es unter beta-1-selektiver Rezeptoren-Blockade nicht zu einer belastungsinduzierten, leistungsbegrenzenden Hypoglykämie mit eventuell paradoxer Kreislaufreaktion, wie es unter gemischter Beta-Rezeptoren-Blockade möglich ist [1, 17, 19, 29, 34, 42, 43, 45].

Literatur

[1]   Aigner, A., Muß, M., Krempler, F., Fenninger, H. und Sandhofer, F.: Einfluß einer akuten β_1-und β_1/β_2-Rezeptorenblockade auf den Kohlenhydrat- und Fettstoffwechsel unter Belastungs-bedingungen. *Dtsch. med. Wschr.* **108**, 293 (1983).

[2]   Assmann, G., Schriewer, H. und Oberwittler, W.: Klinik und Pathobiochemie der High Density Lipoproteine. *Klin. Wschr.* **58**, 757 (1980).

[3]   Bengtsson, C., Lennartsson, J., Lindquist, O., Noppa, H. und Tibblin, E.: *Metabolic effects of diuretics and β-blockers.* Abstracts sixth scientific meeting of the International Society of Hypertension, S. 123, Göteborg, 1979.

[4]   Berglund, G. und Anderson, O.: Beta-blockers or diuretics in hypertension? A six year follow-up of blood pressure and metabolic side effects. *Lancet* I, 744 (1981).

[5]   Bielmann, P. und Leduc, G.: Effects of metoprolol and propranolol on lipid metabolism. *Internat. J. Clin. Pharmac. Biopharm.* **17**, 378 (1979).

[6]   Bielmann, P., Brun, D., Gagné, C., Moorjani, S., Jéquier, J.-C., Bertrand, M. und Lupien, P.-J.: Beta-blockers and their effects on lipoproteins, phospholipids, apoproteins A and B, in whole plasma and the different fractions. *Internat. J. Clin. Pharmacol., Therapy and Toxicol.* **20**, 259 (1982).

[7]   Brewer, Jr., H. B., Schaefer, E. J., Zech, L. A. und Osborne, Jr., J. C.: Lipoproteine: Struktur, Funktion und Stoffwechsel. In: *Lipoproteine und Herzinfarkt*, herausgegeben von H. Greten, P. D. Lang, G. Schettler, — Gerhard Witzstrock-Verlag, Baden-Baden — Köln — New York, 1979.

[8]   Brummelen, van P.: The relevance of intrinsic sympathomimetic activity for β-blocker-induced changes in plasma lipids. *J. Cardiovasc. Pharmacol.* **5**, 51 (1983).

[9]   Chowanetz, W., Miller, K. und Gross, W.: Der Einfluß von Propranolol und Metoprolol auf beta-adrenerge Stoffwechselreaktionen. *Med. Klin.* **74**, 1286 (1979).

[10]   Day, J. L., Simpson, N., Metcalfe, J. und Page, R. L.: Metabolic consequences of atenolol and propranolol in treatment of essential hypertension. *Brit. Med. J.* **1**, 77 (1979).

[11]   Day, J. L.: Adrenerge Mechanismen und ihre Bedeutung für die Plasma-Lipid-Konzentration. *Wien. med. Wschr.* **132**, Sonderheft 2, Seite 19 (1982).

[12]   Deacon, S. P.: The effects of atenolol and propranolol upon lipolysis. *Brit. J. Clin. Pharmac.* **5**, 123 (1978).

[13]   Dressendorfer, R. H., Wade, Ch. E., Hornick, C. und Timmis, G. C.: High-density lipoprotein-cholesterol in marathon runners during a 20-day road race. *JAMA* **247**, 1715 (1982).

[14]   Durrington, P. N. und Cairns, S. A.: Acute pancreatitis: a complication of beta-blockade. *Brit. Med. J.* **284**, 1016 (1982).

[15]   England, J. D. F., Simons, L. A., Gibson, J. C. und Carlton, M.: The effect of metoprolol and atenolol on plasma high density lipoprotein levels in man. *Clin. Exper. Pharmacol. and Physiol.* **7**, 329 (1980).

[16]   Ernst, N., Fisher, M., Smith, W., Gordon, T., Rifkind, B. M., Little, J. A., Mishkel, M. A. und Williams, O. D.: The association of plasma high-density lipoprotein cholesterol with dietary intake and alcohol consumption. *Circulation* **62** (Suppl. IV), 41 (1980).

[17]   Franz, I.-W. und Lohmann, F. W.: Der Einfluß einer chronischen sog. kardioselektiven und nicht kardioselektiven β-Rezeptoren-Blockade auf den Blutdruck, die O_2-Aufnahme und den Kohlen-hydratstoffwechsel. Ergometrische Untersuchungen bei Hochdruckkranken. *Z. Kardiol.* **68**, 503 (1979).

[18]   Franz, I.-W. und Lohmann, F. W.: The effect of β-blockers on metabolism during exercise. in: *Advances in beta-blocker therapy*, Proceedings of an international symposium (editors: H. Roskamm, K.-H. Graefe). Excerpta Medica, Amsterdam-Oxford-Princeton, 1980.

[19]   Franz, I.-W., und Lohmann, F. W.: Unterschiedlicher Einfluß einer chronischen, überwiegend beta-1-selektiven und beta-1-, beta-2-Rezeptorblockade auf den Kohlenhydratstoffwechsel. Ergometrische Untersuchungen bei Hochdruckkranken. *Klin. Wschr.* **58**, 1155 (1980).

[20]   Franz, I.-W., Lohmann, F. W., Koch, G. und Agrawal, B.: Der Einfluß einer chronischen β-Rezeptoren-Blockade auf den Kohlenhydrat- und Fettstoffwechsel und deren hormonelle Regulation bei Hochdruckkranken. *Verhdlg. dtsch. Ges. inn. Med.* **86**, 905 (1980).

[21]   Franz, I.-W., Lohmann, F. W., Koch, G. und Quabbe, H.-J.: Aspects of hormonal regulation of lipolysis during exercise: effects of chronic β-receptor blockade. *Int. J. Sports Med.* **4**, 14 (1983).

[22] Franz, I.-W., Lohmann, F. W. und Röcker, L.: Unterschiedlicher Einfluß einer Langzeittherapie mit β_1-selektiven und β_1-β_2-Rezeptorenblockern auf den Lipidstoffwechsel bei Hochdruckkranken. *Herz-Kreislauf* **16**, 115 (1984).

[23] Frishman, W. et al.: Effects of beta-adrenergic blockade on plasma lipids: A double-blind randomized placebo-controlled multicenter comparison of labetalol and metoprolol in patients with hypertension. *Amer. J. Cardiol.* **49**, 984 (1982).

[24] Gibbons, D. O., Lant, A. F., Ashford, A., Collins, R. F. und Pinder, S.: Comparative effects of acebutolol and practolol on the lipolytic response to isoprenaline. *Brit. J. Clin. Pharmac.* **3**, 177 (1976).

[25] Gündogdu, A. S., Brown, P. M., Juul, S., Sachs, L. und Sönksen, P. H.: Comparison of hormonal and metabolic effects of salbutamol infusion in normal subjects and insulin-requiring diabetics. *Lancet* **II**, 1317 (1979).

[26] Hartung, G. H., Foreyt, J. P., Mitchell, R. E., Vlasek, I. und Gotto, A. M.: Relation of diet to high-density-lipoprotein cholesterol in middle-aged marathon runners, joggers, and inactive men. *New Engl. J. Med.* **302**, 357 (1980).

[27] Hartung, G. H., Foreyt, J. P., Mitchell, R. E., Mitchell, J. G., Reeves, R. S. und Gotto, A. M.: Effect of alcohol intake on high density lipoprotein cholesterol levels in runners and inactive men. *JAMA* **249**, 747 (1983).

[28] Haskell, W. L., Taylor, H. L., Wood, P. D., Schrott, H. und Heiss, G.: Strenuous physical activity, treadmill exercise test performance and plasma-high-density lipoprotein cholesterol. *Circulation* **62** (Suppl. IV), 53 (1980).

[29] Hausmann, L. und Motzkau, D.: Einfluß eines kardioselektiven Beta-Rezeptorenblockers auf Glukoseniveau und Insulinsekretion beim oral behandelten Diabetiker. *Inn. Med.* **8**, 89 (1981).

[30] Helgeland, A., Hjermann, I., Leren, P. und Holme, I.: Possible metabolic side effects of beta-adrenergic blocking drugs. *Brit. Med. J.* **1**, 828 (1978).

[31] Helgeland, A., Hjermann, I., Leren, P., Enger, S. und Holme, I.: High-density lipoprotein cholesterol and antihypertensive drugs: the Oslo study. *Brit. Med. J.* **2**, 403 (1978).

[32] Hooper, Ph. L., Woo, W., Visconti, L. und Pathak, D. R.: Terbutaline raises high-density-lipoprotein-cholesterol levels. *New Engl. J. Med.* **305**, 1455 (1981).

[33] Imura, H., Kato, Y., Ikeda, M., Morimoto, M. und Yawata, K.: Effect of adrenergic-blocking or -stimulating agents on plasma growth hormone, immunoreactive insulin, and blood free fatty acid levels in man. *J. Clin. Invest.* **50**, 1069 (1971).

[34] Janowski, K., Ratzmann, K. P. und Kedor, S.: Konsequenzen adrenerger Rezeptorenblockade für den Kohlenhydrat- und Fettstoffwechsel. *Dt. Gesundh.-Wesen* **38**, 568 (1983).

[35] Kindermann, W., Schmitt, W. M., Biro, G. und Schnabel, A.: Metabolismus und hormonelles Verhalten bei Körperarbeit unter akuter Beta-1-Sympathikolyse. *Z. Kardiol.* **70**, 406 (1981).

[36] Kristensen, B. O.: Effect of long-term treatment with beta-blocking drugs on plasma lipids and lipoproteins. *Brit. Med. J.* **283**, 191 (1981).

[37] Lager, I., Blohmé, G. und Smith, U.: Effect of cardioselective and non-selective β-blockade on the hypoglycaemic response in insulin-dependent diabetics. *Lancet* **3**, 458 (1979).

[38] Lancet, Editorial: Antihypertensive drugs, plasma lipids, and coronary disease. *Lancet* **II**, 19 (1980).

[39] Lehtonen, A. und Viikari, J.: *Long term effects of sotalol on serum lipids.* Abstracts sixth scientific meeting of the International Society of Hypertension, p. 149, Göteborg 1979.

[40] Leren, P., Helgeland, A., Holme, I., Foss, P. O., Hjermann, I. und Lund-Larsen, P. G.: Effect of propranolol and prazosin on blood lipids. *Lancet* **II**, 4 (1980).

[41] Leweling, A.: Betablocker und Plasmalipide – eine Bestandsaufnahme. *Hochdruck* **3**, 29 (1983).

[42] Lohmann, F. W.: Die Beeinflussung des Stoffwechsels durch Beta-Rezeptoren-Blocker. *Klin. Wschr.* **59**, 49 (1981).

[43] Lohmann, F. W.: Beta-Rezeptoren-Blocker. Metabolische Wirkungen und Konsequenzen für die Therapie. *Münch. med. Wschr.* **123**, 1795 (1981).

[44] Lohmann, F. W.: Veränderungen der Serum-Lipide bei der medikamentösen Hochdrucktherapie. *Wien. med. Wschr.* **132**, Sonderheft 2, Seite 6 (1982).

[45] Lohmann, F. W. (Herausgeber): *Beta-Rezeptorenblockade – aktuelle Gesichtspunkte.* Springer-Verlag, Berlin – Heidelberg – New York 1982.

[46] Lohmann, F. W. (Herausgeber): *Stoffwechsel und medikamentöse Hochdruckbehandlung.* Urban & Schwarzenberg, München – Wien – Baltimore 1983.

[47] Maciejko, J. J., Holmes, D. R., Kottke, B. A., Zinsmeister, A. R., Dinh, D. M. und Mao, S. J. T.: Apolipoprotein A-I as a marker of angiographically assessed coronary-artery disease. *New Engl. J. Med.* **309**, 385 (1983).

[48] MacLaren, N. K., Taylor, G. E. und Raiti, S.: Propranolol augmented, exercise-induced human growth hormone release. *Pediatrics* **56**, 804 (1975).

[49] Martyn, Ch., Jellinek, E. H. und Webb, J. N.: Lipid storage myopathy: successful treatment with propranolol. *Brit. Med. J.* **282**, 1997 (1981).

[50] Martignoni, A., Perani, G., Finardi, G., Mastropasqua, E. und Fogari, R.: Effect of mepindolol on serum lipids. *Internat. J. Clin. Pharmacol., Therapy and Toxicol.* **20**, 543 (1982).

[51] Matzkies, F.: Die Bedeutung der Lipoproteine höherer Dichte für die Arterioskleroseforschung. *Klinikarzt* **8**, 822 (1979).

[52] McGonigle, R. J. S., Williams, L., Murphy, M. J. und Parsons, V.: Labetalol and lipids. *Lancet* **I**, 163 (1981).

[53] Merker, R., Schwittek, W., Kladetzky, R.-G. und Kuhn, H.: Serumlipide unter chronischer Behandlung mit Beta-Rezeptoren-Blockern bei Patienten mit koronarer Herzkrankheit. *Z. Kardiol.* **70**, 455 (1981).

[54] Miettinen, T. A., Huttunen, J. K., Ehnholm, Chr., Kumlin, T., Mattila, S. und Naukkarinen, V.: Effect of long-term antihypertensive and hypolipidemic treatment on high density lipoprotein cholesterol and apolipoproteins A-I and A-II. *Atherosclerosis* **36**, 249 (1980).

[55] Mordasini, R., Kaffarnik, H., Schneider, J. und Riesen, W.: Alkohol und Plasmalipoproteine im Akut- und Langzeitversuch. *Schweiz. med. Wschr.* **112**, 1928 (1982).

[56] Newman, R. J.: Comparison of the antilipolytic effect of metoprolol, acebutolol, and propranolol in man. *Brit. Med. J.* **2**, 601 (1977).

[57] Pasotti, C., Capra, A., Fiorella, G., Vibelli, C. und Chierichetti, S. M.: Effects of pindolol and metoprolol on plasma lipids and lipoproteins. *Brit. J. clin. Pharmacol.* **13**, 435 S (1982).

[58] Ponti, G. B., Carnovali, M., Banderali, G. und Missaglia, A.: Effects of labetalol on the lipid metabolism in hypertensive patients. *Current Therapeutic Research* **33**, 466 (1983).

[59] Raptis, S., Rosenthal, J., Welzel, D. und Moulopoulos, S.: Effects of cardioselective and non-cardioselective beta-blockade on adrenaline-induced metabolic and cardiovascular responses in man. *Eur. J. Clin. Pharmacol.* **20**, 17 (1981).

[60] Rössner, S.: Serum lipid changes during treatment with antihypertensive drugs. *Acta Med. Scand.* **205**, (Suppl. 628) 89 (1979).

[61] Rössner, S.: Serum lipoproteins and ischemic vascular disease: On the interpretation of serum lipid versus serum lipoprotein concentrations. *J. Cardiovascul. Pharmacol.* **3** (Suppl. 3), 151 (1981).

[62] Schettler, G.: Pathophysiologie, Klinik und prognostische Bedeutung der Hyperlipoproteinämien. *Dtsch. Ärzteblatt* **77**, 661 (1980).

[63] Schettler, G., Mörl, H., Lohmann, F. W. und Wirth, A. (Herausgeber): *Metabolische und kardioprotektive Effekte durch Beta-Rezeptorenblockade.* Springer-Verlag, Berlin — Heidelberg — New York 1983.

[64] Schimert, G. Ch.: Auswahlkriterien für Betasympathikolytika. *Therapiewoche* **29**, 5857 (1979).

[65] Simonsen, S. und Kjekshus, J. K.: The effect of free fatty acids on myocardial oxygen consumption during atrial pacing and catecholamine infusion in man. *Circulation* **58**, 484 (1978).

[66] Smith, U. (Herausgeber): Adrenergic control of metabolic functions. *Acta Medica Scandinavica*, Supplementum 672, 1983.

[67] Schnabel, A. und Kindermann W.: Lipoprotein-Cholesterin bei unterschiedlicher körperlicher Aktivität. Vergleichende Untersuchungen bei jüngeren und älteren Gesunden sowie Koronarpatienten. *Klin. Wschr.* **60**, 349 (1982).

[68] Stubbe, I., Eskilsson, J. und Nilsson-Ehle, P.: High-density lipoprotein concentrations increase after stopping smoking. *Brit. Med. J.* **284**, 1511 (1982).

[69] Tanaka, N., Sakaguchi, S., Oshige, K., Niimura, T. und Kanehisa, T.: Effect of chronic administration of propranolol an lipoprotein composition. *Metabolism* **25**, 1071 (1976).

[70] Taskinen, M.-R. und Nikkilä, E. A.: Lipoprotein lipase activity of adipose tissue and skeletal muscle in insulin-deficient human diabetes. *Diabetologica* **17**, 351 (1979).

[71] Waal-Manning, H. J.: Metabolic effects of β-adrenoreceptor blockers. *Drugs* **11** (Suppl. 1), 121 (1976).

[72] Wilson, P. W., Garrison, R. J., Castelli, W. P., Feinleib, M., McNamara, P. M. und Kannel, W. B.: Prevalence of coronary heart disease in the Framingham Offspring Study: Role of lipoprotein cholesterol. *Amer. J. Cardiol.* **46**, 649 (1980).

Diskussion

N. N.

Herr Lohmann, Sie haben sehr sorgfältig die Literatur recherchiert. Gibt es aus Ihren Untersuchungen, bzw. aus den Literaturdaten Hinweise dafür, daß es sich um eine dosiskorrelierte Veränderung der Lipoproteinemuster handelt? So wurden doch unterschiedliche Dosierungen eingesetzt, dann könnte man natürlich auch die Empfehlung aussprechen, den Betablocker, der ohnehin dosismäßig bezüglich der Affinitäten relativ hoch dosiert wird, diesen zu reduzieren?

Lohmann

Es gibt wenige Untersuchungen, die zeigen, daß das ähnlich wie bei den Saluretika auch bei der Betarezeptorenblockade ein Dosisproblem ist. Das heißt, daß mit hoher oder zu hoher Dosis auch das Ausmaß dieser reaktiven Veränderungen zunimmt. Aus diesem Grunde ist es ja generell auch üblich geworden, sowohl in der Hypotoniebehandlung, gerade dort, aber auch bei der koronaren Herzkrankheit, ab einer gewissen Grenze die Kombinationstherapie durchzuführen. Aber auch im niederen Dosisbereich zeigen die wenigen Studien doch auch noch die hier geschilderten Unterschiede, so daß sich das also dort nicht nivelliert; das ist nicht ein Problem der hohen Dosis.

N. N.

Herr Lohmann, zwei Feststellungen passen für mich nicht zusammen. Sie sagten: erstens, nach akuter Betablockade wird zwar die Lipolyse unterdrückt und dann kommt sekundär nicht die nicht katecholaminabhängige Lipolyse. Das war die erste Feststellung. Die zweite Feststellung war, daß die Störungen des Lipidstoffwechsels nach Betablockade zwar initial auftreten, in den ersten drei Monaten, daß aber nach 16, oder noch weiteren Monaten nun diese Lipidstoffwechselstörungen wieder zurückgehen. Wie paßt das zusammen?

Lohmann

Das ist wahrscheinlich ein quantitatives Problem. Was ich angedeutet habe, war der Unterschied der Akutwirkung und der chronischen Wirkung. Man kann also aus der Akutwirkung einer Substanz, bei der einmaligen parenteralen Anwendung nicht schließen auf ihre chronischen Auswirkungen bei der Dauertherapie. Zum anderen, das ist z. B. auch sehr diffizil untersucht worden mit Longitudinal-Untersuchungen an kleinen Kollektiven, sind die Veränderungen der Lipoproteine unter Betarezeptorenblockade immer bis 4 Wochen, meistens bis 8 Wochen, nachweisbar. Das hängt davon ab, was für ein Betarezeptorenblocker, und was für eine Dosierung vorliegt. Dabei zeigt sich, daß der gemischte Betarezeptorenblocker, z. B. das Nadolol mit der sehr langen Halbwertzeit auch nach 16 Monaten noch die nahezu gleichstarken Veränderungen zeigt, und zwar wahrscheinlich dadurch, weil durch die komplette und auch über die Tageszeit gesehen, anhaltende ständige Blockade der katecholaminvermittelten Lipolyse, die kompensatorische Gegenregulation intensiver und anhaltender steigert als es bei einem selektiven Blocker in abgeschwächter Form möglich ist. So würden sich diese Veränderungen unter Zugrundelegung der hier geschilderten Mechanismen erklären können, wobei ich sagen muß — das habe ich auch angedeutet, ich habe es Ihnen hier nur vereinfacht und schematisiert darstellen können — die Veränderungen sind im Detail komplexer. Es ist aber so, daß in der Langzeit-Therapie mit Beta-1-selektiver Rezeptorenblockade das notwendige Ausmaß der Gegenregulation geringer sein kann, um die Lipolyse in der Bilanz aufrechtzuerhalten.

Gleichmann

Die Stellungnahme, die Sie abgegeben haben, entspricht voll der Stellungnahme der Hochdruckliga, die derzeit publiziert wird. Ich möchte ergänzen; wir haben zu diesem Thema 2 Punkte herausgestrichen, die Langzeit-Therapie ist das wichtige. Und Langzeit fängt ab 1 Jahr oder länger an. Der zweite Punkt, der noch wichtig erscheint, ist vermutlich der Ausgangswert des Cholesterins. Hain und Schneider haben im vorigen Jahr die Beeinflussung der Fettwerte aus der Hypertension Follow-up-Studie publiziert, die ja bekanntlich über 7 Jahre ging. Sie konnten nachweisen, daß je höher der Cholesterinwert war, um so länger wurden über diesen Zeitraum von 7 Jahren lipidsenkende Effekte beobachtet. Bei Werten um 280 mg % konnte über die 7 Jahre unter der Therapie, die allerdings nicht immer nur Betablocker-Therapie war, eine 20 %ige Lipidsenkung festgestellt werden. Nur bei den Werten unter 200 mg %, wo das Atherogene-Risiko keine entscheidende Rolle spielt, fanden sich diskrete Anstiege. Also, es ist sehr differenziert zu sehen. Man darf sich nicht ein einziges epidemiologisches Datum herausgreifen.

A Controlled Comparison of the Peripheral Vasoconstrictor Effects of Labetalol with a Conventional Beta-Blocker in Raynaud's Phenomenon

G. Holti

University Department of Dermatology, Royal Victoria Infirmary, Queen Victoria Road, Newcastle upon Tyne, NE1 4LP, U.K.

Beta-adrenergic receptors can be separated into beta$_1$-receptors which predominate in the heart and renin secreting renal tissue and beta$_2$-receptors which mediate dilation of vascular and other smooth muscle. 'Nonselective' beta-blockers, such as propranolol or nadolol, affect almost equally cardiac, vascular and bronchiolar function, whereas socalled 'cardioselective' blockers affect arteriolar and bronchial smooth muscle significantly when relatively large doses are given. In individuals with a constitutional or acquired tendency to develop peripheral vascular spasm, evident clinically as cold limbs with or without attacks of Raynaud's phenomenon, intermittent claudication, skin necrosis, loss of ischaemic fingers and even of limbs have been documented as side effects of some of these drugs [1, 2, 8–14].

Predisposed patients, who are prone to develop cold extremities and Raynaud's phenomenon, often stop their medication with beta-blockers on cold days, when their need for these drugs is greatest, because of their side effects.

Different beta-blockers vary widely in their peripheral vasoconstrictor effects. A drug such as labetalol which has alpha- as well as beta-blocking activity may be expected to have less peripheral vasoconstrictor activity than conventional beta-blocking agents.

Purpose of Study

This study was designed to compare under strictly controlled experimental conditions the peripheral vaso-constrictor action of labetalol with that of the most widely used beta-blocking drug propranolol in patients subject to frequent attacks of Raynaud's phenomenon [4, 5, 7].

Labetalol was given at a dose of 100 mg. thrice daily and propranolol 40 mg. with equal frequency.

Methodology

Trial design

A double-blind, randomised, within patient cross-over study, preceded by a 3-week "single-blind" period during which the patients took placebo capsules and a similar single-blind 3-week "wash-out" period between each of the 3-week treatments was chosen. The investigation thus lasted 12 weeks for each patient.
It was commenced early in December during a cold winter and was completed by March. The outside temperatures varied between $-4\,°C$ and $+5\,°C$ during the trial period.

Patients

Twelve patients were admitted to the study and all completed it. They had been selected from about 200 patients with primary and secondary Raynaud's phenomenon because they were reliable attenders of testing sessions, were known to be reliable takers of their tablets and good observers of their symptoms. All had given their informed consent to participate in the evaluation of the 2 drugs and knew that they would not receive any vaso-active drugs during 2 phases of this study.
Their ages ranged from 25—65 years.
Patients with hypertension requiring continuous treatment with drugs were not included. Their systolic blood pressures ranged from 125 mm Hg—170 mm Hg when they felt cold, with a median value of 141 mm Hg and their diastolic pressures from 85 mm Hg—105 mm Hg with a median value of 92.5 mm Hg. When warm their systolic pressures ranged from 120 mm Hg—160 mm Hg with a median value of 136.1 mm Hg and their diastolic pressures from 80 mm Hg—95 mm Hg with a median value of 85 mm Hg.
Patients with symptomatic ischaemic heart disease or diabetes mellitus were not included. Nine female and 3 male patients participated in the study.
Six had seemingly primary Raynaud's phenomenon without any evidence, after repeated and extensive investigations, of an underlying obliterative vascular disease.
The remaining patients had systemic sclerosis, lupus erythematosus or arteriosclerosis obliterans.
Patients' characteristics are set out in Table 1.

Table 1: Patients' characteristics

Number	Raynaud's Phenomenon (RP)	Age (years)	Duration of RP (years)
6	Primary	Range 27—41 Mean 34.5	Range 5—20 Mean 18.1
6	Secondary	Range 50—62 Mean 56.5	Range 8—20 Mean 12.6

Clinical and Biometric Evaluation

At the beginning and the end of the 4 'treatment' periods the trophic state and any vascular discolouration of the patients' extremities were examined, their blood pressure was taken, supine and erect, and the diary cards in which all patients had recorded the fre-

quency and severity of their attacks of Raynaud's phenomenon (R.P), any suspected side-effects of their treatments and any other relevant observations were examined.
The following biometric tests were carried out at each of the 5 testing sessions which took place between 07.30 hours and 09.30 hours since at that time of day attacks of R.P. are commonest and in order to obtain consistent test conditions and blood samples:

1. Immediately on arrival at the hospital and before patients had the opportunity to get warm, all fingertip temperatures were recorded using a copper — tellurite — copper thermopile [3] which gives "steady state" readings within 10 seconds, in order to assess total digital bloodflow.
2. Nutrient skin bloodflow in the fingertips was assessed at a depth of 1.5 mm from the skin surface using a non-invasice thermal clearance probe [6].
3. If R.P. was not present on arrival, it was induced by the patient holding between her/his thumb and fingertips a rectangular metal tray containing ice cubes. Provided patients feel cold and have an oral temperature not above 36 °C, a common finding on a cold morning, the time required to induce R.P. was consistent for each patient under identical experimental conditions.
4. The patients' peripheral vascular tone and functional vascular reserve were assessed by measuring their vascular responses during reactive hyperaemia which was induced after warming patients until their oral temperature had been raised to 37.5 °C.
5. The patients' blood pressure and pulse rate were recorded in the erect and supine position when they were cold and after inducing hyperthermia in order to assess the effect of the two beta-blocking drugs.
6. Blood samples were taken at each testing session in order to monitor any toxic effects attributable to the drugs and for estimations of the plasma viscosity, fibrinogen and serum lipid levels.

Results

Although one half of the patients had Raynaud's phenomenon secondary to an underlying obliterative vascular disease, in the analysis of the data there were no statistically significant differences between this group and the patients with seemingly primary R.P. All twelve patients are therefore presented as one group.

1. Recordings of the pulse rate and blood pressure showed that both beta-blockers in the dose used in this study were of equal therapeutic efficacy and confirmed that all patients had taken their drugs as directed.
2. The blood tests did not indicate any toxic effect of either drug upon any haematological indices, liver function, blood sugar or plasma viscosity.

3. Biometric tests

Table 2: Finger Tip Temperatures "on arrival". Median Temperatures of 12 Patients (°C)

Control 17.3	Labetalol 17.8	t NS
17.6	Propranolol 15.9	5.14 (P < 0.001)

Table 2 shows that while patients took labetalol their fingertip temperatures (mean value of all 10 fingers) were significantly higher when they arrived on cold mornings at the laboratory than they were while taking propranolol when compared with the placebo periods.

Table 3: Time Taken for Induction of Raynaud's Phenomenon. Number of Patients: 12 (Median Time in Seconds)

Control 104.6	Labetalol 95.8	t NS
100.8	Propranolol 33.8	3.53 (P < 0.01)

Table 3 shows that patients taking propranolol developed Raynaud's phenomenon significantly earlier during the dry cold challenge test than during labetalol therapy. While on labetalol they were no more prone to develop R.P. than while on placebo.

Table 4: Digital Temperatures During Reactive Hyperaemia. Number of Patients: 12 Median Temperatures ($^\circ$C)

Control 26.9	Labetalol 26.2	t 1.85 (NS)
27.0	Propranolol 23.3	5.68 (P < 0.001)

Table 4 shows that patients' vascular tone was significantly less impaired by labetalol than by propanolol.

Table 5: Thermal Clearance Rates During Reactive Hyperaemia. Median Readings from All Fingers of 12 Patients (ΔT $^\circ$C)

Control 2.02	Labetalol 2.00	t NS
2.00	Propranolol 2.20	2.87 (P < 0.05)

Table 5 shows that patients taking labetalol did not show during reactive hyperaemia a diminution of their nutrient skin bloodflow, a feature seen in patients taking propranolol, who demonstrated a feeble rise of their skin temperature indicating that their increase in total skin bloodflow was attained by "borrowing" blood from the nutrient flow and by opening up of arterio-venous shunts.

Side-Effects

When, after completion of the study, the trial code was broken it was found that of well known side effects of beta-blockers such as fatigue, headaches, nightmares, "heaviness" of legs, dizziness after ascending stairs rapidly, and diarrhoea, some patients on labetalol were aware of mild alimentary tract manifestations, such as abdominal gurgling and loose motions, but few of the other symptoms, which affected significantly 10 out of 12 patients while taking propranolol.

Conclusions

This controlled comparison of labetalol, which has alpha- as well as beta-blocking action, with the perhaps most widely used beta-blocking drug propranolol, showed that labetalol did not enhance the inherently increased peripheral vascular tone of individuals subject to frequent attacks of Raynaud's phenomenon. It compared very favourably in this respect with propranolol. The skin bloodflow reducing effect of the latter drug, which had been reported by other workers for this and other conventional beta-adrenergic blocking drugs was confirmed.

Other unwelcome side effects of socalled 'cardio-selective' as well as of 'non-cardio-selective' beta-blocking drugs in particular undue fatigue, diminished exercise tolerance, restless sleep, bad dreams and intestinal upsets were not experienced significantly by patients taking labetalol.

Neither propranolol nor labetalol caused toxic effects upon blood parameters, liver function tests, glucose tolerance or urate metabolism.

Acknowledgements

I gratefully acknowledge the help and support of the Medical Department of Allen and Hanburys Limited who arranged the supply of the coded trial drugs. The dedicated and cheerful technical assistance of Mrs. Elizabeth Wells is most gratefully acknowledged. Grateful thanks are due to Dr. K. D. MacRae for his expert statistical analyses. Last but not least I am greatly indebted to the 12 patients for their loyal co-operation in a study which involved prolonged and, in part, uncomfortable testing sessions at "unsocial" hours. Without such loyal co-operation the clinical evaluation of drugs could not be undertaken.

References

[1] Fröhlich, E. D., Tarazi, R. C., and Dunston, H. P.: Peripheral Arterial Insufficiency — A Complication of Beta-Adrenergic Blocking Therapy. *JAMA* **208**, 2471–2472 (1969).

[2] Gokal, R., Dornan, T. L., and Ledingham, J. G. G.: Peripheral Skin Necrosis Complicating Beta-Blockade. *Brit. med. J.* **1**, 721–722 (1979).

[3] Holti, G.: The Copper — Tellurite — Copper Thermopile Adapted as a Skin Thermometer. *Clin. Sci.* **14**, 137–141 (1955).

[4] Holti, G.: Experimentally Controlled Evaluation of Vasoactive Drugs. *Angiology* **29**, 89–94 (1978).

[5] Holti, G.: A Double-Blind Study of the Peripheral Vasoconstrictor Effects of the Beta-Blocking Drug Penbutolol in Patients with Raynaud's Phenomenon. *Curr. Med. Res. Opin.* **6**, 267–270 (1979).

[6] Holti, G. and Mitchell, K. W.: Estimation of the Nutrient Skin Bloodflow using a Segmented Thermal Clearance Probe. *Clin. Exp. Derm.* **3**, 189–198 (1978).

[7] Holti, G.: A Comparison of Two Beta-Blocking drugs in patients with Raynaud's Phenomenon. *The Practitioner* **226**, 781–783 (1982).

[8] Marshall, A. J., Roberts, C. J. C. and Barritt, D. W.: Raynaud's Phenomenon as Side-Effect of Beta-Blockers in Hypertension. *Brit. Med. J.* **I**, 1498–1499 (1976).

[9] McSorley, D. D. and Warren, D. J.: Effects of Propanolol and Metropolol on the Peripheral Circulation. *Brit. Med. J.* **II**, 1598–1600 (1978).

[10] Rodger, J. C., Sheldon, C. D., Lerski, R. A. and Livingstone, W. R.: Intermittent Claudication Complicating Beta-Blockade. *Brit. Med. J.* **I**, 1125 (1976).

[11] Smith, R. S. and Warren, D. J.: Effect of Beta-Blocking Drugs on Peripheral Bloodflow in Intermittent Claudication. *J. Cardiovasc. Pharm.* **4**, 2—4 (1982).

[12] Vale, J. A., Van De Petite and Price, T. M. L.: Peripheral Gangrene Complicating Beta-Blockade. *Lancet* **II**, 412 (1977).

[13] Vale, J. A. and Jefferys, D. B.: Peripheral Gangrene Complicating Beta-Blockade. *Lancet* **I**, 1216 (1978).

[14] Zacharias, R. J., Cowen, K. J., Prest, J., Vickers, J., and Wall, B. G.: Propranolol in Hypertension — A Study of Long Term Therapy, 1964—1970. *Am. Heart J.* **83**, 755—761 (1977).

Discussion

Franz

In my opinion there are no good reasons to give propranolol or to use beta-receptor-blockade in such patients. If those patients are suffering from hypertension, I would prefer calcium antagonists. So do you have any results on this aspect with calcium antagonists?

Holti

I couldn't agree more. None of these patients were suffering from hypertension. I use these patients entirely in order to demonstrate clearly the vasoconstrictor effect of propranolol compared with labetalol, but I have in fact treated patients with quite severe Raynaud's-phenomenon with labetalol, and their peripheral vasoconstrictor manifestation did not deteriorate. They could tolerate labetalol, but I agree with you entirely, nifedipine or prazosin are preferable.

N. N.

There is no doubt at all, reserpine is a highly effective drug, but its side-effects are just unacceptable. I had one patient who attempted suicide on two occasions, and who had to be taken off reserpine.

Holti

I have never carried out a controlled trial of reserpine against these drugs, but I have certainly measured frequently the peripheral vasodilator effect of reserpine giving intravenously and intraarterially. There is no doubt at all, reserpine is a highly effective drug, but its side-effects are just unacceptable. I had one patient who attempted suicide on two occasions, and who had to be taken off reserpine.

Pharmacokinetic Glossary of Labetalol

N. Rietbrock, B. G. Woodcock

Department of Clinical Pharmacology, University Clinic Frankfurt, Theodor-Stern-Kai 7,
D-6000 Frankfurt, FRG

Physico-chemical properties

Owing to the presence of an amide group in the molecule labetalol is more
polar than propranolol and therefore has relatively low lipid solubility [1].

Chloroform/water partition coefficient

Labetalol	1.2 : 1
Propranolol	9 : 1
Oxprenolol	10 : 1

Labetalol contains 2 optical centres and clinical preparations consist of
equal proportions of the resulting 4 optical isomers. Most of the beta-adrenoceptor activity is associated with the RR isomer whereas the alpha-blocking
activity is present mainly in the SR isomer [2].

Absorption

Following oral doses of 100–200 mg peak concentrations in blood are
attained sometimes as early as 20 minutes and usually within 2 hours [3].

Bioavailability

Labetalol administered orally is well absorbed but undergoes substantial first
pass metabolism during passage across the liver. The extent of presystemic
metabolism varies widely between subjects. In middle-aged hypertensive
patients the bioavailability was 11 % to 86 % with an average value of 31 %—
33 % [3, 4].
The bioavailability of labetalol is moderately increased from 26 % in the
fasting state to 36 % when administered with food. Food slows the rate of
absorption. In one study peak blood levels occurred at 3 hours after the

dose when taken with food, in comparison to 1 hour after the dose when taken in the fasting state [5].

Distribution

The apparent distribution volume of labetalol (V_d) is higher than that of most conventional β-blocking drugs. The drug has therefore relatively more affinity to tissue proteins than plasma proteins in comparison with the other β-blockers.
In hypertensive patients the average value for V_d was 392 liters with individual values ranging from 188 to 747 liters [3].
High levels of labetalol are found in lung, liver and kidney but not in brain [1].

Plasma protein binding

In human blood labetalol is 50 % bound to plasma proteins [1].

Elimination

Less than 5 % of labetalol is excreted in the urine following oral application. Elimination occurs predominantly by metabolism in the liver notably by hydroxylation and conjugation and significant quantities of active metabolites have not been detected. The most important conjugate is an 0-glucuronide (on the secondary alcohol group) with small quantities of 0-phenyl-glucuronide, N-glucuronide and a glucuronide formed following hydroxylation [1].
The metabolites are excreted in the faeces (12 % to 27 %) and in the urine (55 % to 60 %) [1].
Following intravenous administration there is a bi- or tri-exponential decline in labetalol plasma concentrations. Reported values for the elimination halflife (terminal) range from 3.1 to 4.9 hours [3, 5, 6, 7]. In 12 hypertensives the range was 1.7 hours to 6.1 hours [3].
Labetalol is concentrated in red blood cells. The red-cell : plasma concentration ratio is 1.8 : 1 [8]. This value enables the plasma clearance of approximately 1500 ml/min to be converted to blood clearance, 1100 ml/min [3]. The hepatic extraction, taking liver blood flow as 25 % of cardiac output, is estimated to be 80–90 % [9]. The high value for systemic clearance indicates that the clearance of labetalol will be dependent on liver blood flow.

Plasma concentrations and therapeutic range

Clinical experience has confirmed that postural hypotension occurs in some patients receiving high doses of labetalol and this is acknowledged to be the drug's major dose-limiting side-effect. This points to the importance of an optimal plasma concentration range, below which the drug's hypotensive effect may be sub-optimal and above which postural hypotension may require reduction of the dose. This means that with labetalol the therapeutic concentration range will be dependent, to some extent, on the vasodilatation response induced by alpha-blockade in the individual patient.

During long-term administration labetalol accumulates to produce steady-state levels which are 1.7 times higher than those predicted from the single-dose pharmacokinetic parameters [10].

In 12 subjects stabilised on a dose of 200 mg labetalol twice daily, mean steady-state concentrations varied over 5-fold, from 36 ng/ml to 183 ng/ml [11]. This variability is probably due to differences in absorption and clearance. When the dosage of labetalol covers a large enough range (200 mg daily to 1200 mg daily) there is a clear relationship between the plasma drug concentration and the fall in blood pressure, especially in the upright position [8].

Age

There is some evidence that the bioavailability of labetalol increases with increasing age [12]. In the 30—40 year-olds bioavailability was 30 % whereas in the 80 year-olds it was 60—70 % and there was a trend towards longer halflives in the older patients.

Chronic liver disease

In patients with liver cirrhosis the bioavailability of labetalol was 63 % in comparison with 33 % in controls. Plasma concentrations were also considerably higher and this was reflected in a greater fall in blood pressure in these patients. The average dose of labetalol in patients with chronic liver disease may be about half that of subjects with normal liver function [6].

Chronic renal disease

The plasma clearance and terminal elimination halflife of labetalol in patients with severe renal impairment (creatinine clearance 6 ml/min) was not appreciabley different from patients with normal renal function (creatinine clearance greater than 84 ml/min). No modification of the dose of labetalol is required in the presence of renal function impairment [13, 14].

Pregnancy

No clinically significant differences in clearance or halflife of labetalol have been observed in pregnant subjects so that the dosage regimens appropriate for pregnant patients are probably similar to those recommended for normal non-pregnant subjects [15].
The concentration of labetalol in fetal plasma is less than the corresponding maternal plasma drug concentration. Infant to maternal blood concentrations varied from 0.3 to 0.5 over a wide dosage range [16].
The concentration of labetalol in breast milk is substantially less than in maternal plasma. Areas under plasma and breast milk concentration curves (0–12 h) were in the ratio 1.5 : 1. Individual measurements made on breast milk gave concentrations of only 20–40 % of those in maternal plasma [16, 17].

References

[1] Martin, L. E.; Hopkins, R. and Bland, R.: Metabolism of labetalol by animals and man. *British Journal of Clinical Pharmacology* 3 (Suppl. 3): 695–710 (1976).
[2] Brittain, R. T.; Drew, G. M. and Levy, G. P.: The α- and β-adrenoceptor blocking potencies of labetalol and its individual stereoisomers in anaesthetized dogs and in isolated tissues. *British Journal of Pharmacology* 77: 105–114 (1982).
[3] McNeil, J.J.; Anderson, A. E. and Louis, W. J.: Pharmacokinetics and pharmacodynamic studies of labetalol in hypertensive subjects. *British Journal of Clinical Pharmacology* 8: 157S–161S (1979).
[4] Louis, W. J.; Christophidis, N.; Brignell, M.; Bijayasekaran, V.; McNeil, J. J. and Vajda, F. J. E.: Labetalol: Bioavailability, drug plasma levels, plasma renin and catecholamines in acute and chronic treatment of resistant hypertension. *Australian and New Zealand Journal of Medicine* 8: 602–609 (1978).
[5] Daneshmend, T. K.; Homeida, M. and Roberts, C. J. C.: The effect of hepatosplenic schistosomiasis on the pharmacokinetics of metronidazole and labetalol (abstract). *British Journal of Clinical Pharmacology* 14: 152P–153P (1982).
[6] Homeida, M.; Jackson, L. and Roberts, C. J. C.: Decreased first-pass metabolism of labetalol in chronic liver disease. *British Medical Journal* 2: 1048–1050 (1978).
[7] Kanto, J.; Allonen, H.; Kleimola, T. and Mantyla, R.: Pharmacokinetics of labetalol in healthy volunteers. *International Journal of Clinical Pharmacology, Therapy and Toxicology* 19 (No. 1): 41–44 (1981).
[8] McNeil, J. J.: Ph. D. Thesis, University of Melbourne (1981).
[9] McNeil, J. J.; Louis, W. J.: Clinical pharmacokinetics of labetalol. *Clinical Pharmacokinetics* 9: 157–167 (1984).
[10] McNeil, J. J.; Anderson, A. E. and Louis, W. J.: An analysis of the blood pressure response to labetalol in hypertensive patients. *Clinical Sciences* 61: 449S–452S (1981).
[11] McNeil, J. J.; Anderson, A. E.; Louis, W. J. and Raymond, K.: Labetalol steady-state pharmaco-

kinetics in hypertensive patients. *British Journal of Clinical Pharmacology* **13** (Suppl. I): 75S–80S (1982).

[12] Kelly, J. G.; McGarry, K.; O'Malley, K. and O'Brien, E. T.: Bioavailability of labetalol increases with age. *British Journal of Clinical Pharmacology* **14**: 304–305 (1982).

[13] Wood, A. J.; Ferry D. G. and Bailey, R. R.: Elimination kinetics of labetalol in severe renal failure. *British Journal of Clinical Pharmacology* **13** (Suppl. I): 81S–86S (1982).

[14] Walstad, R. A.; Nilsen, O. G.; Berg, K. J. and Wessel-Aas, T.: The pharmacokinetics and clinical effects of one single dose of labetalol in patients with normal and impaired renal function. *Acta Pharmacologica et Toxicologica* **49**: 54 (1981).

[15] Rubin, P. C.; Butters, L.; Kelman, A. W.; Fitzsimmons, C. and Reid, J. L.: Labetalol disposition and concentration-effect relationships during pregnancy. *British Journal of Clinical Pharmacology* **15**: 465–470 (1983).

[16] Michael, C. A.: Use of labetalol in the treatment of severe hypertension during pregnancy. *British Journal of Clinical Pharmacology* **8** (Suppl. 2): 211S–215S (1979).

[17] Leitz, F.; Bariletto, S.; Gural, R.; Jaworsky, L.; Patrick J. and Symchowicz, S.: Secretion of labetalol in breast milk of lactating women. *Federation Proceedings* **42**: 378 (1983).

III Balanced Alpha/Beta Blockade in the Therapy of Hypertension

Änderung der Hämodynamik und die Pharmakotherapie des Hochdrucks

P. Lund-Johansen
Cardiology Section, Medical Department, 5016 Haukeland Hospital, Bergen, Norway

Zusammenfassung

Vom hämodynamischen Gesichtspunkt aus ist die adäquate Reaktion auf eine antihypertensive Therapie die Wiederherstellung eines normalen Kreislaufsystems. Bei den meisten Patienten mit leichter bis mittelschwerer essentieller Hypertonie, bei denen eine medikamentöse Behandlung angezeigt erscheint, besteht die wesentliche hämodynamische Störung in einem erhöhten peripheren Gesamtwiderstand und einem normalen oder verminderten Herzzeitvolumen. Im Laufe von 10—17jährigen Kontrolluntersuchungen unbehandelter Hypertoniker wurde eine allmähliche Zunahme des peripheren Gesamtwiderstands und eine Verringerung des Herzzeit- und Schlagvolumens sowie ein Anstieg des arteriellen Mitteldrucks festgestellt.
Die hämodynamischen Reaktionen auf eine medikamentöse Langzeittherapie wurden bei 250 Männern mit leichter bis mittelschwerer essentieller Hypertonie im WHO-Stadium I in Ruhe und unter Belastung untersucht. Es wurde eine signifikante Reduktion des peripheren Gesamtwiderstandes unter Diuretika, Nifedipin und Verapamil registriert, jedoch erhöhte keine dieser Substanzen ein vermindertes Herzzeit- oder Schlagvolumen.
Eine bessere Normalisierung der zentralen Hämodynamik ließ sich durch Prazosin erzielen, das eine Herabsetzung des peripheren Gesamtwiderstandes und eine Zunahme von Herzzeit- und Schlagvolumen, besonders bei Belastung, bewirkte. Dagegen ging die Behandlung mit β-Blockern mit einer chronischen Reduktion von Herzzeitvolumen und Herzfrequenz einher. Der periphere Gesamtwiderstand sank gewöhnlich nicht unter prätherapeutische Werte ab. Die Abnahme des Herzzeitvolumens ging mit einem Anstieg der arteriovenösen O_2-Differenz parallel.
Bei 14 Patienten mit einem behandlungsresistenten Hochdruck fand sich eine stark ausgeprägte Erhöhung des peripheren Gesamtwiderstandes. Captopril führte zu einer Senkung des peripheren Gesamtwiderstandes in Ruhe, unter Belastung auch zu einer Erniedrigung des Herzzeitvolumens. Während einer 5jährigen Langzeitbehandlung mit β-Blockern blieb die antihypertensive Wirkung erhalten, aber ohne weitere Senkung des peripheren Gesamtwiderstandes. Dagegen bewirkte eine 5jährige Therapie mit Labetalol einen allmählichen Abfall des Gesamtwiderstandes unter das Niveau vor der Behandlung sowie eine allmähliche Zunahme des Herzzeitvolumens.

Vom hämodynamischen Gesichtspunkt aus ließe sich die adäquate Reaktion auf eine antihypertensive Therapie als Wiederherstellung normaler Kreislaufverhältnisse sowohl in

Ruhe als auch unter Belastung definieren. Eine nicht-adäquate Reaktion wäre das Ausbleiben dieser Wirkung selbst wenn der Blutdruck gesenkt würde.

Bei der Mehrzahl der Patienten, bei denen eine medikamentöse Hochdruckbehandlung erforderlich erscheint, ist die wesentliche Störung in einem erhöhten peripheren Gesamtwiderstand [1—3] zu sehen. Eine solche Erhöhung findet sich im allgemeinen in den meisten Stromgebieten wie der Niere, den Organen im Bauchraum und der Haut, bei fortgeschrittener Hypertonie auch in der Skelettmuskulatur [2, 4]. Das Herzzeitvolumen ist in der Regel normal oder vermindert, und das Schlagvolumen ist subnormal. Bei Muskeltätigkeit findet sich gewöhnlich ein subnormales Herzzeit- und Schlagvolumen, und zwar sogar bei einem leichten Hypertonus im jüngeren Alter [1].

Bei einer unbehandelten Hypertonie sind die Spontanveränderungen durch ein allmähliches Absinken von Herzzeit- und Schlagvolumen und durch einen Anstieg des peripheren Gesamtwiderstandes in Ruhe und bei Muskeltätigkeit charakterisiert [1]. Die Blutdruckveränderungen können variieren. Bei den meisten Patienten mit einem leichten oder mittelschweren fixierten Hochdruck (nicht bei Grenzfällen) steigt der Blutdruck in einem Zeitraum von 10—17 Jahren an. Bei einer 10-Jahres-Kontrolle von 29 Patienten mit leichtem Hochdruck sank das Herzzeitvolumen um 20 % unter Ruhebedingungen. Der periphere Gesamtwiderstand erhöhte sich um 30 % [1]. Acht dieser Probanden wurden nach 17 Jahren einer dritten hämodynamischen Verlaufskontrolle unterzogen. Die nach 10 Jahren festgestellten Veränderungen waren inzwischen fortgeschritten und sind aus Abbildung 1 ersichtlich.

In der nachfolgenden Übersicht soll in erster Linie erörtert werden, wie die am häufigsten verordneten Antihypertonika bei Langzeitbehandlung die zentrale Hämodynamik bei den typischen Patienten mit leichter bis mittelschwerer essentieller Hypertonie beeinflussen. Es wird weiter diskutiert, ob eine inadäquate Blutdrucksenkung einer schweren hämodynamischen Störung und/oder einer ungeeigneten Medikamentenwahl zuzuschreiben ist. Die Erörterung beschränkt sich auf Diuretika, α- und β-Blocker (allein oder kombiniert), Calcium-Antagonisten und den Converting-Enzym-Hemmer Captopril.

Antihypertensive Langzeitbehandlung und Änderung der Hämodynamik

Über mehrere Jahre haben wir die hämodynamischen Reaktionen auf eine medikamentöse Langzeitbehandlung an 250 Männern mit leichter bis mittelschwerer essentieller Hypertonie im WHO-Stadium I (diastolischer Druck 100—120 mmHg) kontrolliert. Vor der Behandlung wiesen praktisch alle Patienten einen erhöhten peripheren Gesamtwiderstand (> 2800 dyn s cm^{-5} m^{-2}) in Ruhe und auch unter Belastung auf. Das Herzzeitvolumen war normal oder mäßig herabgesetzt, das Schlagvolumen war in Ruhe durchweg normal und unter Belastung um etwa 20 % vermindert. Unter Belastung war die arteriovenöse O_2-Differenz im allgemeinen um 10—15 % erhöht [1].

Diuretika (Thiazide und Tienylsäure (Ticrynaten))

Vor etwa 20 Jahren haben Conway und Lauwers nachgewiesen, daß eine Blutdrucksenkung in den ersten Tagen einer Thiazidtherapie mit einem Abfall des Herzzeitvolumens ohne Änderung des peripheren Gesamtwiderstandes einhergeht. Eine mehrmonatige Langzeittherapie verursachte jedoch eine Senkung des peripheren Gesamtwiderstandes auf Normalwerte und eine allmähliche Zunahme des Herzzeitvolumens. Etwa 10 Jahre später

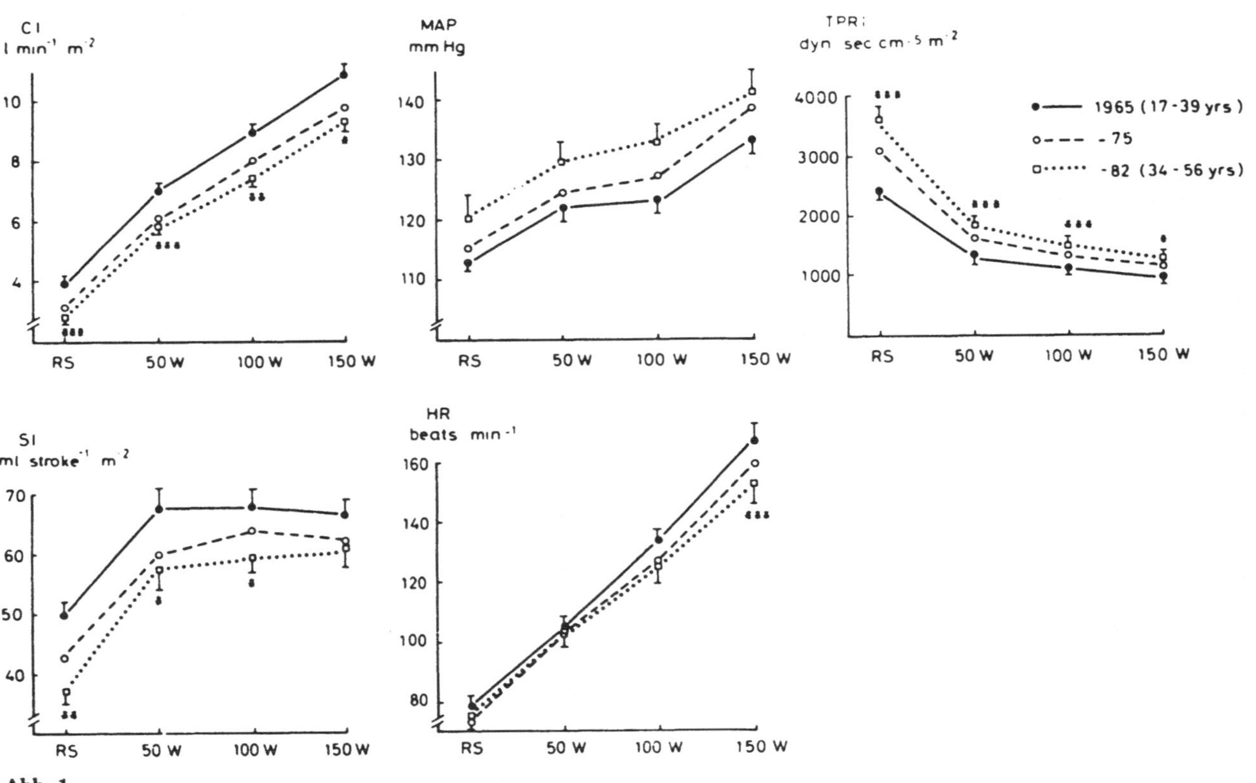

Abb. 1

Zentrale Hämodynamik bei männlichen Patienten mit unbehandeltem essentiellem Hochdruck. 1. Untersuchung 1965 (Alter 17–39 Jahre), sodann erneut 1975 und 1982 untersucht (Alter 34–56 Jahre). RS = sitzende Position in Ruhe. W = Watt. CI = Herzindex. MAP = mittlerer artieller Druck. TPRI = peripherer Gesamtwiderstandsindex. SI = Schlagvolumenindex. HR = Herzfrequenz. Die Sternchen geben die statistischen Differenzen zwischen der 1. und der letzten Prüfung an: * = p < 0.05, ** = p < 0.01, *** = p < 0.001.

wurden diese Ergebnisse in unserer Klinik bestätigt. Dabei wurde auch gezeigt, daß das Blutdruckniveau unter Belastung vorwiegend durch dieselben Mechanismen — eine Senkung des peripheren Gesamtwiderstandes ohne Herzzeitvolumenreduktion — aufrechterhalten wurde. Die Reaktion der Herzfrequenz auf Belastung blieb unbeeinflußt [6]. Eine gleichartige hämodynamische Reaktion war später mittels Tienylsäure nachweisbar [7]. Demnach dürften die Thiaziddiuretika und Tienylsäure mindestens eine partielle Korrektur der hämodynamischen Störungen bewirken; ,,partiell'' deshalb, weil das verminderte Schlag- und Herzzeitvolumen unter Belastung nicht korrigiert wird [5—8].

β-Blocker

Gut dokumentiert sind unterschiedliche hämodynamische Reaktionen auf die verschiedenen Typen von β-Blockern in Ruhe. Dagegen sind die hämodynamischen Reaktionen bei Muskeltätigkeit im großen und ganzen dieselben, besonders bei Langzeitbehandlung [9—13]. Wir haben 7 verschiedene β-Blocker bei 89, sämtlich nicht vorbehandelten Patienten mit leichter bis mittelschwerer essentieller Hypertonie geprüft [14]. Die typische Reaktion auf die Langzeitbehandlung mit β-Blockern ohne sympathomimetische Eigenwirkung war eine Blutdrucksenkung um etwa 15—20 % sowie eine Senkung von Herzfrequenz und Herzzeitvolumen um etwa 20—25 % in Ruhe. Unter Belastung stieg das Schlagvolumen kompensatorisch an, und die Herzzeitvolumenverminderung war etwas geringer (10—15 %). Der periphere Gesamtwiderstand sank nicht unter das Niveau vor Behandlung. Abbildung 2 zeigt die Ergebnisse innerhalb eines Jahres bei einer mit Atenolol behandelten Hypertonikergruppe [14a].

β-Blocker mit starker sympathomimetischer Eigenwirkung (z.B. Pindolol) führten gewöhnlich zu einer Blutdrucksenkung in Ruhe bei geringerer Herzfrequenz- und Herzzeitvolumensenkung als β-Blocker ohne sympathomimetische Eigenwirkung. Der periphere Gesamtwiderstand blieb auf dem Vorbehandlungsniveau oder lag leicht darunter. Unter Belastung (Erhöhung des Sympathikotonus) war die Blutdrucksenkung ausgeprägt, aber geringer als unter β-Blockern ohne sympathomimetische Eigenwirkung. Das Schlagvolumen stieg (im Vergleich zum Zeitraum vor Behandlung) an, der periphere Gesamtwiderstand sank leicht unter dieses Niveau.

Die meisten Untersucher berichten über die gleichen hämodynamischen Änderungen [10—14], aber einige Berichte lauten anders. So wurden Patienten beschrieben, die auf eine Langzeitbehandlung mit β-Blockern mit einem Anstieg des Herzzeitvolumens und einer starken Senkung des peripheren Gesamtwiderstandes reagierten [15, 16]. Bei Patienten mit leichter bis mittelschwerer essentieller Hypertonie ist dieses Reaktionsmuster selten. Abbildung 3 zeigt die individuellen Änderungen des Herzindex. Man sieht, daß der Herzindex bei den meisten Patienten absinkt; dies am stärksten bei denen mit den höchsten Ausgangswerten, obwohl auch bei ziemlich niedrigen Ausgangswerten erhebliche Indexsenkungen vorkamen. Abbildung 4 zeigt, daß bei Patienten dieser Kategorie relativ wenige mit einer Senkung des Gesamtwiderstandes reagierten. Gemäß Tabelle 1 war die Anzahl der Patienten mit einer mindestens 10%igen Senkung des peripheren Gesamtwiderstandes in Ruhe und unter Belastung relativ klein.

Die meisten Untersuchungen haben ergeben, daß eine Langzeittherapie mit β-Blockern den O_2-Verbrauch (V_{O_2}) in Ruhe und bei Belastung nur gering beeinflußt [14]. Da der Herzindex erniedrigt ist (gewöhnlich 20—25 %), bedeutet dies, daß die arteriovenöse O_2-Differenz entsprechend erhöht ist. Die Bedeutung dieses Phänomens ist unbekannt.

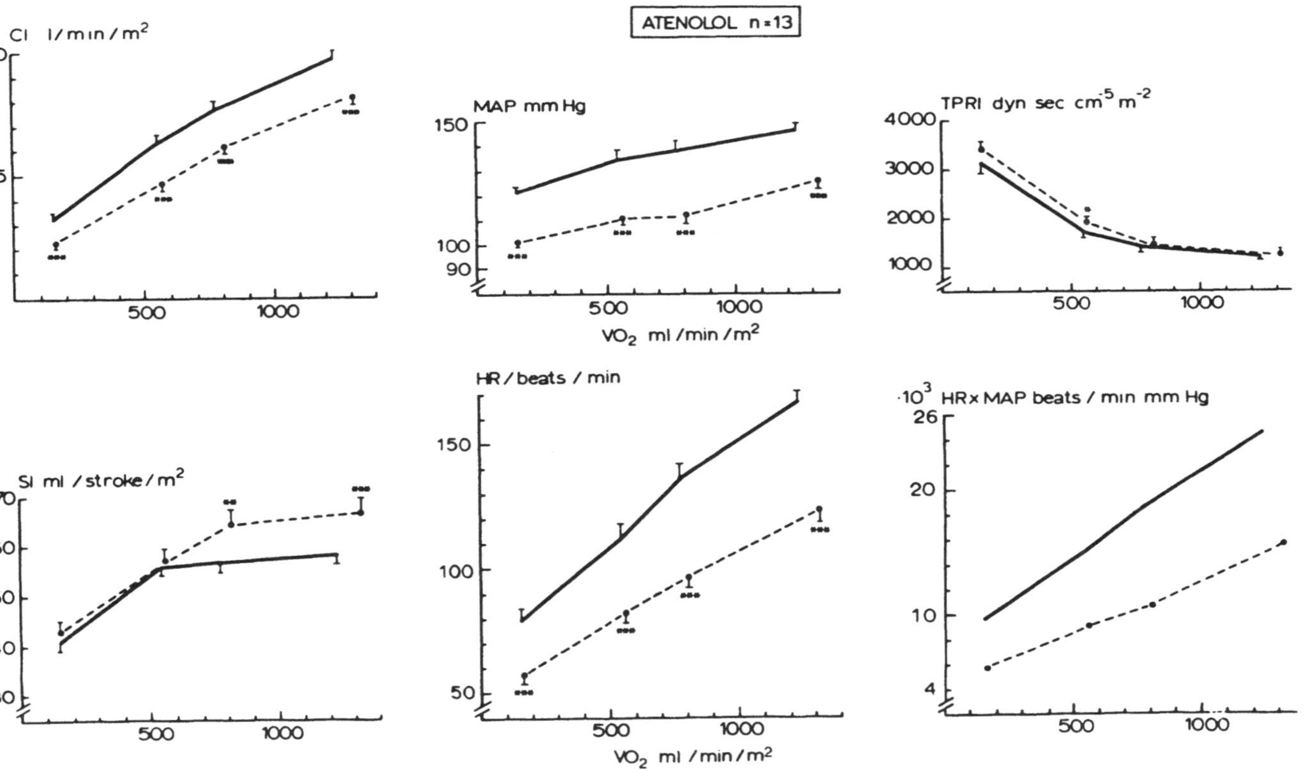

Abb. 2

Hämodynamische Veränderungen nach 1 Jahr Atenolol-Behandlung bei 13 männlichen Patienten mit essentieller Hypertonie. V_{O_2} = O_2-Verbrauch. Sonst wie Abb. 1. ———— = vor der Behandlung. ———— = während der Behandlung. Man beachte den posttherapeutischen Anstieg des Schlagvolumenindex unter Belastung, der die Herzfrequenzsenkung teilweise ausgleicht [14a].

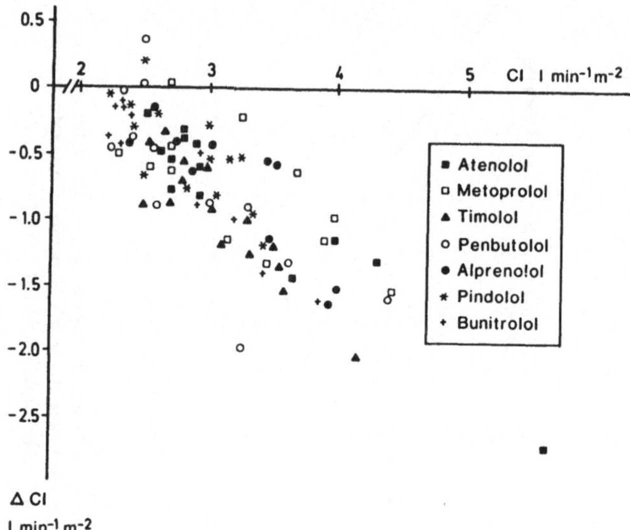

Abb. 3

Die Veränderungen des Herzindex im Vergleich zum Index vor der Behandlung in sitzender Position in Ruhe bei 89 männlichen Patienten mit leichter bis mittelschwerer Hypertonie unter Behandlung mit verschiedenen β-Blockern [14].

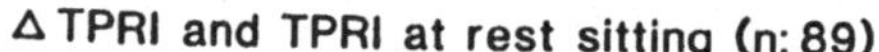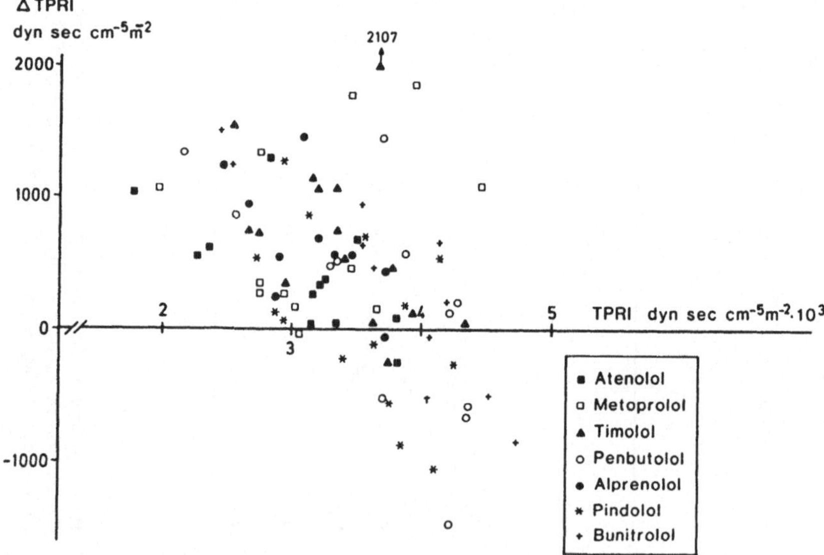

Abb. 4

Die Veränderungen des peripheren Gesamtwiderstandsindex im Vergleich zum Wert vor der Behandlung bei Langzeit-β-Blockade [14].

Tabelle 1: Individuelle Änderungen des peripheren Gesamtwiderstands-Indexes ΔTPRI > 10 % in Ruhe (sitzend) und unter 2 Belastungsstufen bei 89 Männern mit leichter bis mittelschwerer Hypertonie unter Behandlung mit verschiedenen β-Blockern

Substanz	n
Atenolol	1 von 13
Metoprolol	1 von 12
Timolol	0 von 16
Penbutolol	4 von 13
Alprenolol	1 von 10
Bunitrolol	0 von 11
Pindolol	3 von 14
Total	10 von 89 $\hat{=}$ 11 %

Zwar reagieren viele Patienten auf die Einleitung einer β-Blockertherapie mit Muskel-müdigkeit sowie kalten Händen und Füßen, aber diese Beschwerden gehen — wenigstens bei Patienten mit leichter bis mittelschwerer Hypertonie — oft unter der Langzeitmedikation zurück, wenn auch kalte Extremitäten (wahrscheinlich aufgrund einer Verminderung der peripheren Durchblutung) in kalten Klimazonen ein nicht zu unterschätzendes Problem darstellen können. Jedenfalls ist bei Patienten unter Langzeitbehandlung mit β-Blockern —hämodynamisch gesehen — die normokinetische hypertone Zirkulation durch ein normotones, aber hypokinetisches System ersetzt worden. Es ist natürlich bedeutsam, daß das Produkt aus Blutdruck und Herzfrequenz unter β-Blockerbehandlung erheblich verringert ist, besonders bei muskulärer Belastung, bei der es zu einer 40%igen oder noch stärkeren Senkung kommen kann. Diese Reaktion ist natürlich vor allem bei Patienten mit gestörter Koronardurchblutung erwünscht.

α-Blocker (Prazosin)

Die Untersuchungen über Prazosin stimmen darin überein, daß der Blutdruck sowohl akut als auch auf Dauer ausschließlich über eine Herabsetzung des peripheren Gesamt-widerstandes gesenkt wird [17—19]. Herzfrequenz und Herzzeitvolumen bleiben in Ruhe unverändert. Bei Belastung steigt das Herzzeitvolumen aufgrund einer Erhöhung des Schlagvolumens und eines leichten, aber nichtsignifikanten Anstieges der Herzfrequenz an. Eine Senkung des peripheren Gesamtwiderstandes ist ein recht konstanter Befund. Die Ergebnisse unserer 1-Jahresstudie vermittelt Abbildung 5. Danach normalisiert Prazosin bei der Mehrzahl der Patienten mit leichter bis mittelschwerer essentieller Hypertonie den Kreislauf. Eine Herabsetzung der renalen oder peripheren Durchblutung fand sich nicht [19]. Bei Patienten mit pathologischem Koronarkreislauf sollte jedoch festgehalten werden, daß die Arbeitsbelastung des Herzens weit weniger gemindert wird als durch β-Blocker, da nur der Blutdruck, nicht aber die Herzfrequenz sinkt.

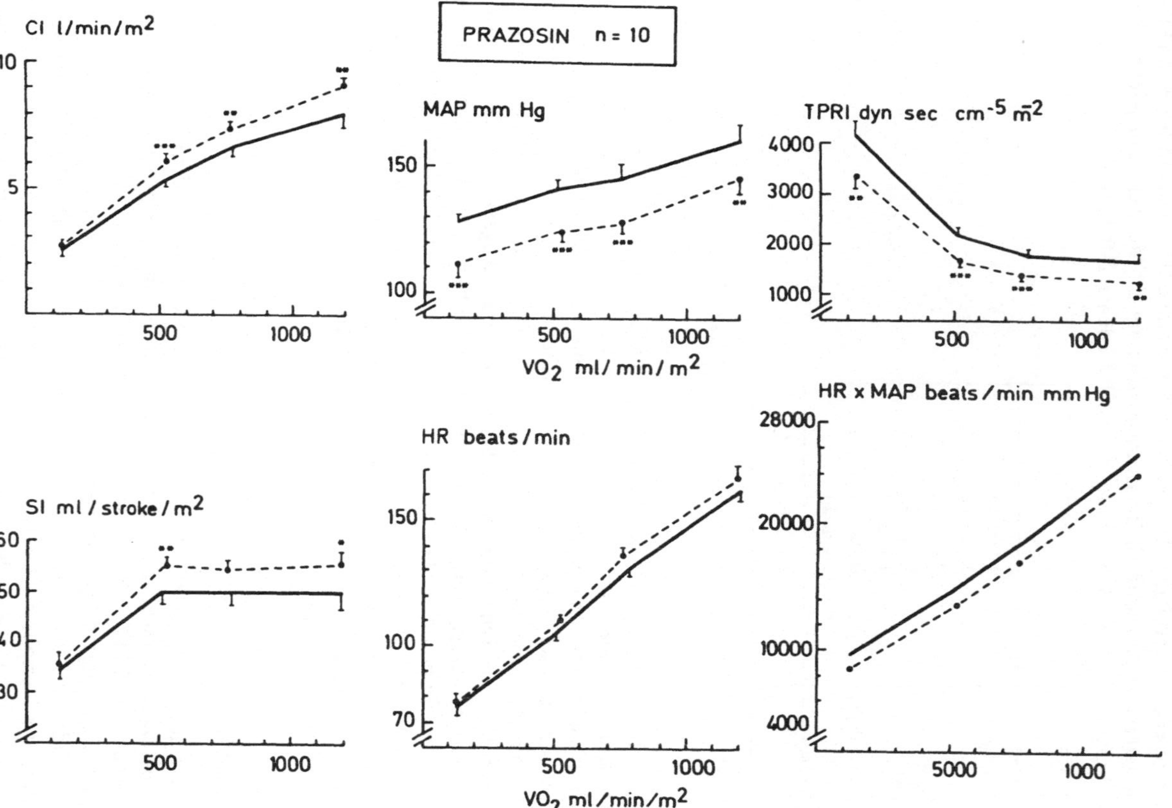

Abb. 5

Hämodynamische Veränderungen unter 1 Jahr Prazosin-Therapie bei 10 männlichen Patienten mit essentieller Hypertonie. Man beachte die erhebliche Senkung des peripheren Gesamtwiderstandsindex und den signifikanten Anstieg des Herzindex unter Belastung, ferner die geringe Verkleinerung des Produktes aus Herzfrequenz und mittlerem arteriellem Druck. Sonst wie Abb. 2 [18].

Kombination von α- und β-Blockern (Prazosin + β-Blocker, Labetalol)

Bei adäquatem Verhältnis zwischen α- und β-Blockade läßt sich oft eine wesentliche Blutdrucksenkung erzielen, die teils auf einer Erniedrigung des peripheren Gesamtwiderstandes, teils auf einer Senkung des Herzzeitvolumens beruht [20]. Zu erwarten wäre auch eine Schlagvolumenreduktion; die Senkung des Herzzeitvolumens bei Belastung ist geringer als unter reiner β-Blockade.
Labetalol bewirkt — wie zu erwarten — vergleichbare Änderungen, da diese Substanz sowohl α- als auch β_1- und β_2-Rezeptoren blockiert [21–24]. In unseren Untersuchungen betrug die Senkung im Mittel 23 %. Unter Belastung war das Herzzeitvolumen weit weniger vermindert als unter Therapie mit β-Blockern [23].

Calcium-Antagonisten (Verapamil und Nifedipin)

In den letzten Jahren wurden die Calcium-Antagonisten in die Hochdrucktherapie eingeführt [25–29]. Diese Substanzen senken den Blutdruck über eine Reduktion des peripheren Gesamtwiderstandes. Bei Langzeitbehandlung erniedrigte Nifedipin in Retardform [29] den Ruheblutdruck um 17 % ohne wesentliche Veränderungen des Herzzeit- und Schlagvolumens und der Herzfrequenz (Abb. 6). Verapamil bewirkte eine etwa gleiche Senkung des peripheren Gesamtwiderstandes, aber auch eine 10%ige Senkung der Herzfrequenz, was jedoch durch eine Erhöhung des Schlagvolumens kompensiert wurde. Das Herzzeitvolumen blieb unverändert.
Die Calcium-Antagonisten halten also (wie die Diuretika) den Blutdruck mittels partieller Korrektur der hämodynamischen Störungen niedrig. „Partiell" deshalb, weil das unternormale Zeitvolumen bei Belastung nicht korrigiert wird.

Hämodynamische Reaktionen auf medikamentöse Langzeitbehandlung

Da mindestens einige der hämodynamischen Anomalien bei fixierter Hypertonie auf Strukturveränderungen an Herz und Widerstandsgefäßen beruht, wäre zu hoffen, daß eine Dauerregulierung des Blutdrucks eine Rückbildung dieser Veränderungen bewirkt und im Verlaufe der Langzeittherapie auch die weitere Normalisierung der zentralen Hämodynamik fördert. Wir haben Gruppen von Patienten untersucht, die mit verschiedenen β-Blockern (Alprenolol, Atenolol oder Metoprolol) sowie mit Labetalol behandelt und nach 3–5 Jahren hämodynamisch untersucht wurden. Die Ergebnisse der Atenolol-Studie sind aus Abbildung 7 ersichtlich. Die zentrale Hämodynamik blieb von 1 Jahr bis 5 Jahre nach Therapiebeginn praktisch unverändert. Enttäuschend war das Ausbleiben einer Herzzeit- und Schlagvolumenerhöhung oder einer Senkung des peripheren Gesamtwiderstandes. Andererseits war keine eindeutige Verschlechterung eingetreten [30]. Unter Alprenolol und Metoprolol war es zu ähnlichen Veränderungen gekommen. Die Herabsetzung der Arbeitsbelastung des Herzens blieb bestehen.
Neuerdings haben wir eine Kontrolluntersuchung an 15 Patienten mit mäßigem Hochdruck beendet, die 6 Jahre mit Labetalol behandelt worden waren. Die Reaktionen waren etwas anders als bei einer Langzeitbehandlung mit β-Blockern. Der Blutdruck blieb während dieser 6 Jahre reguliert und änderte sich nicht wesentlich. Jedoch war der periphere Gesamtwiderstand in Ruhe und bei Belastung gefallen, und lag nach den 6 Jahren unter dem nach 1 Behandlungsjahr (Abb. 8). Der Herzindex war nach 6 Jahren etwas höher als

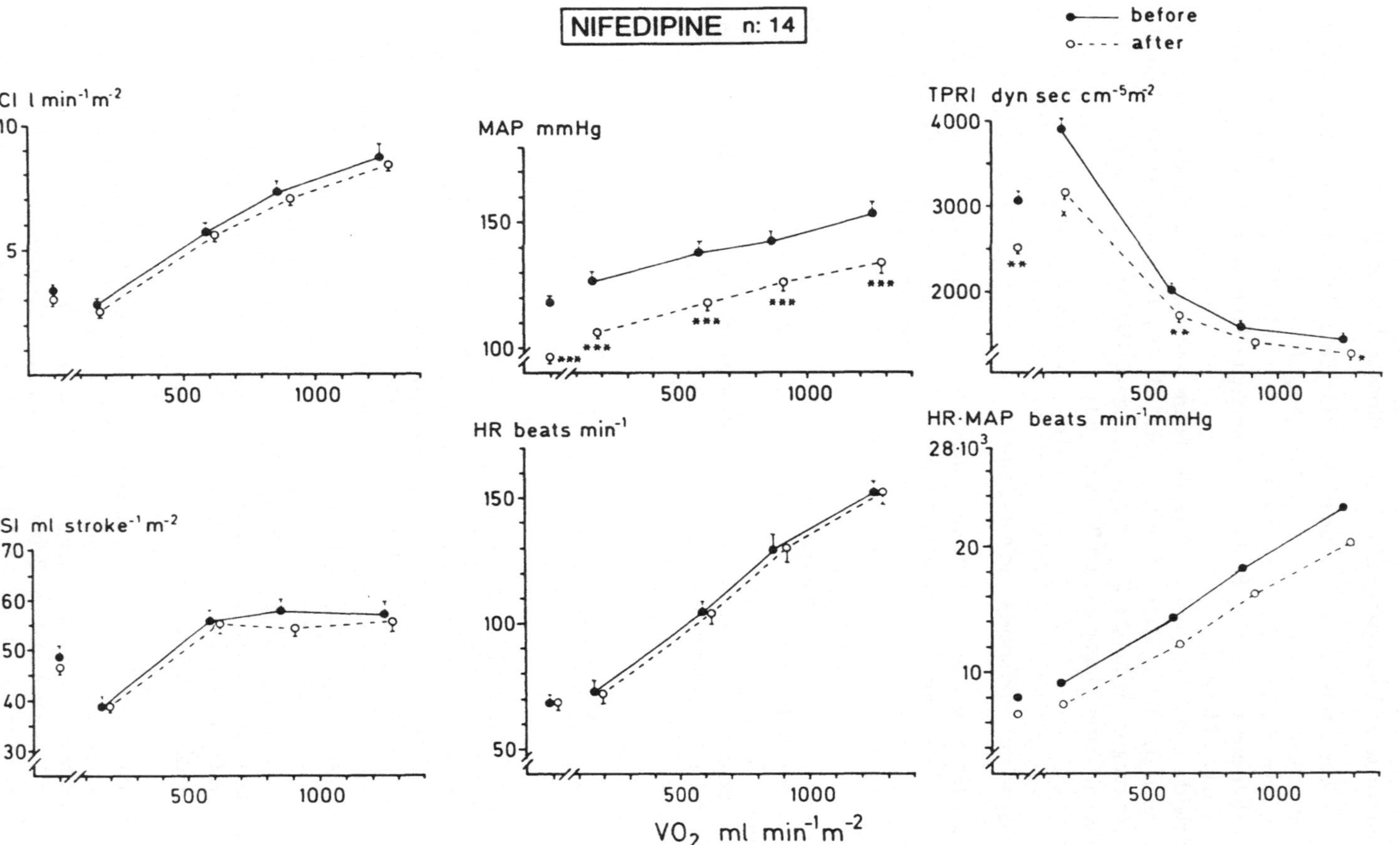

Abb. 6

Hämodynamische Veränderungen unter Langzeitbehandlung mit Retard-Nifedipin bei 14 männlichen Patienten mit essentieller Hypertonie. Man beachte die Herabsetzung des peripheren Gesamtwiderstandsindex sowie das Fehlen von Veränderungen des Herzzeit- und Schlagvolumenindex sowie der Herzfrequenz.

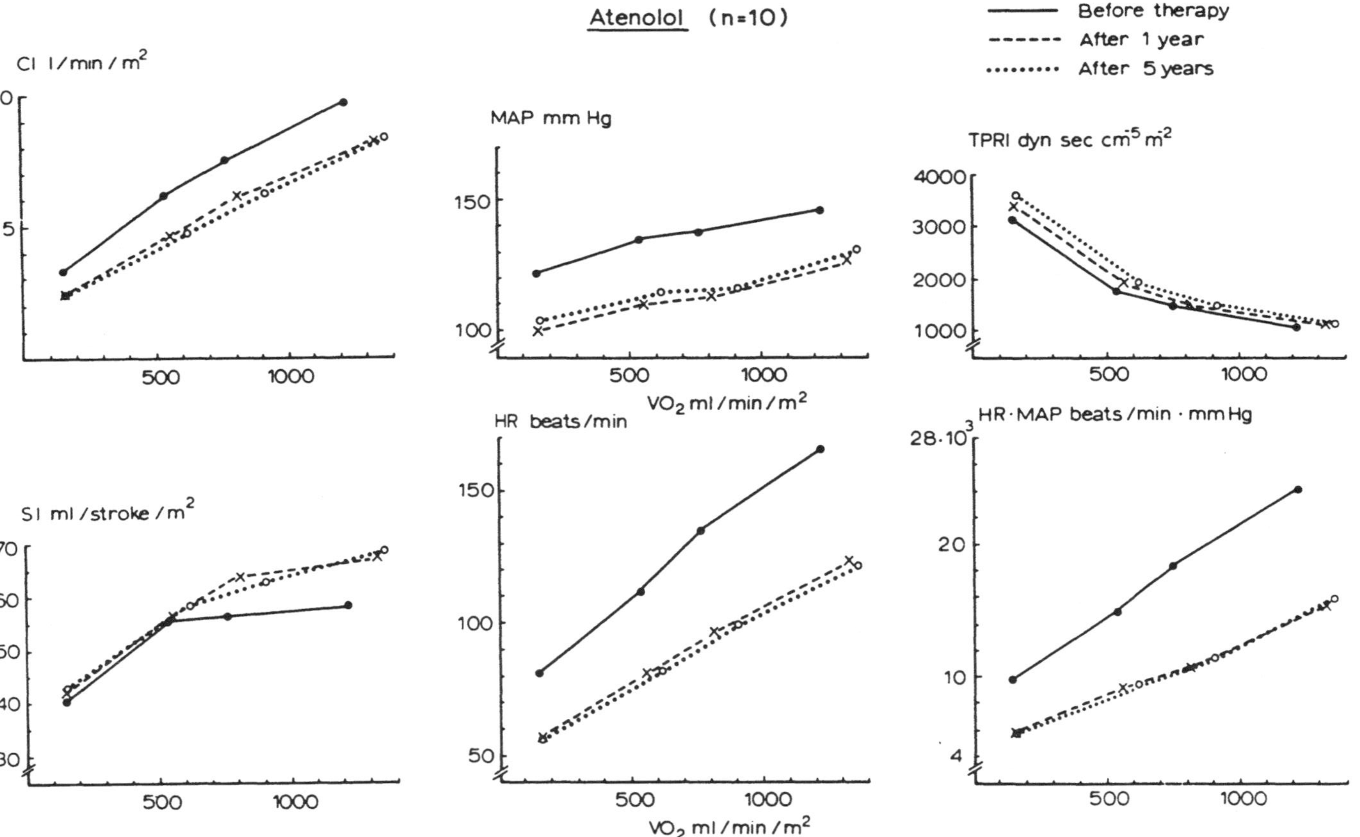

Abb. 7
Veränderungen von Herzindex, mittlerem arteriellem Druck und peripherem Gesamtwiderstandsindex bei 10 männlichen Patienten unter Atenolol-Langzeitbehandlung vor der Therapie und nach 1 und 5 Jahren. Angegeben sind Mittelwerte [30].

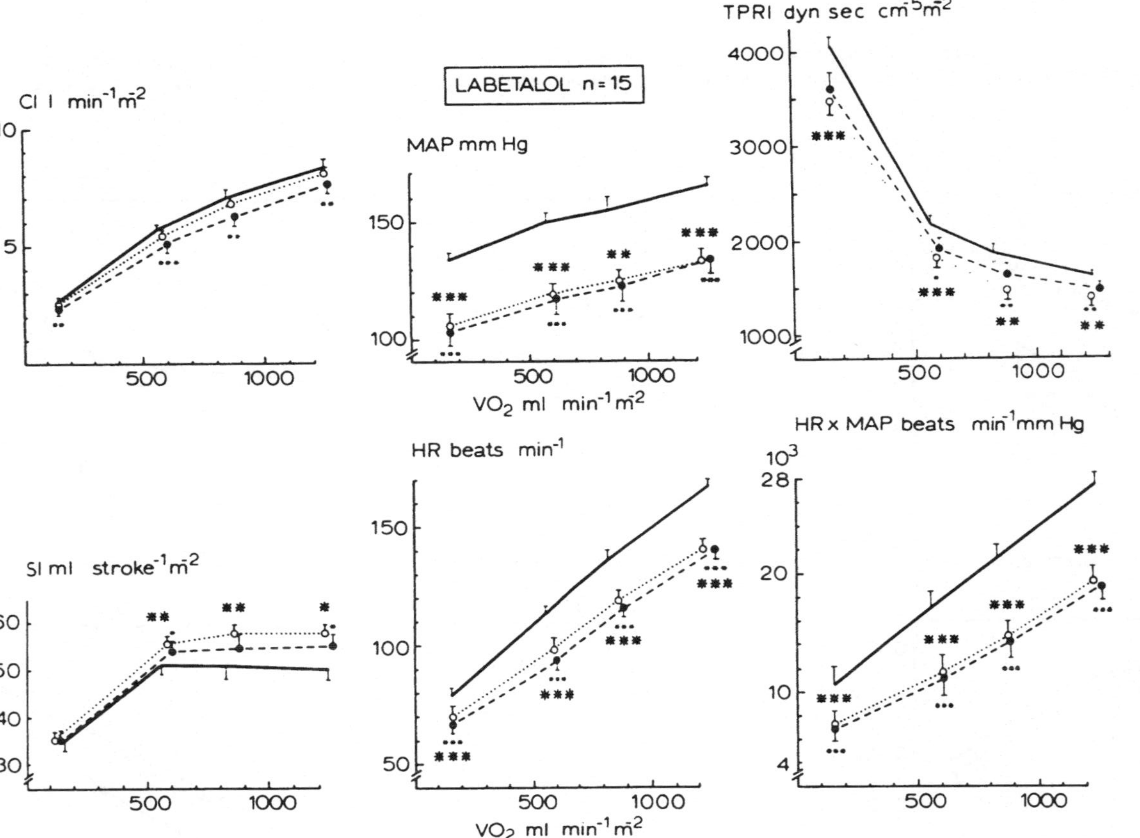

Abb. 8

Hämodynamische Veränderungen unter 6jähriger Labetalolbehandlung bei 15 männlichen Patienten. Werte vor (———) und nach 1 (———) und 6 Jahren (···) Therapie. Angegeben sind Mittelwerte und Standardfehler des Mittelwertes. Kleine Sternchen: Differenzen zwischen der 1. und 2. Untersuchung. Große Sternchen: ebenso zwischen der 1. und 3. Untersuchung. Man beachte die allmähliche Senkung des peripheren Gesamtwiderstandsindex und die leichte Zunahme von Schlagvolumen- und Herzindex in den 5 Jahren zwischen der 2. und 3. Untersuchung.

nach 1 Jahr, aber die Unterschiede zwischen der 1- und 6-Jahresbehandlung waren statistisch nicht signifikant. Insgesamt indes sprechen die Ergebnisse für eine größere Normalisierung der zentralen Hämodynamik unter Labetalol-Dauertherapie, verglichen mit der β-Blocker-Langzeittherapie.

Hämodynamische Charakteristika und Reaktionen bei Patienten mit schwerer, therapieresistenter Hypertonie

Anderson et al. [31] haben eine Patientengruppe untersucht, die sich therapieresistent gegenüber herkömmlichen Antihypertonika (Dreifachtherapie mit Diuretika, β-Blockern und Vasodilatantien) verhielten. Wurde die Behandlung ausgesetzt und stieg der Blutdruck an, so bestand die charakteristische hämodynamische Störung in einem ausgeprägten Anstieg des peripheren Gesamtwiderstandes, kombiniert mit einem subnormalen Schlag- und Herzzeitvolumen. Der Blutdruck war hoch (etwa 230/140 mmHg in Ruhe). Bei einer ähnlichen Patientengruppe haben wir diese hämodynamischen Charakteristika in Ruhe und unter leichter Belastung bestätigt (Omvik und Lund-Johansen 1983, unveröff. Ergebnisse). Da der hohe Widerstand − abgesehen von Strukturveränderungen in den Widerstandsgefäßen − theoretisch auch auf einer Hyperaktivität im Renin-Angiotensin-System (nicht bestimmt) beruhen konnte, wurden die Patienten mit Captopril und einem Diuretikum behandelt. Die meisten reagierten mit einem erheblichen Blutdruckabfall, in einigen Fällen auf praktisch normotone Werte. In Ruhe war der Blutdruck infolge einer Senkung des peripheren Gesamtwiderstandes bei geringer Änderung des Herzzeitvolumens erniedrigt. Unter Belastung kam es auch zu einer Senkung des Herzzeitsvolumens. Ähnliche Reaktionen in Ruhe wurden auch von anderen Autoren berichtet [32−33].

Schlußfolgerung

Die meisten der üblicherweise verschriebenen Antihypertonika können den Blutdruck regulieren, oft jedoch nur durch eine partielle Korrektur der hämodynamischen Störungen. Insbesondere die β-Blocker führen in der Regel nur zu einem Herzzeitvolumen unter der Norm in Ruhe und unter Belastung natürlich zu einer subnormalen Herzfrequenz. Die arteriovenöse O_2-Differenz ist unter Belastungsbedingungen erhöht. Eine bessere Normalisierung der zentralen Hämodynamik läßt sich durch Diuretika und Calcium-Antagonisten erzielen, dies allerdings in der Regel ohne vollständige Normalisierung des Herzzeitvolumens. Nach unserer Erfahrung wurde die beste Normalisierung der zentralen Hämodynamik mit dem α-Blocker Prazosin erreicht.
Unter der 5−6jährigen Langzeitbehandlung verhinderten die β-Blocker eine weitere Abnahme des Schlagvolumens und einen weiteren Anstieg des peripheren Gesamtwiderstandes und unterdrücken daher anscheinend die sonst bei unbehandelten Patienten zu erwartenden Veränderungen. Die Langzeittherapie unter kombinierter α- und β-Blockade (mit Labetalol) führte zu einer allmählichen Erniedrigung des peripheren Gesamtwiderstandes und zu einem leichten Anstieg des Herzzeitsvolumens in Ruhe und unter Belastung. So könnte die Kombination von α- und β-Blockade bessere Ergebnisse erbringen als β-Blocker allein.
In dieser kurzen Übersicht wurden nur die typischen Reaktionen von Patienten mit leichter bis mittelschwerer essentieller Hypertonie besprochen. Die meisten dieser Patienten scheinen die durch die β-Blockade bedingte chronische Verringerung des Herzzeitvolu-

mens erstaunlich gut zu vertragen, im allgemeinen sogar unter nur geringer Einschränkung ihrer körperlichen Tätigkeit.

In besonderen Untergruppen von Patienten kann indes jedoch die Verordnung eines falschen Antihypertonikums Fehlreaktionen auslösen: d.h. Sinken des Herzindex bei Patienten mit Hochdruck und peripheren Gefäßstörungen. Bei Patienten mit sehr schwerem, therapieresistenten Hochdruck sind manchmal Converting-Enzym-Hemmer besonders wirksam, die dann die zentrale Hämodynamik über eine Senkung des peripheren Gesamtwiderstandes wenigstens teilweise normalisieren.

Zum Schluß sei betont, daß zwar die Reaktionen auf Antihypertonika vom hämodynamischen Gesichtspunkt aus stark variieren, daß aber andere Wirkungen dieser Substanzen für das klinische Ergebnis natürlich bedeutsamer sein können. Hat man es jedoch mit relativ jungen Patienten mit leichter bis mittelschwerer essentieller Hypertonie zu tun, bei denen eine jahrelange (vielleicht lebenslängliche) Therapie erforderlich sein kann, so erscheint die Wiederherstellung normaler Kreislaufverhältnisse ein logischer therapeutischer Weg.

Literatur

[1] Lund-Johansen, P.: State of the art review. Haemodynamics in essential hypertension. *Clin. Sci.* 59 : 343, 1980.

[2] Birkenhäger, W. H., de Leeuw, P. W., Schalekamp, M. A. D. H.: *Control Mechanisms in Essential Hypertension.* Amsterdam, New York, Oxford, Elsevier Biomedical Press, 1982.

[3] Bühler, F. R.: Pathophysiology of primary hypertension: role of adrenoceptors in the transformation from an early high cardiac output into a later high arteriolar resistance phase. In: *Hypertensive Cardiovascular Disease: Pathophysiology and Treatment*, edited by Amery, A. The Hague, Boston, London, Martinus Nijhoff Publishers, 1982, p 164.

[4] Folkow, B.: Physiological aspects of primary hypertension. *Physiol. Rev.* 62 : 347, 1982.

[5] Conway, J., Lauwers, P.: Hemodynamic and hypotensive effects of long-term therapy with chlorothiazide. *Circulation* 21 : 21, 1960.

[6] Lund-Johansen, P.: Hemodynamic changes in long-term diuretic therapy of essential hypertension. *Acta Med. Scand.* 187 : 509, 1970.

[7] Lund-Johansen, P.: Hemodynamic and metabolic long-term effects of tienilic acid in essential hypertension. *Acta Med. Scand.* (Suppl 646): 106, 1980.

[8] Van Brummelen, P., Man in't Veld, A. J., Schalekamp, M. A. D. H.: Hemodynamic changes during long-term thiazide treatment of essential hypertension in responders and nonresponders. *Clin. Pharmacol. Ther.* 27 : 328, 1980.

[9] Clark, B. J.: Beta-adrenoceptor-blocking agents: Are pharmacologic differences relevant? *Am. Heart J.* 104 : 2334, 1982.

[10] Man in't Veld, A. J., Schalekamp, M. A. D. H.: How intrinsic sympathomimetic activity modulates the haemodynamic responses to beta-adrenoceptor antagonists. A clue to the nature of their antihypertensive mechanism. *Br. J. Clin. Pharmacol.* 13 : 245, 1982.

[11] Tarazi, R. C., Dustan, H. P.: Beta-adrenergic blockade in hypertension. *Am. J. Cardiol.* 29 : 633, 1972.

[12] Tarazi, R. C., Fouad, F. M., Bravo, E. L.: Total peripheral resistance and beta-adrenergic blockade. In: *Frontiers in Hypertension Research*, edited by Laragh, J. H., Bühler, F. R., Seldin, D. W. Berlin, Heidelberg, New York, Springer Verlag 1981, p. 454.

[13] Svendsen, T. L., Carlsen, J. E., Hartling, O., McNair, A., Trap-Jensen, J.: A comparison of the acute haemodynamic effects of propranolol and pindolol at rest and during supine exercise in man. *Clin. Sci.* 59 : 465, 1980.

[14] Lund-Johansen, P.: Central hemodynamic effects of beta-blockers in hypertension. A comparison between atenolol, metoprolol, timolol, penbutolol, alprenolol, pindolol and bunitrolol. *Eur. Heart J.* (Suppl. 4): D1–D12, 1983.

[14a] Lund-Johansen, P.: Hemodynamic long-term effects of a new beta-adrenoceptor blocking drug atenolol (ICI 66082) in essential hypertension. *Br. J. Clin. Pharmacol.* 3:445–451, 1976.

[15] Atterhøg, J. H., Duner, H., Pernow, B.: Hemodynamic effects of pindolol in hypertensive patients. *Acta Med. Scand.* (Suppl 606):55, 1977.

[16] Guazzi, M., Polese, A., Fiorentini, C., Olivari, M. T., Magrini, F.: Cardiac performance and beta-adrenergic blockade in arterial hypertension. *Am. J. Med. Sci.* 273:63, 1977.

[17] Smith, I. S., Fernandes, M., Kim, K. E., Swartz, C., Onesti, G.: A three-phase clinical evaluation of prazosin. In: *Prazosin – Clinical Symposium Proceedings*, edited by McGraw-Hill. Post-Graduate Medicine, 1975, p 53.

[18] Lund-Johansen, P.: Haemodynamic changes at rest and during exercise in long-term prazosin therapy of essential hypertension. In: *Prazosin – Evaluation of a New Antihypertensive Agent*, edited by Cotton, D. W. K., Amsterdam, Excerpta Medica, 1974, p 43.

[19] de Leeuw, P. W., Wester, A., Stienstra, R., Falke, H. E., Birkenhäger, W. H.: Hemodynamic and endocrinological studies with prazosin in essential hypertension. In: *Recent Advances in Hypertension and Congestive Heart Failure – Prazosin*, edited by Lund-Johansen, P., Mason, D. T., Amsterdam, Excerpta Medica, 1978, p 11.

[20] Lund-Johansen, P.: Haemodynamic long-term effects of prazosin plus tolamolol in essential hypertension. *Br. J. Clin. Pharmacol.* 4:141, 1977.

[21] Koch, G.: Haemodynamic effects of combined alpha- and beta-adrenoceptor blockade after intravenous labetalol in hypertensive patients at rest and during exercise. *Br. J. Clin. Pharmacol.* (Suppl) 3:725, 1976.

[22] Omvik, P., Lund-Johansen, P.: Acute hemodynamic effects of labetalol in severe hypertension. *J. Cardiovasc. Pharmacol.* 4:915, 1982.

[23] Lund-Johansen, P., Bakke, O. M.: Haemodynamic effects and plasma concentration of labetalol during long-term treatment of essential hypertension. *Br. J. Clin. Pharmacol.* 7:169, 1979.

[24] Fagard, R., Lijnen, P., Amery, A.: Response of the systemic pulmonary circulation to labetalol at rest and during exercise. *System. Pulm. Circ.* (Suppl):13S, 1982.

[25] Doyle, A. E., Anavekar, S. N., Oliver, L. E.: A clinical trial of verapamil in treatment of hypertension. In: *Calcium Antagonism in Cardiovascular Therapy: Experience with verapamil*, edited by Zanchetti, A., Krikler, D. M. Amsterdam, Excerpta Medica, 1981, p 252.

[26] de Leeuw, P. W., Smout, A. J. P. M., Willemse, P. J., Birkenhäger, W. H.: Effects of verapamil in hypertensive patients. In: *Calcium Antagonism in Cardiovascular Therapy: Experience with verapamil*, edited by Zanchetti, A., Krikler, D. M. Amsterdam, Excerpta Medica, 1981, p 233.

[27] Lund-Johansen, P.: Hemodynamic long-term effects of verapamil in essential hypertension at rest and during exercise. *Acta Med. Scand.* (Suppl. 676): 86–102, 1983.

[28] Olivari, M. T., Bartorelli, C., Polese, A., Fiorentini, C., Moruzzi, P., Guazzi, M. D.: Treatment of hypertension with nifedipine, a calcium antagonistic agent. *Circulation* 59:1056, 1979.

[29] Lund-Johansen, P., Omvik, P.: Haemodynamic effects of nifedipine in essential hypertension at rest and during exercise. *J. Hypertension, 1983. In press.*

[30] Lund-Johansen, P.: Hemodynamic consequences of long-term beta-blocker therapy: A 5-year follow-up study of atenolol. *J. Cardiovasc. Pharmacol.* 1:487–495, 1979.

[31] Anderson, O., Hansson, L., Sivertsson, R.: Primary hypertension refractory to triple drug treatment: a study on central and peripheral hemodynamics. *Circulation* 58: 615, 1978.

[32] Tarazi, R. C., Bravo, E. L., Fouad, F. M., Omvik, P., Cody, R. J. jr.: Hemodynamic and volume changes associated with captopril. *Hypertension* 2:576, 1980.

[33] Fagard, R., Bulpitt, C., Lijnen, P., Amery, A.: Response of the systemic and pulmonary circulation to converting-enzyme inhibition (captopril) at rest and during exercise in hypertensive patients. *Circulation* 65:33, 1982.

Discussion

Mann

Do you have any explanations for the finding of Tarazi and Dustan showing a decrease in total peripheral resistence over long-term, and your finding with atenolol? You pointed out an increase in total peripheral resistence after one year.

Lund-Johansen

First I must point out that the figure of Tarazi is based on those patients who responded with a marked fall in the blood pressure. He had a much larger group of patients, but he excluded those who did not have a nice fall in the blood pressure. That is one thing which must be taken into consideration. If you look at his figure you will see that after 19-months application total peripheral resistence during rest-supine is slightly below pre-treatment level. But the difference is not statistically significant. The major point also is that in his studies he has this chronic reduction in the cardiac pump function. I think that is the most important fact we should take into consideration, and which could be responsible for many of the unpleasant side-effects of the beta-blockers mentioned by Holti.

Borchard

Have you any explanation for the difference between the two beta-blockers timolol and atenolol on the stroke-index during exercise?

Lund-Johansen

No, I have no easy way to explain that. When we look at the data, there is no doubt that with timolol we have no increase in the stroke volume after one year in contrast to what we had with atenolol. Why it is so I cannot tell you. May be you could have the theory that timolol would have a greater depressive effect on the cardiac pump function than atenolol. That could be one explanation.

Giessler

You chose, I think, four dosages for your labetalol trial. Why did you do that?

Lund-Johansen

Well, what we did was to start with 100 mg twice a day, aiming at a casual blood pressure 140/90 without side-effects. Then we went up to 400 mg twice daily as the highest dose. In a few patients we tried to increase the dose further, then we had at least temporary side-effects and we went back to 800 mg daily. During the 6-year-period three patients had a thiazide diuretic as I showed, and then their blood pressure was satisfactorily controlled.

Haemodynamic Responses to Combined Alpha-Beta-Receptor Blockade with Labetalol in Relation to the Pathophysiological Mechanisms of Hypertension

G. Koch

Department of Clinical Physiology, Centrallasarettet, Karlskrona, Sweden, and
Department of Physiology, Free University of Berlin, West-Berlin, F.R.G.

Summary

Increased peripheral vascular resistance is the most important pathophysiological mechanism and the cause of elevated blood pressure in virtually all forms of systemic hypertension. Both structural changes in response to increased wall stress and functional alterations in the vascular smooth muscle cell itself appear to contribute to the elevated resistance. Left ventricular filling pressures gradually rise and cardiac output gradually declines reflecting progressive left ventricular function impairment. As important mediators of the vasoconstrictor responses, α-adrenoceptors play an essential of not predominant role in the initiation and/or maintenance of high resistance and pressure.

In contrast to β-receptor blockade alone, combined α-β-receptor blockade lowers blood pressure predominantly by α-receptor mediated reduction of the systemic vascular resistance, both when induced acutely and, in particular, during longterm administration. Cardiac output is maintained at pretreatment levels, as are left ventricular filling pressures.

Since a well-balanced blockade of both α- and β-receptors counteracts the pathophysiological changes causing and/or maintaining hypertension, and tends to restore cardiovascular dynamics towards normal, combined α-β-receptor blockade with labetalol appears to be a logical and rational therapeutic approach to hypertension.

Zusammenfassung

Bei praktisch allen Formen von Hypertonie ist ein erhöhter Strömungswiderstand vorwiegend im Bereich der präkapillären Widerstandsgefäße die wichtigste pathophysiologische Veränderung und Ursache des erhöhten Blutdrucks. Sowohl reaktive strukturelle Veränderungen auf den erhöhten Druck und die gesteigerte Wandspannung als auch funktionelle Veränderungen der glatten Gefäßmuskulatur selbst sind an der Widerstandserhöhung beteiligt. Im Laufe der Hochdruckkrankheit kommt es aufgrund der überhöhten Druckbelastung zu einer Funktionseinschränkung der linken Kammer, die sich u.a. in steigenden Füllungsdrucken und abnehmendem Herzminutenvolumen äußert. Als wichtigsten Vermittlern der Vasokonstriktion scheint den α-Rezeptoren für die Entstehung bzw. der Aufrechterhaltung des hohen Widerstandes und Druckes eine entscheidende Rolle zuzukommen.

Im Gegensatz zu alleiniger β-Rezeptorenblockade erfolgt die Blutdrucksenkung bei kombinierter α-β-Blockade hauptsächlich durch eine Verminderung des peripheren Widerstandes über die α-Rezeptoren. Dies gilt insbesondere bei Langzeitbehandlung. Nur bei akuter intravenöser Gabe von Labetalol ist das Herzminutenvolumen geringfügig erniedrigt, insbesondere im Stehen und bei Belastung. Nach Langzeitbehandlung sind Herzminutenvolumen und Füllungsdrucke der linken Kammer unverändert im Vergleich zu den entsprechenden Werten vor Therapiebeginn.

Wie an den hämodynamischen Effekten deutlich wird, stehen die α- und β-Rezeptoren-blockierenden Wirkungen von Labetalol in einem günstigen ausgewogenen Verhältnis. Eine kombinierte α-β-Blockade wirkt im Gegensatz zu alleiniger β-Blockade den der Hypertonie zugrunde liegenden pathophysiologischen Veränderungen entgegen und hat somit einen normalisierenden Einfluß auf die Hämodynamik. Daher erscheint eine kombinierte α-β-Rezeptorenblockade eine sinnvolle und logische Behandlungsform der arteriellen Hypertonie.

Introduction

It is to-day well established that increased peripheral vascular resistance is the cause of elevated blood pressure in virtually all forms of systemic hypertension. Both structural changes at the arteriolar level in response to increased wall stress and functional alterations in vascular smooth muscle itself [12] appear to contribute to the elevated resistance. These changes not only imply increased vascular resistance under basal vasoconstrictor tone but also result in a hyperreactivity of these vessels, with an exaggerated constrictor response to a given smooth muscle activation. The consequent rise in transmural pressure in turn intensifies the structural changes creating a positive feedback interaction [5]. However, adaptive hypertrophic wall changes in response to the increased pressure load, occur not only in the precapillary resistance vessels but also in the conduit arteries and, in particular, in the left ventricle resulting in subsequent progressive left ventricular function impairment [12].

Rationale for combined α-β-receptor blockade

The changes occurring in the vascular bed and the left ventricle are the most important and decisive pathophysiological mechanisms in the hypertensive process. Therefore the most logical therapeutic approach would evidently consist in reversing the elevated vascular resistance towards normal and in appropriately reducing left ventricular systolic load. Since the responses to vasoconstrictor stimuli and noradrenaline in the precapillary resistance vessels are mainly mediated through α-adrenoceptors, blockade of the α-receptors would appear, at least on theoretical grounds, to be the most logical and efficient way of lowering precapillary resistance and of counteracting the vicious circle ensuing from the interaction of intravascular pressure rise, functional excitatory influences and structural changes.

The combination of an α-receptor antagonist with a β-receptor blocking agent appears rational for two main reasons: First, in contrast to β-receptor blockade alone, blood pressure can be expected to be lowered predominantly by a reduction of systemic vascular resistance, while a possible baroreceptor mediated reflex increase of cardiac output would be attenuated or prevented by the β-blocking component. Second, the activation of the renin-angiotensin system generally seen after vasodilatation and/or α-receptor blockade would be supressed; the additional reduction of blood pressure often achieved by adding a β-receptor antagonist to a vasodilator has actually been postulated to be dependent on a renin-suppressing action of the β-receptor antagonist in this situation [18].

Hemodynamic effects of combined α-β-blockade with labetalol

Labetalol constitutes a unique compound in this context since it combines in the same molecule an α-adrenoceptor blocking action, predominantly at the postsynaptic (α_1) site, with β-adrenoceptor antagonistic properties [3]. The β-receptor antagonist component is non-selective but has membrane stabilizing properties. Based on observations of its effect on fetal lung maturation, labetalol has recently been claimed to possess intrinsic sympathetic activity, mainly with respect to β-2-adrenoceptors [19].

This report summarizes the hemodynamic effects of combined α-β-blockade by labetalol in hypertensive patients as established in previous studies [7, 8]. Emphasis is laid on its effects on left ventricular dynamics as analysed at rest in the supine and upright postures as well as during steady state exercise. Both the effects of acute intravenous administration and of longterm oral treatment are evaluated.

Thirteen patients (12 men and 1 woman, mean age 52 years) participated in the acute investigation. Nine male patients agreed to be studied again after almost two years of treatment with oral labetalol in an average dose of 900 mg daily. Throughout the investigations identical methods were used: blood pressures in the brachial artery and in the pulmonary circulation were recorded via catheters that had been introduced percutaneously; cardiac output was measured according to the Fick principle. On each occasion, the patients were studied at rest in the supine and upright position and during steady state bicycle ergometer exercise in the seated position with two different work loads, corresponding to approximately 60 and 120 Watts.

The intravenous administration of labetalol induced a significant fall in systemic blood pressure under all conditions (Fig. 1, 2). After longterm oral treatment, the antihypertensive effect was slightly attenuated (Fig. 1, 2), in particular in the upright position. However, there was no statistically significant difference between the degree of pressure reduction in the two situations [8]. On acute administration, the blood pressure reduction was due to a decrease of both cardiac output (Fig. 3) and total peripheral resistance (Fig. 4), while it was entirely and solely due to a reduction of vascular resistance after longterm treatment (Fig. 4): cardiac output had reverted to pre-treatment values (Fig. 3). The arterio-mixed venous oxygen difference changed inversely with the alterations of cardiac output (Fig. 4). The rise in cardiac output after longterm treatment was due to an increase in stroke volume which entirely counterbalanced the fall in heart rate (Fig. 3). This effect was particularly marked in the upright position. After long-term oral treatment, the stroke volume in the upright position was actually of the same order as the supine stroke volume prior to treatment (Fig. 3). This explains why postural hypotension, which frequently occurred after the acute administration of labetalol, had practically disappeared during the course of oral treatment.

It is evident that the hemodynamic pattern induced by labetalol is significantly different from that seen after β-receptor blockade alone, in particular with respect to cardiac output and systemic vascular resistance. All hemodynamic evaluations of the effect of different β-receptor antagonists using reliable invasive methods have shown that they reduce

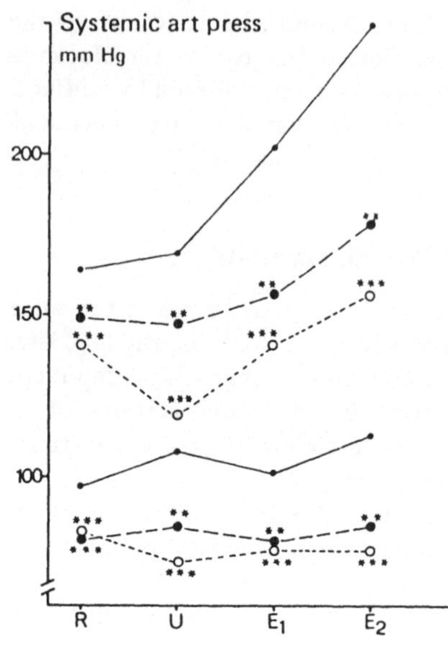

Fig. 1

Systolic and diastolic systemic arterial blood pressures at rest in the supine (R) and upright (U) positions and during steady state exercise with two loads (E_1, E_2) corresponding to approximately 60 and 120W respectively, before (●——————●) and after intravenous administration, 50 mg (○— — — — —○) of labetalol and after longterm treatment (●— — — — —●) with labetalol. **: $p < 0.01$, ***; $p < 0.001$.

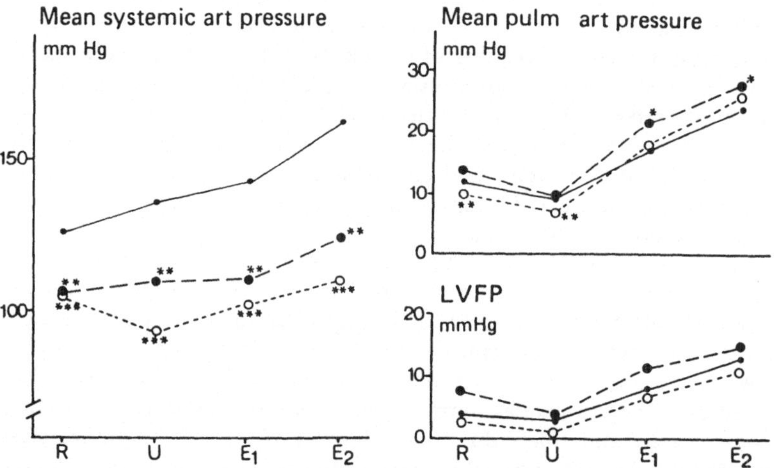

Fig. 2

Mean systemic arterial pressures, mean pulmonary artery pressures and left ventricular filling pressures (LVFP) under resting and exercise conditions before and after intravenous administration of labetalol and after longterm treatment. Abbreviations and symbols as in Fig. 1 *; $p < 0.05$.

cardiac output and raise, or tend to raise, systemic vascular resistance [11, 13]. The particular hemodynamic effects of labetalol can only be explained by a substantial α-receptor blocking effect in addition to the β-receptor antagonistic action.

The tendency of labetalol to induce orthostatic hypotension in the acute experiment can also only be explained by additional α-receptor blockade and suggests that the α-blocking effect is not confined to the precapillary resistance vessels but extends also

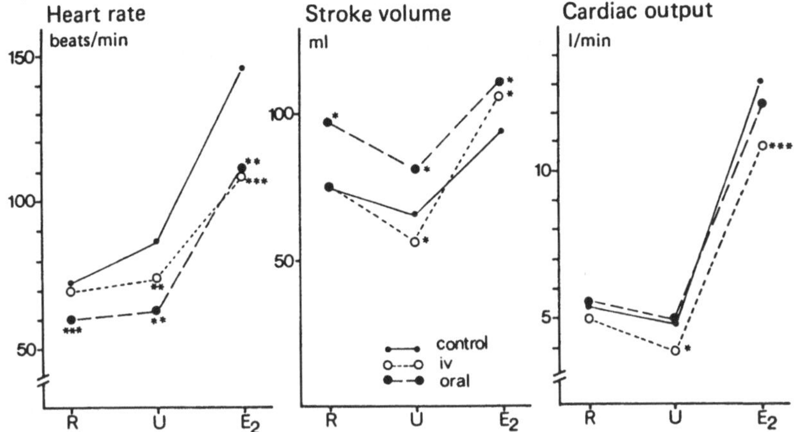

Fig. 3

Heart rate, stroke volume and cardiac output at rest supine (R) and upright (U) and during exercise (E_2, approximately 120 W) before and after intravenous administration of labetalol and after longterm treatment. Symbols as in Fig. 1.

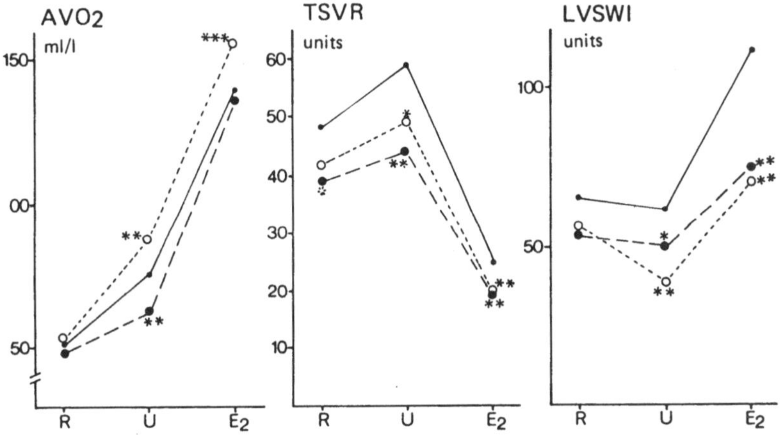

Fig. 4

Arterio-mixed venous oxygen difference (AVO_2), total systemic vascular resistance (TSVR) and left ventricular stroke work index at rest supine (R) and upright (U) and during exercise (E_2, approximately 120 W) before and after intravenous administration of labetalol and after longterm treatment. Symbols as in Fig. 1.

to the postcapillary vessels. In the erect position, this would allow a shift of blood volume from the intrathoracic to the extrathoracic compartment of the capacitance system. Increased venous distensibility after acute intravenous administration of labetalol has actually been described [1]. The attenuation of symptoms and signs of postural hypotension in the course of treatment suggests that the α-adrenoceptor blocking effect of labetalol on the capacitance vessels may be modulated during longterm oral treatment.

It is well established that pharmacological interventions including α- and β-receptor agonists and antagonists, may induce functionally significant changes in the density and/or responsiveness of both α- and β-receptors [4].

In view of the early interference of the hypertensive process with left ventricular function, it is of special interest to analyse more closely the effects of combined α-β-receptor blockade by labetalol on left ventricular dynamics. From Fig. 2 it is evident that intrapulmonary pressures, including left ventricular filling pressures, are not significantly altered whilst stroke volume is substantially raised (Fig. 3). This clearly suggests that the negative intropic effect of the β-receptor blocking component is counterbalanced by the concomitant α-receptor blockade. While this might not be essential in the young and middle-aged hypertensive with largely intact circulatory function, this property should represent an important advantage to the patient exhibiting, or prone to, deterioration of cardiac function. It is well established that β-receptor blockers may have negative effects on left ventricular dynamics in this type of patient, while beneficial effects on preload are generally observed when a suitable vasodilator is added (cf. [10]).

Concerning left ventricular oxygen requirements as evaluated from the pressure-rate product (Fig. 5) and left ventricular stroke work (Fig. 4) combined α-β-receptor blockade appears to have at least the same beneficial effects as β-receptor blockers alone suggesting its usefulness in ischemic heart disease with exercise induced angina. This has recently been established in a comparative study using metoprolol as the β-receptor antagonist [15]. It is important to stress that the increase of stroke work from resting to exercise conditions is not altered by labetalol.

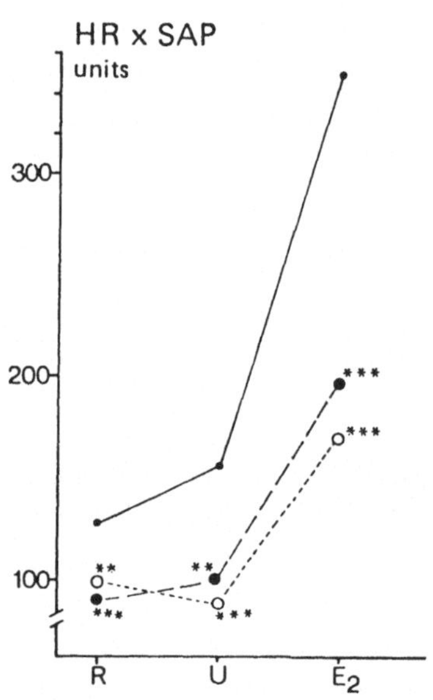

Fig. 5

Product of heart rate and arterial systolic pressure at rest supine (R) and upright (U) and during exercise (E$_2$, approximately 120 W) before and after intravenous administration of labetalol and after longterm treatment. Symbols as in Fig. 1.

Central hemodynamics and regional perfusion

The results presented and those reported subsequently [16] clearly indicate that combined α-β-receptor blockade is a means to reduce high blood pressure in a "physiological" way, namely by restoring the pathophysiological hemodynamic alterations of the hypertensive disorder. Whether this is an important advantage over less "physiological" regimens such as β-receptor blockade alone with respect to life expectancy, quality of life and cardiovascular events has, however, not been clearly established. Most probably, the type of study necessary to provide this kind of information will or can never be undertaken. However, studies of the effects of treatment on organ perfusion give indirect evidence that a regimen which does not significantly lower cardiac output may indeed be advantageous. Thus renal blood flow has been shown to be reduced after the acute administration of labetalol, metoprolol and pindolol [13, 14] approximately in proportion to the changes in cardiac output. Reduction of glomerular filtration rates subsist during long-term treatment with propanolol [6]. No information is available on the renal effects of chronic treatment with labetalol; since cardiac output is restored to pretreatment values it appears, however, reasonable to expect renal blood flow to be restored in a similar way. Indeed, Thompson et al. [20] have shown that glomerular filtration rate in terms of creatinine clearance was unchanged in those patients whose initial clearance was 30 ml/min or more, and only marginally decreased in patients with initial clearances below 30 ml/min.

Liver blood flow has been found to fall more than would be expected from the reduction in systemic arterial pressure during prolonged β-adrenoceptor blockade with propranolol [21, 22] thus indicating an increase in hepatic vascular resistance. Studies of the response of skeletal muscle blood flow to chronic β-receptor blockade [21, 22] show that similar reductions in perfusion also occur in the vascular bed of the working muscle. Furthermore, many clinical observations indicate that the incidence of leg symptoms attributable to reduced muscle flow is higher with β-receptor blockers inducing significant reductions in cardiac output, than with agents having but minor or no effects on cardiac output [2]. This supports the view that regional perfusions follow the changes in central hemodynamics. There is probably one exception to this rule: judging from the results obtained in primates, it appears that cerebral blood flow is relatively less reduced than blood flow in other vascular beds [17].

Conclusions

Combined α-β-adrenoceptor blockade lowers blood pressure predominatly by α-receptor-mediated reduction of the systemic vascular resistance, both when induced acutely and, in particular, during long-term administration. Due to its β-receptor blocking component any increase of cardiac output is inhibited: cardiac output is usually maintained at pretreatment levels, as are left ventricular filling pressures. The hemodynamic action of combined α-β-blockade thus contrasts distinctly with that of β-receptor blockade alone which usually results in a further rise of systemic vascular resistance and of left ventricular filling pressures, and in a reduction of cardiac output.

Since a well-balanced blockade of both α- and β-receptors counteracts the pathophysiological changes responsible for, and maintaining, hypertension, and tends to restore cardiovascular dynamics towards normal, combined α-β-receptor blockade appears a logical and rational therapeutic approach to hypertension.

References

[1] Bahlmann, J., Brod, J., Hubrich, W., Cschovan, M. & Pretschner, P.: Effect of an α- and β-adrenoceptor blocking agent (labetalol) on haemodynamics in hypertension. *Br. J. Clin. Pharmac*, Suppl. 8, 113S—117S (1979).

[2] Bjerle, P., Fransson, L., Koch, G., Lindström, B.: Pindolol and labetalol in hypertension: comparison of their antihypertensive effects with particular respect to conditions in the upright posture and during exercise. *Current Therapeutic Research* 27: 4, 516 526 (1980).

[3] Brogden, R. N., Heel, R. C., Speight, T. M., Avery, G. S.: Labetalol: A review of its pharmacology and therapeutic use in hypertension. *Drugs* 15, 251—273 (1978).

[4] Brunner, H.: Modulation of sympathetic tone at the neuroeffector level. In: Modulation of sympathetic tone in the treatment of cardiovascular diseases (F. Gros, ed.), pp 3—14, Bern, Hans Huber Publishers, 1978.

[5] Folkow, B.: Cardiovascular structural adaption; its role in the initiation and maintenance of primary hypertension. *Clin. Sci. Mol. Med.* 55: 3—12 (1978).

[6] Ibsen, H., Sederberg-Olsen, P.: Changes in glomerular filtration rate during long-term treatment with propranolol in patients with arterial hypertension. *Clin. Sci. Mol. Med.* 44, 129—131 (1973).

[7] Koch, G.: Acute hemodynamic effects of an α- and β-receptor blocking agent (AH 5158) on the systemic and pulmonary circulation at rest and during exercise in hypertensive patients. *Am. Heart J.* 93, 585—591 (1977).

[8] Koch, G.: Hemodynamic adaption at rest and during exercise to long-term antihypertensive treatment with combined α- and β-adrenoreceptor blockade by labetalol. *Br. Heart J.* 41, 192—198 (1979).

[9] Koch, G.: Effects of cardioselective beta-receptor blockade and of combined alpha-beta-receptor blockade on renal dynamics and on adrenergic activity. Abstracts, 6th Scientific Meeting of the International Society of Hypertension, Göteborg, p. 145, (1979).

[10] Koch, G.: Beta-receptor and calcium blockade in ischemic heart disease: effects on systemic and pulmonary hemodynamics and on plasma catecholamines at rest and during exercise. In: 4th International Adalat Symposium. New Therapy of Ischemic Heart Disease (P. Puech, R. Krebs, eds.) pp. 131—141, Amsterdam, Oxford, Princeton, Exercepta Medica 1980.

[11] Koch, G.: Hemodynamic changes after acute and long-term combined α-β-adrenoreceptor blockade with labetalol as compared with β-receptor blockade. *J. Cardiovasc. Pharmacology* 3, Suppl. 1, S30—S39 (1981).

[12] Koch, G.: Rationale for combined α-β-adrenoceptor blockade: haemodynamic considerations. *Acta Med. Scand.* Suppl. 605, 87—92 (1982).

[13] Koch, G., Franz, J.-W., Gubba, A., Lohmann, F. W.: Beta adrenoceptor blockade and physical activity: cardiovascular and metabolic aspects. *Acta Med. Scand. Suppl.* 672, 55—62 (1983).

[14] Koch, G.: Vergleichende Untersuchungen über die Wirkung einer kardioselektiven und nicht-kardioselektiven Beta-Rezeptoren-Blockade auf Glomerulusfiltration, renale Durchblutung und Salz-Wasser-Dynamik. *Therapiewoche* 33: 45, 5985 (1983).

[15] Koch, G.: Beta-adrenoceptor blockers, calcium antagonists and combined alpha-beta-blockade in coronary heart disease: hemodynamic profiles. In: Balanced alpha-beta-blockade of adrenoceptors (N. Rietbrock, B. G. Woodcock, eds.) pp. 170—176. This volume.

[16] Lund-Johansen, P.: Short- and long term (six-year) hemodynamic effects of labetalol in essential hypertension. *Am. J. Medicine* 74, 24—31 (1983).

[17] Nies, A. S., Evans, G. H., Shand, D. G.: Regional hemodynamic effects of beta-adrenergic blockade with propranolol in the unanesthetized primate. *Am. Heart J.*, 85, 97—102 (1973).

[18] Pettinger, A. A. and Mitchell, M. C.: Renin release, saralasin and the vasodilator β-blocker drug interaction in man. *New Eng. J. Med.* 292, 1214—1216 (1975).

[19] Riley, A. J.: Clinical pharmacology of labetalol in pregnancy. *J. Cardiovasc. Pharmacol.* 3, Suppl., S53—S58 (1981).

[20] Thompson, F. D., Joekes, A. M., Hussein, M. M.: Monotherapy with labetalol for hypertensive patients with normal and impaired renal function. *Br. J. Clin. Pharmac.* 8, 129S—133S (1979).

[21] Trap-Jensen, J., Clausen, J. P., Noer, I. I., Mogensen, A., Christensen, M. J., Krogsgaard, A. R., Larsen, O. A.: Regional hemodynamic changes during exercise in essential hypertension before and after prolonged beta-receptor blockade. *Scand. J. Clin. Lab. Invest*, 35, Suppl. 143, 60 (1975).

[22] Trap-Jensen, J., Clausen, J. P., Noer, I., Larsen, O. A., Krogsgaard, A. R., Christensen, N. J.: The effects of beta-adrenoceptor blockers on cardiac output, liver blood flow and skeletal muscle blood flow in hypertensive patients. *Acta Physiol. Scand.* 98, Suppl. 440 30 (1976).

Discussion

Mergin

Mich würde interessieren, ob bei der Langzeittherapie die äußeren Bedingungen wirklich unverändert waren? Es war ein Übergewicht von 10 kg im Schnitt. Bleibt das wirklich 20 Monate unbeeinflußt?

Koch

Uns ging es bei dieser Studie um die haemodynamischen Mechanismen. Ich weiß nicht ob das 10 kg waren. Auf jeden Fall waren die äußeren Bedingungen unverändert, und die Untersuchungen wurden in genau identischer Weise wiederholt.

Heinecker

Sie sagen, daß Sie bis zu Dosen von 2.400 mg gegangen sind. Sind Sie wirklich davon überzeugt, daß diese massiven Dosen notwendig sind? Sie müssen ja eine komplette Blockade der Alpha- und Betarezeptoren dadurch erreicht haben.

Koch

Häufiger haben wir dreimal 2 X 400 mg Tabletten gegeben. Nur 1 oder 2 Patienten haben diese sehr hohen Dosen bekommen. Warum haben die Dosen so sehr geschwankt? Der Grund war, daß wir nur Patienten zu sehen bekommen, die auf konventionelle Therapie nicht angesprochen haben. Denen haben wir Labetalol gegeben. Das war 1974 und 1975. Wir waren erstaunt, wie gering die Nebenwirkungen waren. Wir haben Nebenwirkungen gesehen in Form einer ausgeprägten Orthostase beim Akutversuch. Von 13 Personen sind beim Stehen 4 Leute in die Knie gegangen. Alle blutchemischen Werte waren unverändert.

Greeff

Sie sagen, daß der Hochdruck zum Teil die Ursache der Erhöhung des peripheren Widerstandes ist. Meine Frage ist nun, wenn Sie 20 Monate lang behandeln, können Sie dann absetzen oder können Sie die Dosis reduzieren? Das müßte dann eigentlich möglich sein. Haben Sie das einmal ausprobiert? Wann haben Sie gemessen nach der Medikation?

Koch

Es ist so gewesen, daß wir in den ersten 6 Monaten die Dosen gesteigert haben. Wir wußten ja damals gar nichts. Wir haben gedacht, 50 mg intravenös gibt einen ausgeprägten Effekt. Dann haben wir angefangen, 50 mg per oral zu geben. Das hat keinen Erfolg gezeigt. Dann haben wir die Dosis allmählich weiter erhöht. Nach 6 Monaten Behandlung haben wir in den folgenden 16−20 Monaten die Dosis wieder herabgesetzt.

Haemodynamic Stress Reaction in Essential Hypertension and Effect of a Combined α- and β-Blockade

J. Bahlmann

Krankenhaus Oststadt Hannover, FRG

Summary

The α/β-blockade after labetalol reduces blood pressure by vasodilatation in essential hypertensives at rest. The emotionally induced rise of systolic, diastolic and mean blood pressure, heart rate, cardiac index and forearm blood flow is significantly lessend by the combined α/β-blockade existing after an acute administration of labetalol.
Forearm blood volume and venous distensibility are significantly greater during stress under labetalol. The attenuated circulatory response to an emotional stress should be beneficial in treating hypertensive patients.

In the resting position blood flow to the skeletal muscles averages 20 % of the cardiac output. Both increase steeply during emotional stress and physical exercise. Even the anticipation of stressful conditions will greatly enhance cardiac output and muscular blood flow as an active part in a possible need to respond by fight or flight.
This circulatory adjustment to an emotional stress was investigated in normotensive and hypertensive subjects. Additionally, the modifying effect of a combined α- and β-blockade on the haemodynamic stress reaction was examined.

Methods

The central haemodynamic parameters were studied by direct intravascular measurements and cardiac output by dye-dilution. For regional haemodynamics plethysmography of the forearm was combined with a radionuclide technique as described previously [1, 3]. Blood flow to the hand was excluded during the measurements. The haemodynamic parameters were measured during three 10 min resting periods and the following emotional stress induced by a mathematical exercise whereby the subject subtracts the same two-digit number from different four-digit-numbers continuously for 5 min under strenuous conditions.
Six normotensive subjects and an initial group of 12 essential hypertensive patients without medication were investigated [3].
The effect of an α- and β-blockade by labetalol on the stress reaction was examined in a second group of 7 essential hypertensives [2]. This experimental design was chosen to prevent an adaptation to the stress procedure. As in the first group there was no medication given for at least three weeks before the study. The essential hypertensives of the

second group were also investigated during three resting periods followed by labetalol and in the new steady state after 10—15 min the haemodynamic parameters were measured again over three 10 min periods and thereafter the same stress procedure was undertaken. Labetalol was given i.v. aiming at a 10 % reduction of blood pressure. This was achieved on average with a dose-rate of 1 mg/kg of body weight (range 0.1— 1.6 mg/kg).

Results

Normotensives and Untreated Essential Hypertensives

The circulatory response to this stress procedure was essentially the same in normotensive subjects and untreated essential hypertensives. This was proven statistically [3]. The results will therefore be considered together. The main influence on the arterial side of the circulation (Fig. 1) is a rise in the blood pressure caused by the higher cardiac

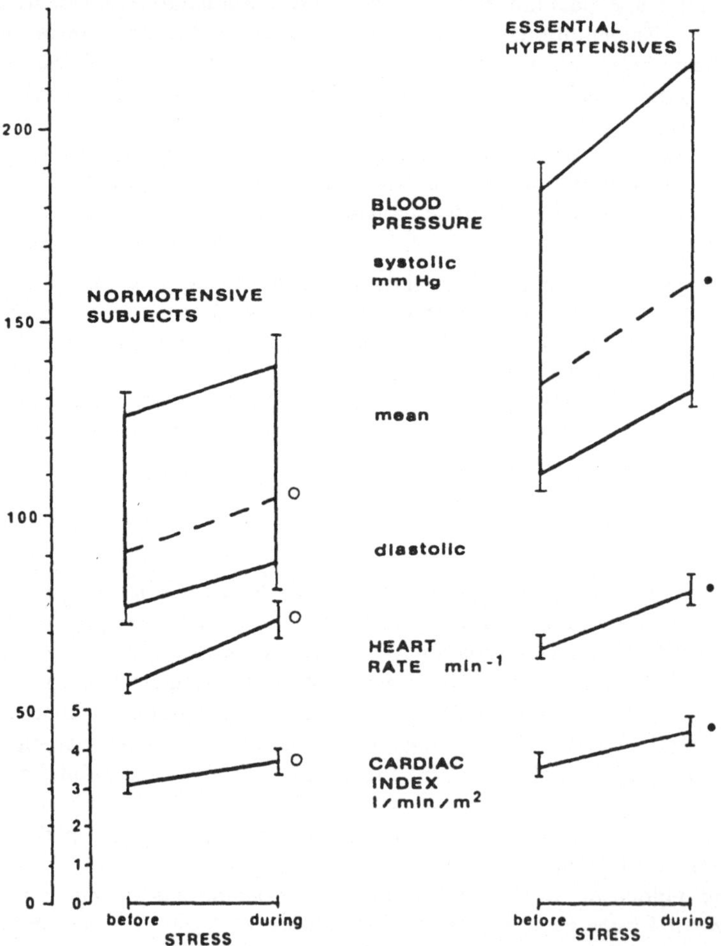

Fig. 1 Effect of emotional stress on central haemodynamics in normotensive subjects (n = 6) and essential hypertensive patients (n = 12); mean ± S.E.M.; open circles p < 0.05, closed circles p < 0.01

output following an increase in heart rate. Stroke volume is not significantly changed. In essential hypertensives — on a percentage basis — the blood pressure rises more than in normotensive subjects but only the higher systolic pressure reaching significance. The total peripheral vascular resistance remains nearly the same, but this is an overall result of balanced changes sometimes in opposite directions in different vascular regions.
The muscle blood flow and other regional haemodynamic parameters were studied in the forearm (Fig. 2, upper panel). Forearm blood flow rose significantly during the in-

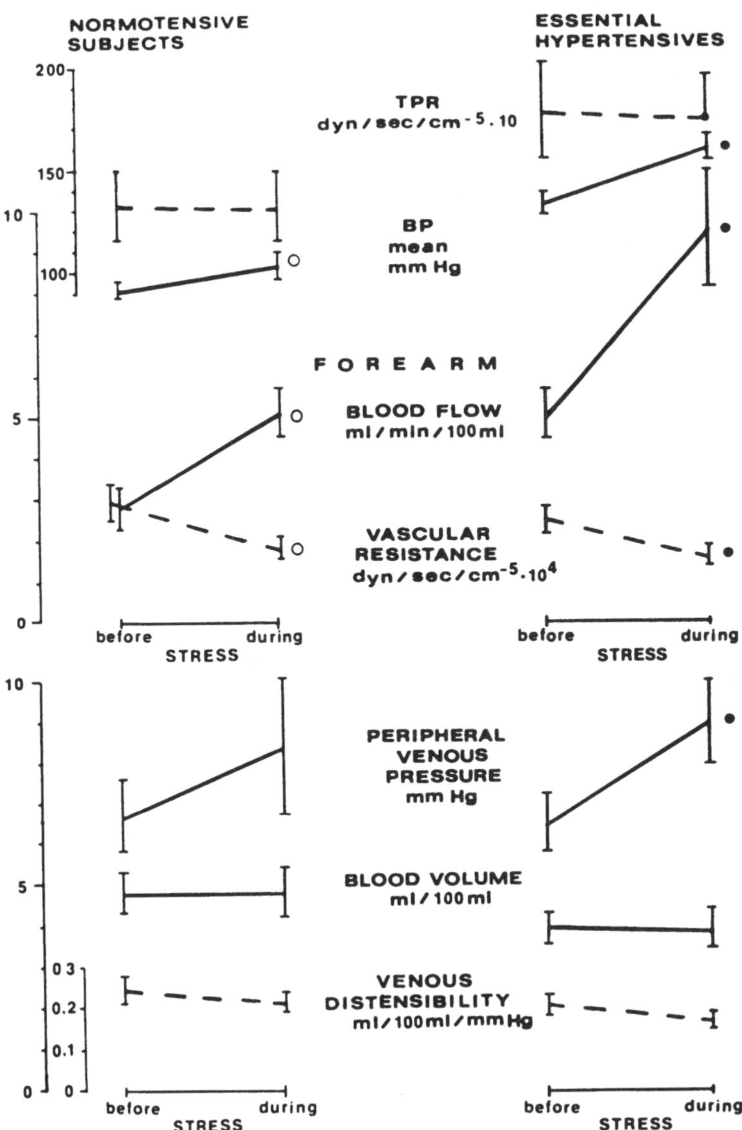

Fig. 2 Effect of emotional stress on toal peripheral vascular resistance (TPR), mean blood pressure (BP) and haemodynamics of the forearm in normotensives (n = 6) and essential hypertensives (n = 12)

rease in arterial perfusion pressure, which is indicated by the mean blood pressure. In addition, a fall of the regional vascular resistance occurred in face of the unchanged total peripheral vascular resistance.

The venous circulation showed an increase in the peripheral venous pressure of the forearm (Fig. 2, lower panel). There, the volume of blood remained unchanged and the venous distensibility had a tendency to decrease. The central venous pressure also increased.

Combined α- and β-Blockade in Essential Hypertensives

The results of the labetalol-treated group of 7 patients with essential hypertension and the previously discussed control group of 12 essential hypertensives are demonstrated in

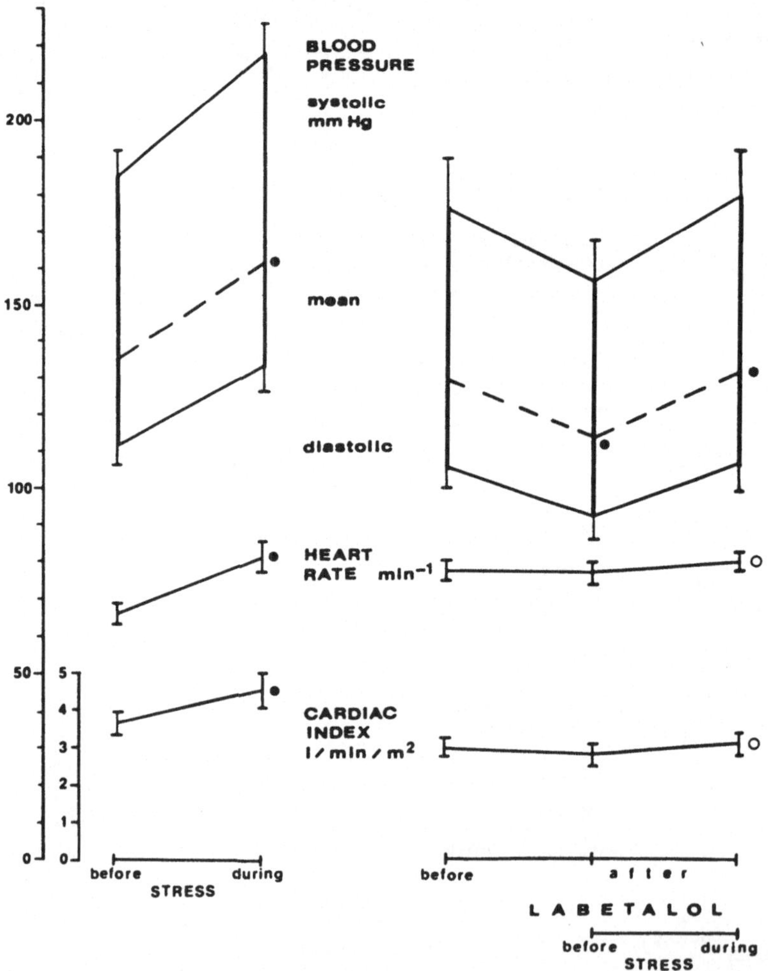

Fig. 3 Central haemodynamic changes during emotional stress in essential hypertension: Untreated group (left side) of 12 hypertensives (same patients as in Fig. 1 and 2). Labetalol-treated group (right side) of 7 hypertensives with acute effects of α/β-blockade at rest (before stress) and during stress

116

Fig. 3. It is obvious that starting levels were slightly different for blood pressure, heart rate, cardiac output and total peripheral vascular resistance. Labetalol reduced the blood pressure significantly by lowering the total peripheral vascular resistance. Cardiac output, stroke volume and heart rate did not change significantly. Under resting conditions labetalol acutely reduces blood pressure by α-blockade. β-blockade prevents the increase in heart rate or even reduces it. This is in agreement with other investigations [7, 9, 15]. It should be noted that stress still produced a significant rise in blood pressure, heart rate and cardiac output but to a lesser extent — especially in the latter two parameters — than in the controls.

In the forearm the same significant fall of the regional vascular resistance was observed after labetalol (Fig. 4). It dropped parallel to the total peripheral vascular resistance. The lowered perfusion pressure (mean blood pressure) and the simultaneous vasodilatation were responsible for the slight increase in forearm blood flow. Blood volume and venous distensibility decreased only slightly and insignificantly. The blood vessels of the forearm reacted differently to stress after labetalol. The vascular resistance was not further lowered by the emotional stimulation. This is the reason for the much smaller increase in the forearm blood flow compared to the steep rise in the untreated group. Peripheral venous pressure increased significantly but also to a lesser extent. The forearm blood volume and venous distensibility reached higher values after labetalol. These were only significant when compared to the untreated hypertensives (first group).

Discussion

The pattern of haemodynamic changes during stress results largely from central sympathetic discharge represented by in α- and β-mediated sympathetic stimulation. This stimulation increases cardiac output parallel to the rise in heart rate. Normally, an increase of the cardiac output increases the total peripheral vascular resistance because the increased blood flow through tissues causes an autoregulatory vasoconstriction. In emotional stress this is offset by a fall in the arteriolar resistance of the skeletal muscle, where the blood flows rapidly from the arteries to the veins. This increased local blood flow enhances venous return and increases right atrial pressure. The increase in peripheral venous pressure impedes venous return partially but the increase in venous tone prevents venous pooling and contributes to the continuing high venous return necessary for the stimulated cardiac output.

There is evidence from experimental work in animals that neuronally released and humorally transported norepinephrine has different effects on adrenergic receptors in the arterial bed. Humoral norepinephrine stimulates both α- and β-receptors; norepinephrine from nerve terminals does not produce significant β-stimulation [6]. On the other hand, epinephrine in physiological concentration stimulates β-receptors. Central cardiovascular response to stress in man correlated significantly with plasma levels of norepinephrine and epinephrine as an index of sympathetic neuronal function [12]. The vasodilatation in skeletal muscle of man during emotional stress is apparently the effect of a β-adrenergic stimulation [8]. The increase and redistribution of cardiac output during stress was also confirmed by aversive conditional stimulation in monkeys [13]. In these as well as in man β-blockade prevented the stress-induced increase in blood flow to skeletal muscles [8, 13]. Resting muscle blood flow fell after non-selective β-blockade [11], probably due to unopposed α-activity. This was not observed after the combined blockade (Fig. 4).

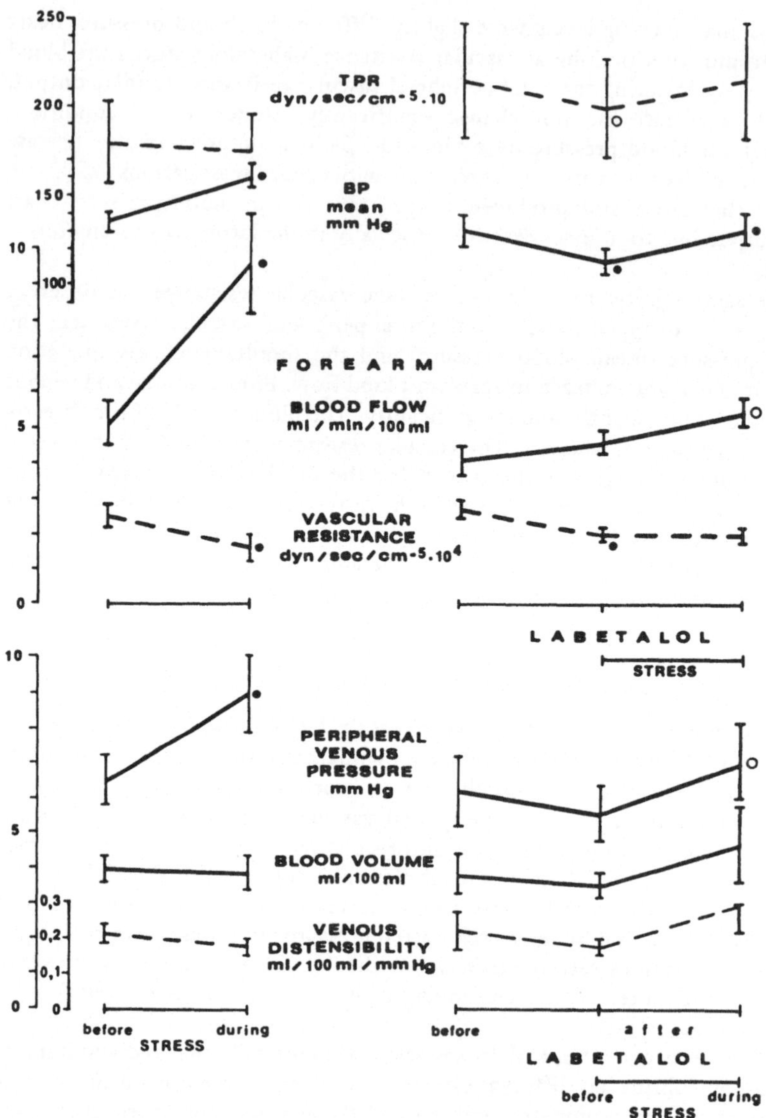

Fig. 4 Total peripheral vascular resistance (TPR), mean blood pressure (BP) and forearm haemodynamics without and with α/β-blockade by labetalol (see legend of Fig. 3)

α- and β-blockade using labetalol modifies the circulatory response to an emotional stress by a significantly diminished increase in heart rate and cardiac index through its β-blocking component. The usual increase in muscular blood flow is almost stopped by the β-blockade. This prevents a further stress-induced fall of the regional vascular resistance. This is in agreement with results obtained after β-blockade which influences the haemodynamic changes provoked by mental arithmetic similarly [8], but in our and other investigations the emotional blood pressure rise was not abolished. In our case the smaller

118

increase in cardiac output was partly compensated for by a higher total peripheral vascular resistance. This enabled the blood pressure to reach the level before labetalol. The cold pressor response was not reduced by β-blockade but labetalol did so by its α-blocking component [10].

The pressure effects of infused norepinephrine and epinephrine were antagonized by labetalol in normotensives accompanied by a reduction in heart rate and cardiac output [14]. This circulatory pattern is not comparable to the effect of labetalol on the haemodynamics during emotional stress emphasizing the different action of neuronally and humorally released catecholamines.

α- and β-adrenoceptors have also been demonstrated in veins; adrenergic nerve stimulation increases wall tension mediated by α-receptors and β-stimulation causes venous relaxation proportional to the initial degree of wall tension [16]. Infused norepinephrine and epinephrine have a constrictor action on forearm veins [5] pointing to the more pronounced α-mediated effects of catecholamines on veins and β-blockade enhances the constrictor response to both [16]. Labetalol antagonized this constrictor response to norepinephrine but also the dilator action of isoprenaline in hand veins [4].

In the present investigation venous parameters of essential hypertensives were not significantly influenced after labetalol under resting conditions but during emotional stress peripheral venous pressure increased to a lesser degree and forearm blood volume was significantly higher. This can be explained by the increased venous distensibility after labetalol. The venous response was altered despite the smaller changes of the regional blood flow which makes passive changes unlikely.

These results suggest that after acute labetalol administration a predominant α-blockade of the venous smooth muscle contributes to the increased venous capacitance during stress. This may well be a first dose effect since during long-term administration postural hypotension becomes less or disappears [15].

References

[1] Bahlmann, J., Brod, J., Cachovan, M.: Stress-induced changes of the venous circulation. *Contr. Nephrol.* **30**, 43–48 (1982).

[2] Bahlmann, J., Brod, J., Hubrich, W., Pretscher, P.: Beeinflussung der hämodynamischen Streßreaktion bei Hypertonikern durch eine kombinierte α- und β-Blockade mit Labetalol. *Dtsch. Med. Wschr.* **105**, 1414–1418 (1980).

[3] Brod, J., Cachovan, M., Bahlmann, J., Bauer, G. E., Celsen, B., Sippel, R., Hundeshagen, H., Feldmann, U., Rienhoff, O.: Haemodynamic changes during acute emotional stress in man with special reference to the capacitance vessels. *Klin. Wschr.* **57**, 555–565 (1979).

[4] Collier, J. G., Dawnay, N. A. H., Nachev, C., Robinson, B. F.: Clinical investigation of an antagonist at α- and β-adrenoceptors — AH 5158 A. *Brit. J. Pharmac.* **44**, 286–293 (1972).

[5] Eckstein, J. W., Hamilton, W. K.: The pressure-volume responses of human forearm veins during epinephrine and norepinephrine infusions. *J. Clin. Invest.* **36**, 1663–1670 (1957).

[6] Glick, G., Epstein, S. E., Wechsler, A. S., Braunwald, E.: Physiological differences between the effects of neuronally released and bloodborne norepinephrine on beta adrenergic receptors in the arterial bed of the dog. *Circ. Res.* **21**, 217–227 (1967).

[7] Koch, G.: Haemodynamic effects of combined α- and β-adrenoceptor blockade after intravenous labetalol in hypertensive patients at rest and during exercise. *Brit. J. Clin. Pharmacol.* **3** Suppl. 3, 725–728 (1976).

[8] Konzett, H., Strieder, N., Ziegler, E.: Die Wirkung eines β-Receptorenblockers auf emotionell bedingte Kreislaufreaktionen, insbesondere auf die Durchblutung des Unterarmes. *Wien. Klin. Wschr.* **80**, 953–959 (1968).

[9] Lund-Johansen, P., Bakke, O. M.: Haemodynamic effects and plasma concentrations of labetalol during long-term treatment of essential hypertension. *Brit. J. Clin. Pharmacol.* **7**, 169–174 (1979).

[10] Maconochie, J. G., Richards, D. A., Woodings, E. P.: Modification of pressor responses induced by "cold". *Brit. J. Clin. Pharmacol.* **4**, 389 P (1977).

[11] McSorley, P. D., Warren, D. J.: Effects of propranolol and metoprolol on the peripheral circulation. *Brit. Med. J.* **2**, 1598–1600 (1978).

[12] Nestel, P. J.: Blood-pressure and catecholamine excretion after mental stress in labile hypertension. *Lancet* **I**, 692–694 (1969).

[13] Randall, D. C., Cottrill, C. M., Todd, E. P., Price, M. A., Wachtel, C. C.: Cardiac output and blood flow distribution during rest and classical aversive conditioning in monkey. *Psychophysiology* **19**, 490–497 (1982).

[14] Richards, D. A., Prichard, B. N. C., Hernándes, R.: Circulatory effects of noradrenaline and adrenaline before and after labetalol. *Brit. J. Clin. Pharmacol.* **7**, 371–378 (1979).

[15] Wallin, J. D., O'Neil, W. M.: Labetalol: Current research and therapeutic status. *Arch. Intern. Med.* **143**, 485–490 (1983).

[16] Webb-Peploe, M. M., Shepherd, J. T.: Beta-receptor mechanisms in the superficial limb veins of the dog. *J. Clin. Invest.* **48**, 1328–1335 (1969).

Discussion

Palm

Sie sagten, daß für die haemodynamischen Veränderungen durch Streß die zirkulierenden Katecholamine der Grund wären. Ich möchte das bezweifeln. Es sind nicht die zirkulierenden Katecholamine, sondern es sind die lokal freigesetzten, denn die zirkulierende Katecholaminkonzentration ist viel zu niedrig.

Bahlmann

Es ist genauso wie Sie sagen, daß das Indiz der gemessenen Noradrenalin- und Adrenalin-Werte natürlich nicht die lokalen Veränderungen an den Nervenendigungen widerspiegelt, sondern hauptsächlich von einem zentralen, neuronal vermittelten sympathischem Stimulus vermittelt wird.

Combined Alpha/Beta Blockade with Acebutolol and Prazosin

I.-W. Franz

Departments of Cardiology and Sports Medicine, Klinikum Charlottenburg, Free University of Berlin, 1000 Berlin 33, FRG

Summary

1. The cardiovascular risk of hypertension depends not only on blood pressure under resting conditions, but particularly on blood pressure increases induced by daily physical and emotional activity.
2. Therefore, the ability of the β_1-receptor antagonist acebutolol (400 mg/day) and of the α_1-receptor antagonist prazosin (4 mg/day) to reduce exercise-induced increases in blood pressure and pressure-rate product during and after standardized ergometric work (50—100 watts) was compared in an intrapatient study including 24 outpatients with arterial hypertension (WHO stage 1—2) aged 29—55 years.
3. Both drugs resulted in a significant reduction of systolic ($p < 0.01$) and diastolic ($p < 0.001$) blood pressure at rest.
4. However, systolic blood pressure ($p < 0.001$) and pressure-rate product ($p < 0.001$) during exercise were only significant reduced by acebutolol. The strongest blood pressure lowering effect under all conditions could be proved for the combination of prazosin and acebutolol.
5. From these findings it is concluded that: (1) β-adrenoreceptor-blocking agents are the drugs of first choice in the baseline therapy of mild to moderate arterial hypertension, and (2) prazosin potentiates the antihypertensive effect of β-blocking agents.
6. This therapeutic regimen is recommended especially for hypertensives with ischemic heart disease, because prazosin fails to reduce pressure-rate product as a measure of myocardial O_2-consumption.

Zusammenfassung

1. Das kardiovaskuläre Risiko der Hypertonie wird neben der Ruheblutdruckerhöhung auch wesentlich durch überhöhte Blutdruckanstiege während körperlicher und emotionaler Belastungen bestimmt.
2. Deshalb wurde bei 24 ambulanten Patienten mit einer essentiellen Hypertonie des Stadium I—II (20 ♂, 4 ♀) und einem Alter von 29—55 Jahren ($\bar{x}$ 43,3 ± 7 Jahre) die Wirkung einer jeweils sechswöchigen Therapie mit 4 mg des α_1-Rezeptorenblockers Prazosin und 400 mg des β_1-Rezeptorenblockers Acebutolol sowie deren Kombination (n = 8) auf den Blutdruck und das Doppelprodukt vor, während und nach Ergometrie (50—100 Watt) vergleichend untersucht.

3. Unter Ruhebedingungen wurde der systolische (p < 0,01) und der diastolische (p < 0,001) Blutdruck durch Prazosin und Acebutolol signifikant und annähernd gleich stark gesenkt.
4. Während der Ergometrie ergab sich jedoch unter Prazosin kein signifikanter Einfluß auf den systolischen Blutdruck und das Doppelprodukt als Maß für den myokardialen O_2-Verbrauch. Demgegenüber bewirkte Acebutolol eine signifikante Senkung des systolischen Blutdruckes (p < 0,001) und des Doppelproduktes (p < 0,001). Der diastolische Belastungsblutdruck wurde allerdings durch beide Substanzen gleich stark und signifikant (p < 0,001) gesenkt.
5. Der stärkste antihypertensive Effekt konnte zu allen Untersuchungszeitpunkten durch die Kombination aus Acebutolol und Prazosin erzielt werden, wobei sich die Wirkung der Einzelsubstanzen nicht nur addierte, sondern potenzierte.
6. Zur Basisbehandlung der leichten bis mittleren Hypertonie müssen deshalb β-Rezeptorenblocker als Medikamente der ersten Wahl empfohlen werden, wobei allerdings die blutdrucksenkende Wirkung durch die zusätzliche Prazosingabe erheblich verstärkt werden kann. Diese Behandlungsempfehlung gilt ganz besonders für Hypertoniker mit gleichzeitiger koronarer Herzkrankheit, da durch Prazosin das Doppelprodukt bei Belastung nicht gesenkt wird.

Introduction

The use of β-receptor blockers is widespread in the treatment of arterial hypertension, whereas prazosin, an α_1-receptor blocking agent, is a relatively new antihypertensive drug [4]. The comparison of antihypertensive studies [1, 4, 7, 10, 11, 14, 15, 17, 21, 22, 28, 33] with different kinds of β-receptor blockers and prazosin show a similar blood pressure lowering effect under resting conditions in patients with mild to moderate arterial hypertension. Assessment of antihypertensive therapy, based only on values at rest, is, however, of limited usefulness, because measurements of blood pressure at rest obviously involve uncertainty as to the presence of a pathologically elevated blood pressure increase in response to daily physical and mental stress [3, 8, 13, 18, 19, 20, 27, 35]. The cardiovascular risk of hypertension, however, depends not only on blood pressure under resting conditions but particularly on blood pressure increases induced by daily physical and emotional activity [8, 18, 20, 31, 32, 35]. Therefore, antihypertensive drugs must be expected not only to regulate blood pressure at rest but also to adequately reduce these pressure changes [9, 10, 11, 14, 21, 22, 24, 26, 28, 29, 33], which are sufficiently controlled under β-receptor blockade [6, 7, 10]. However, there is little information as to the capacity of prazosin to decrease blood pressure during ergometric exercise [1, 21]. Therefore, the capacity of the α_1-receptor-blocking agent prazosin to reduce blood pressure at rest and during exercise was investigated in comparison with the beta receptor blocker acebutolol.

As prazosin has been classified as vasodilator, a logical combination therefore might be with a β-receptor blocking agent. For this reason the purpose of the study was also to investigate the hypotensive effects of an α_1-receptor blockade in combination with a β_1-receptor blockade.

Methods

Patients

Twenty-four outpatients, 20 men and 4 women aged 29 to 55 years (mean 43.3 ± 6.5), participated in the study after having given written consent. Clinical evaluation indicated that all had stage 1 to 2 essential hypertension using criteria given by the World Health Organization in 1959. None had ischemic heart disease or other diseases and none had previously received antihypertensive treatment. Blood pressures, when measured according to the Riva-Rocci-Korotkoff cuff method, were between 167 ± 22 and 108 ± 10 mmHg at rest supine and 215 ± 23 and 126 ± 12 mmHg during ergometric exercise at 100 watts (612 kpm min^{-1}). The study only included patients who had hypertensive blood pressure values, both under resting conditions and during exercise [9].

Treatment protocol

After the initial pretreatment study, the patients were randomly allotted to two groups. Treatment was then started with a single morning dose of 400 mg of oral acebutolol in one group (I) and 4 mg of prazosin (2 mg in the morning, 2 mg at noon) in the other group (II) with a crossover change after 6 weeks. Eight patients with insufficient blood pressure responses continued the study for a further 6 week treatment period with a daily dose of 400 mg acebutolol and 4 mg prazosin.

Exercise test

At the control examination and after each 6-week treatment period the patients were studied under identical conditions using an identical technique according to the Proposal for the International Standardization of Ergometry [1]. In particular the patients exercised at the same time, on each occasion that is between 3 and 5 p.m. approximately eight or two hours after the last administration of acebutolol and prazosin, respectively. Exercise was performed in a reclined sitting position on a bicyle ergometer (ERG 301^R, Robert Bosch, Berlin) with a pedal frequency of 50 cycles/min, starting at 50 watts with a 10 watt increment every minute to a maximum of 100 watts.

Blood pressure and heart rate measurements

Casual blood pressure readings were taken after 5 minutes of rest in the supine position and in the standing position 1 minute after rising, values being the mean of two measurements respectively. During exercise and 5 minutes thereafter readings were taken every minute according to the Riva-Rocci-Korotkoff cuff method (diastolic pressure corresponding to Korotkoff phase 4). All readings were made by the same investigator using the same calibrated mercury manometer. The heart rate was obtained from the electrocardiogram, which was recorded in the last 10 seconds of every minute.

Statistics

Data in the text are expressed as mean ± standard deviation. Statistical significance was assessed with Student's t-test for paired samples.

Results

Blood pressure

Acebutolol and prazosin resulted in a significant ($p < 0.01$–$p < 0.001$) and almost identical reduction in blood pressure at rest. Under resting supine conditions pretreatment values of $167 \pm 22/108 \pm 10$ mmHg, were significantly higher compared with the blood

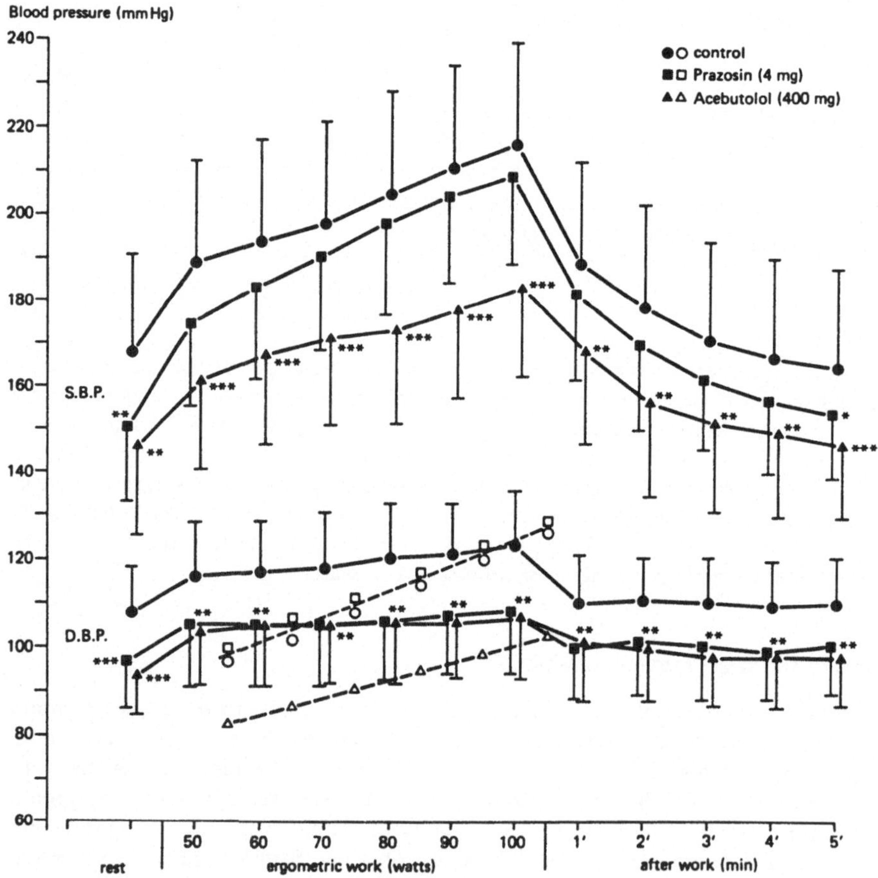

Fig. 1

Systolic (S.B.P.) and diastolic (D.B.P.) blood pressures (mean ± SD) at rest and during and after exercise in 24 hypertensives before and after 6-week treatment periods with 400 mg acebutolol and 4 mg prazosin.

pressure response under the action of acebutolol (146 ± 23/94 ± 9 mmHg) and prazosin (150 ± 77/96 ± 11 mmHg). However, prazosin failed to reduce systolic blood pressure during exercise significantly (Fig. 1), whereas with acebutolol a significant decrease was observed compared with the pretreatment values (p < 0.001). The diastolic blood pressure during and after exercise was significantly (p < 0.001) reduced by both drugs.

Heart rate

Heart rate was practically unaltered after therapy with prazosin both at rest and with exercise. Acebutolol resulted in significantly (p < 0.001) decreased heart rates at rest (16.5 percent reduction) and during (19.1 percent reduction) and after (19.0 percent reduction) ergometric work (p < 0.001).

Pressure-rate product

Pressure-rate product as a measure of myocardial O_2-consumption [30] prior to therapy revealed at 100 watts a 36.5 percent increase (26804 mmHg $\cdot$ min^{-1}, compared with age-matched normotensives; 19640 mmHg $\cdot$ min^{-1}; 12). This marked increase in myocardial O_2-consumption was not significantly reduced by prazosin either at rest or during (at 100 watts 25856 mmHg $\cdot$ min^{-1}) and after ergometer exercising. In contrast treatmemt with the beta-receptor blocker produced a highly significant (p < 0.001) reduction in double product not only at rest (26.6 percent) but particularly during ergometer exercising (at 100 watts 18544 mmHg $\cdot$ min^{-1}; 44.5 percent reduction) into the normal range and produced a rapid decrease after ergometric work in the first recovery minute (27.7 percent).

Additive effect of β-receptor blocker and α_1-adrenergic blocking agent

Acebutolol and prazosin alone dit not achieve a sufficient reduction in blood pressure in thirty-three percent (n = 8) at rest and during and after exercise, Fi.g 2, however, shows that prazosin significantly enhanced the antihypertensive effect of acebutolol before, during and after exercise.
Fig. 3 clearly demonstrates that there was not only an additive effect of acebutolol and prazosin, but that the antihypertensive efficiency of the β-receptor blocker was potentiated by the additional use of an α_1-adrenergic blocking agent.

Discussion

Not all drugs with an antihypertensive effect at rest do, in fact, reduce exercise-induced blood pressure increases. It has been shown that α-methyldopa [33], clonidine [21], reserpine [26] and also diuretics [10, 14] fail to reduce blood pressure response to exercise and reveal a significantly and distinctly reduced effect compared with β-receptor blockers. However, hypertensive patients are endangered not only by higher blood pressures at rest but especially by larger increases in blood pressure during exercise and a delayed return to baseline levels after work [3, 8, 13, 18, 19, 20, 27, 29, 35]. The vascular risk of hypertension is, therefore, satisfactorily indicated by the blood pressure values measured during

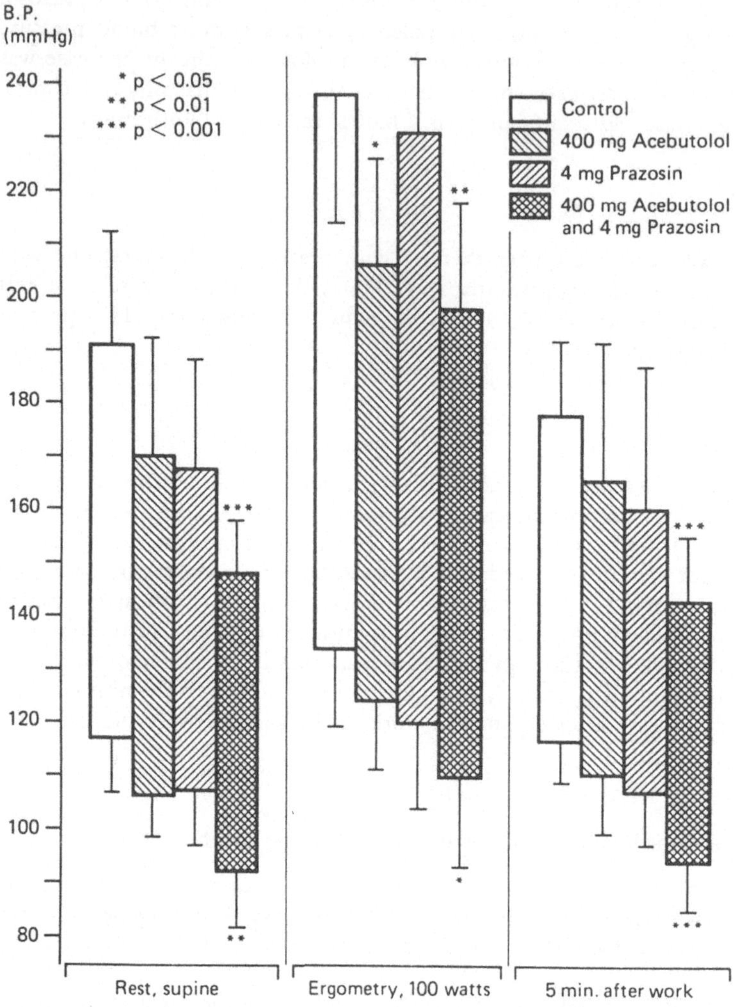

Fig. 2
Systolic and diastolic blood pressures (B.P.; mean ± SD) at rest and during and after exercise in eight
hypertensives before (control) and after 6-week treatment periods with 400 mg acebutolol, 4 mg
prazosin and their combination.

and after ergometric work, because (1.) the risk of arterial hypertension and its vascular
complications [8, 18, 20, 29, 31, 32] is mainly dependant on the intensity, frequency and
duration of the increases in blood pressures produced by daily physical and emotional
stress, and (2.) there is a close correlation between elevated blood pressure increases during
daily activities and during ergometric exercise [8, 25, 27]. In the assessment of antihypertensive drugs the response to exercise should, therefore, also be analysed.

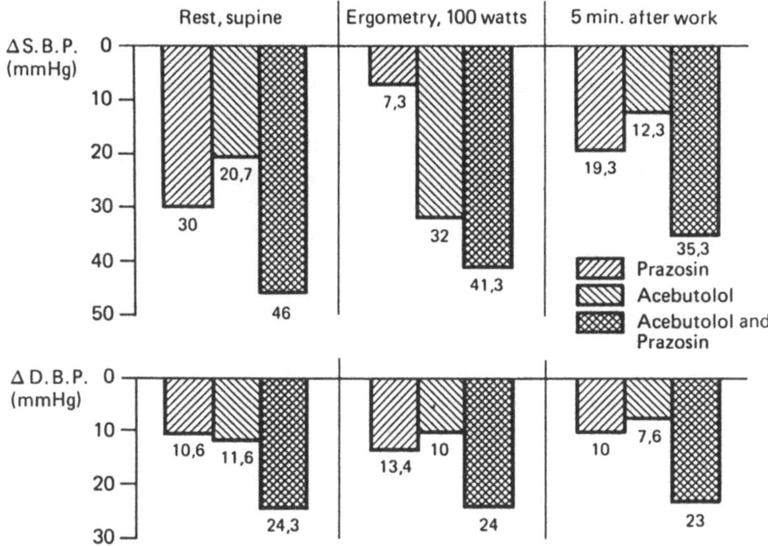

Fig. 3

The decrease in systolic (S.B.P.) and diastolic (D.B.P.) blood pressures compared with control values under the actions of prazosin, acebutolol and their combination in eight hypertensives, at rest and during and after work.

The adequate and significant reduction of systolic blood pressure to values within the limits of normotension at 100 watts [13] under β-receptor blockade with acebutolol is a finding consistant with previous data [10, 11, 14, 15, 22, 26, 28]. It is particularly noteworthy that the blood pressure decreasing effects of the β-receptor blocker acebutolol and the α_1-adrenergic blocking agent prazosin were almost identical at rest, however, prazosin failed to reduce systolic blood pressure during ergometric work. The findings clearly demonstrate that a decrease in blood pressure by an antihypertensive therapy at rest does not mean that the blood pressure is also sufficiently decreased during exercise [9].

Taking into consideration that pathologically elevated systolic blood pressure increases lead to a marked incrementation in myocardial oxygen consumption [30] with an enhanced risk of an acute coronary event [34], β-receptor blockers might be of advantage, especially in hypertensives with ischemic heart disease. Myocardial oxygen consumption depends not only on the systolic blood pressure but also on the heart rate, which was significantly reduced under acebutolol but practically unaltered after therapy with prazosin.

For the management of hypertension it should be noted in particular that prazosin and acebutolol potentiated each other with regard to antihypertensive effects, especially during and after exercise, and revealed a stronger effect compared with the combination of β-receptor blockers and diuretics [10, 14].

Implications

β-receptor blockers should be the drug of first choice in the baseline therapy of mild hypertension, because they are also effective on blood pressure increases during daily physical and emotional stress [6, 7, 24]. They are recommended especially for hypertensives with coronary heart disease who are physically active on the job or are engaged in a rehabilitative, cardiac training program. The additional use of an α_1-adrenergic blocking agent, however, potentiates the antihypertensive effect of β-receptor blockers and this combination can be recommended for the treatment of moderate and severe hypertension [1, 5, 16, 23].

References

[1]   Äärynen, M., Mäkelä, M., Hämeenaho, P., Mattila, M. J.: Prazosin enhances the antihypertensive effects of beta-blockers during isometric and dynamic exercise. *Ann. Clin. Research.* **13**, 71—75 (1981).

[2]   Agreement of the Research Committee of the ICSPE for the International Standardization. In: Mellerowicz, H., Hansen, G. ed. *IIth International Seminar of Ergometry.* Berlin: Ergon, 1968: 314.

[3]   Bachmann, K., Zerzawy, R., Riess, P. J., Zölch, K. A.: Blutdrucktelemetrie — kontinuierliche, direkte Blutdruckmessung im Alltag und beim Sport. *Dtsch. Med. Wschr.* **95**, 741—743 (1970).

[4]   Colucci, W. S.: Alpha-adrenergic receptor blockade with prazosin. *Ann. Intern. Med.* **97**, 67—76 (1982).

[5]   De Divitis, O., Petitto, M., Di Somma, S., Capunano, V., Fazio, S.: Prazosin and minoxidil combined with atenolol and chlorthalidone: Double-blind comparison in the treatment of severe arterial hypertension. *Curr. Therap. Research.* **29**, 235—249 (1981).

[6]   Eliasson, K., Hjemdahl, P., Hylander, B., Kahan, T., Lins, L.-E.: *Circulatory and sympatho-adrenal responses to stress after long-term beta blockade.* Abstract Ninth Scientific Meeting of the International Society of Hypertension, Mexico City, 1982.

[7]   Floras, J. S., Fox, P., Hassan, M. O., Jones, J. K., Sleight, P., Turner, K. L.: Assessment of the antihypertensive effect of atenolol with 24 h ambulatory monitoring of blood pressure. *Clin. Sci.* **57**, 387 (1979).

[8]   Floras, J. S., Hassan, M. O., Sever, P. S., Jones, J. V., Osikowska, B., Sleight, P.: Cuff and ambulatory blood pressure in subjects with essential hypertension. *Lancet* **II**, 107—109 (1981).

[9]   Franz, I.-W., Lohmann, F. W.: Ergometry in the assessment of antihypertensive treatment. *Dtsch. Med. Wschr.* **38**, 1487—1491 (1978).

[10]   Franz, I.-W.: Differential antihypertensive effect of acebutolol and the fixed combination hydrochlorothiazide/amiloridhydrochloride on elevated exercise blood pressures in hypertensive patients. *Am. J. Cardiol.* **46**, 301—305 (1980).

[11]   Franz, I.-W., Lohmann, F. W., Koch, G.: Excessive plasma dopamine increase at rest and during exercise after long-term beta-adrenoreceptor blockade in hypertensive patients. *Br. Heart J.* **44**, 25—29 (1980).

[12]   Franz, I.-W., Mellerowicz, H.: Ergometric investigations of the tension-time-index and of the PWC_{170} in patients with borderline and stable hypertension in comparison with normals. *Z. Kardiol.* **69**, 587—591 (1980).

[13]   Franz, I.-W.: Assessment of blood pressure response during ergometric work in normotensive and hypertensive patients. *Acta med. Scand.* Suppl. 670, 35—47 (1982).

[14]   Franz, I.-W.: The effect of beta-receptor antagonists and diuretics and their combination on blood pressure and pressure-rate product during ergometric work in hypertensive patients. *Z. Kardiol.* **71**, 129—137 (1982).

[15]   Franz, I.-W., Lohmann, F. W., Koch, G.: Effects of chronic antihypertensive treatment with acebutolol and pindolol on blood pressures, plasma catecholamines and oxygen uptake at rest and during submaximal and maximal exercise. *J. Cardiovasc. Pharmacol.* **4**, 180—186 (1982).

[16]   Franz, I.-W.: The effects of prazosin and acebutolol and their combination on blood pressure and pressure-rate product during ergometric work in hypertensive patients. *Z. Kardiol.* **72**, 746—754 (1983).

[17] Graham, R. M., Mulvihill-Wilson, J.: Clinical pharmacology of prazosin used alone or in combination in the therapy of hypertension. *J. Cardiovasc. Pharmacol.* **2**, Suppl. 3, 387—398 (1980).

[18] Krönig, B.: *Blutdruckvariabilität bei Hochdruckkranken.* Heidelberg: Hüthig, 1976.

[19] Littler, W. A., Honour, A. J., Pugsley, J., Sleight, P.: Continuous recording of direct arterial pressure in untreated patients: its role in the diagnosis and management of high blood pressure. *Circulation.* **51**, 1101—1106 (1975).

[20] Littler, W. A., Watson, R. D. S.: Circulation variation in blood pressure. *Lancet* **I**, 995—996 (1978).

[21] Lund-Johansen, P.: Central hemodynamics in essential hypertension at rest and during exercise. Spontaneous changes and effects of diuretics, beta-receptor blockers and vasodilators. In: Franz, I.-W. (ed.): *Exercise blood pressure in hypertensive patients.* Berlin, Heidelberg, New York: Springer, 1981: 107.

[22] Lund-Johansen, P.: Hemodynamic consequences of long-term beta-blocker therapy: a 5 year follow-up study of atenolol. *J. Cardiovasc. Pharmacol.* **1**, 487—495 (1979).

[23] Marshall, A. J., Barritt, D. W., Pocok, J., Heaton, S. T.: Evaluation of beta blockade, bendrofluazide, and prazosin in severe hypertension. *Lancet* **I**, 271—275 (1977).

[24] Mc Allister, R. G.: Effects of adrenergic receptor blockade on the responses to ergometric handgrip: Studies in normal and hypertensive subjects. *J. cardiovasc. Pharmacol.* **1**, 253—256 (1979).

[25] Neuss, H., Schulte, W., Friedrich, G., Rüddel, H., Schirmer, G., v. Eiff, A. W.: Relationship between blood pressure reactions on an ergometric and an emotional stress test. *Klin. Wschr.* **59**, 47 (1981).

[26] Patyna, W. D.: The effects of a reserpine-diuretic combination and of β-receptor blockers on blood pressure at rest and during exercise. In: Franz, I.-W. (ed.): *Exercise blood pressure in hypertensive patients.* Berlin, Heidelberg, New York: Springer, 1981: 139.

[27] Pickering, T. G., Harsfield, G. A., Kleinert, H. D., Blank, S., Laragh, J. H.: Blood pressure during normal daily activities, sleep and exercise. *JAMA* **247**, 992—996 (1982).

[28] Reybrouck, T., Amery, A., Billiet, L.: Hemodynamic response to graded exercise after chronic beta-adrenergic blockade. *J. Appl. Physiol.* **42**, 133—138 (1977).

[29] Rowlands, D. B., Ireland, M. A., Stallard, T. J., Glover, D. R., McLeay, R. A. B., Watson, R. D. S., Littler, W. A.: Assessment of left-ventricular mass and its response to antihypertensive treatment. *Lancet* **II**, 467—470 (1982).

[30] Sarnoff, S., Case, J. R. B., Stainky, W. N., Macruz, R.: Hemodynamic determinants of oxygen consumption of the heart with special reference to the tension-time-index. *Am. J. Physiol.* **192**, 148—152 (1958).

[31] Sokolow, M., Wardegar, P., Kain, H. K., Huiman, A. T.: Relationship between level of blood pressure measured casually and by portable recorders and severity of complications in essential hypertension. *Circulation* **34**, 279 (1966).

[32] Sokolow, M., Perloff, D., Cowan, R.: *A 10-year prospective study of the incidence of cardiovascular events in hypertensive patients utilizing ambulatory blood pressure measurements.* Abstract Ninth Scientific Meeting of the International Society of Hypertension, Mexico City: 1982.

[33] Stoker, J. B. N., Greeharan, R. J., Linden, J., Barbour, M. P., Lorimer, A. R., Hillis, W. S., Lawrie, T. D. V.: Effects of exercise in hypertension controlled with metoprolol or methyldopa. *Clin. Sci.* **57**, 391—392 (1979).

[34] Strauer, B. E.: *Das Hochdruckherz.* Springer, Berlin, Heidelberg, New York: 1979.

[35] Taylor, S. H.: The circulation in hypertension. In: Burley, D. M., Birdwood, G. F. B., Fryer, J. H., Taylor, S. H.: *Hypertension — its nature and treatment.* London: Metropolis Press, 1975: 29.

Discussion

Rietbrock, N.
Wie sind Sie zu diesem Dosenverhältnis gekommen? Gibt es eventuell ein günstigeres Dosenverhältnis? Dieses war ein Verhältnis 1 : 100.

Franz
Die Frage ist berechtigt. Wir haben uns entschlossen, eine mittlere Dosis eines Betablockers mit einer mittleren Dosis eines Vasodilators zu vergleichen. Es ist uns gelungen, daß die gewählten Dosen unter Ruhebedingungen eine gleichstarke Senkung des Blutdruckes erzielten. Ich gebe Ihnen vollkommen recht, hätte man vielleicht die Dosis erhöht, wobei man dann natürlich auch bei der leichteren Hochdruckform in Bereiche kommt, wo doch der Blutdruckabfall unter Prazosin doch erheblich zunimmt, dann hätte es vielleicht zusätzlich einen etwas stärkeren Effekt ausgegeben. Aber ich glaube, daß die prinzipielle Aussage sich nicht geändert hätte. Dafür sprechen eigentlich auch die Untersuchungen, die wir heute gesehen haben von Lund-Johansen. Er hat noch höhere Dosen angewendet.

Schulz
Sie sagten, Sie hätten eine Potenzierung und keine Addition gefunden. Es ging eigentlich bis auf 1 mm genau auf, daß es eine Addition war. Warum nehmen Sie keinen Kalciumantagonisten anstatt des Betablockers?

Franz
Nach diesem Konzept haben wir viele Antihypertensiva untersucht, unter gleichen Bedingungen. Ich kann sagen, daß die additive Wirkung zwischen Betablocker und Diuretikum keinesfalls so ausgeprägt ist, sondern wesentlich geringer ist. Ich darf vielleicht die zweite Frage gleich in diesem Zusammenhang beantworten. Wenn man Betablocker und Kalciumantagonisten bei Hochdruckpatienten untersucht, dann ist es in der Tat so, daß man praktisch zu identischen Ergebnissen kommt. Das heißt, daß auch hier die Wirkung sehr ausgeprägt ist, und auch die Kombination eines Betarezeptorenblockers mit einem Kalciumantagonist geht über die Wirkung eines Betablockers mit einem Diuretikum hinaus.

Vöhringer
Haben Sie Nebenwirkungen während Ihrer beinahe 5-monatigen Untersuchungszeit gefunden? Gab es bei den Prazosin-Patienten insbesondere compliance-Probleme?

Franz
Wir haben keine schwerwiegenden Nebenwirkungen gefunden. Wir haben bei 2 Patienten die Therapie beenden müssen. Unter Prazosin, wegen einer sehr stark verstopften Nase, die eine Weiterführung der Therapie, auch in der Kombination, nicht zuließ, und unter Betablocker bei einem Patienten, weil möglicherweise eine spastische Bronchitis induziert wurde. Was wir unter Prazosin an Nebenwirkungen besonders gehört haben, war ein Phänomen, das man schwer beschreiben kann. Der Patient sagt, sein Herz schlägt schneller sowie morgendlicher kurzfristiger Schwindel bei Lagewechsel.

Vöhringer
Und die Compliance?

Franz
Wir machen deswegen diese Untersuchungen grundsätzlich nur samstags, an einem arbeitsfreien Tag. Wir bestellen sämtliche unserer Patienten in kleinen Gruppen und unterrichten sie über das, was wir machen. Ich glaube, daß wir durch dieses Konzept eine sehr hohe Zuverlässigkeit haben.

Clinical Pharmacology of Labetalol in Elderly Hypertensives

K. O'Malley, K. McGarry, W. G. O'Callaghan, E. O'Brien, J. G. Kelly

Department of Clinical Pharmacology, Royal College of Surgeons in Ireland, St. Stephens Green, Dublin 2;
and
The Blood Pressure Clinic, The Charitable Infirmary, Jervis Street, Dublin 1, Ireland

Introduction

Most estimates suggest that approximately one half of all drugs prescribed are intended for those over 60 years of age. Furthermore, this group bears the brunt of adverse reactions, perhaps due in part to the disproportionately large volume of prescribing. In addition, however, there are many differences both in pharmacokinetics and pharmacodynamics of drugs in the elderly, and while the pharmacokinetics alterations with ageing have been reasonably well described changes in pharmacodynamics are poorly understood. Sensitivity to drugs is thought to be increased in some cases e.g. those acting on the central nervous system and anticoagulants but responsiveness is decreased with other drugs such as beta adrenoceptor blocking drugs and agonists.

In the present work we have examined the pharmacokinetics of labetalol in the elderly and in addition have examined the blood pressure lowering and renal haemodynamic effects of this drug in elderly hypertensives. In order to carry out this work we initially had to devise an assay for the drug and we describe this also.

Assay of Labetalol

Most published studies in which measurement of plasma labetalol concentrations have been employed have used a spectrofluorometric technique [1]. More recently a high performance liquid chromatographic assay for labetalol has been described [2]. Since labetalol competitively antagonizes both alpha and beta adrenoceptors and since its metabolites in man are inactive [3], a radioreceptor assay might provide a sensitive and specific method for its estimation in biological materials. We have developed such an assay, based on the ability of labetalol, extracted from plasma, to inhibit the binding of ^{3}H dihydroalprenolol (DHA) to beta adrenoceptors.

A cardiac membrane preparation served as the source of beta adrenoceptors. A fresh sheep's heart was sliced and homogenized in 4 volumes of Hanks Balanced Salt Solution (HBSS). The homogenate was centrifuged at 2,000 g for 5 min and the supernatant filtered through two layers of muslin. The filtrate was centrifuged at 30,000 g for 30 min. The resulting pellet was washed and resuspended in HBSS. This was then divided and placed in glass screw-capped bottles. All the above steps were carried out at 4 °C. The stock preparations were stored at −80 °C and remained usable for at least 6 months.

Samples of plasma (0.5 ml or 1 ml) were made alkaline by adding an equal volume of normal ammonia solution and labetalol extracted by shaking with 5 ml diethyl ether for 10 min. The specimens were centrifuged to separate the phases, 4 ml of the organic layer removed and evaporated to dryness in glass conical bottomed tubes. Dried extracts were reconstituted with 300 µl of HBSS and used directly in the binding assay. To each tube were added 100 µl of HBSS containing 0.6 pmole of DHA (102 Ci/mmole) and 100 µl of HBSS containing 10 mg cardiac membranes. These amounts were chosen to result in binding of 10—20 % of added radioactivity, producing of the order of 4,000 counts/min in the zero calibration standard. Tubes were vortex-mixed and incubated at

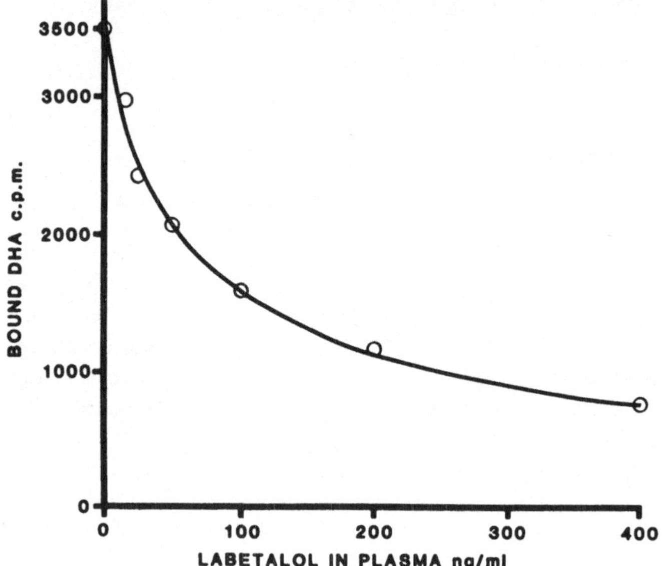

Fig. 1

Binding of ^{3}H DHA to cardiac membranes versus concentration of labetalol in plasma (Ref. [30]).

room temperature for 30 min. The incubation was ended by adding 2 ml ice-cold buffer with immediate filtration through Whatman GFC filters. After washing, the radioactivity in the filters was determined by liquid scintillation counting in a Triton X100/toluence-based cocktail. Calibration standards containing labetalol in the concentration range 0—400 ng/ml were carried through the same procedure on each day and a typical calibration curve is illustrated (Fig. 1). All samples were assayed in duplicate. The useful range of the assay was 5—400 ng/ml using 0.5 ml plasma specimens.

Labetalol Pharmacokinetics in the Elderly

Labetalol is subject to presystemic metabolism by the liver [4]. Its oral bioavailability accordingly varies widely with resulting large variations in blood concentrations after oral administration [5, 6]. We have examined the effects of age on the bioavailability and elimination of labetalol.

Observations were made in ten, drug-free mild-to-moderate hypertensive patients. The study had previously been approved by the Hospital Ethics Committee and each patient gave informed consent. Labetalol was administered to each person on two occasions, once orally and once intravenously. The doses were administered in random order, separated by at least one week. The oral dose was 200 mg except in the two oldest and one young subject, when 100 mg was given. Three subjects received an intravenous dose of 1 mg/kg and 0.5 mg/kg was given to the remaining seven. Blood samples for estimation of plasma labetolol concentrations were taken over a period of 11 hours following administration of the drug. The plasma specimens were stored at $-20\,^{\circ}$C prior to assay by the radioreceptor method described above. From the results for each patient were calculated the elimination half life of labetalol by linear least squares regression analysis of the terminal part of the log concentration-time graph and the area under the plasma concentration-time curve by the trapezoidal rule. Plasma clearance was calculated by dividing the intravenous dose by the area under the plasma concentration-time curve extrapolated to infinity ($Cl = DOSE/AUC_{\infty}$). The apparent volume of distribution was calculated as $Vd = Cl \times t_{1/2}/0.693$. Bioavailability was calculated from the ratio of the areas under the oral and intravenous plasma concentration-time curves, extrapolated to infinity and corrected for dose differences.

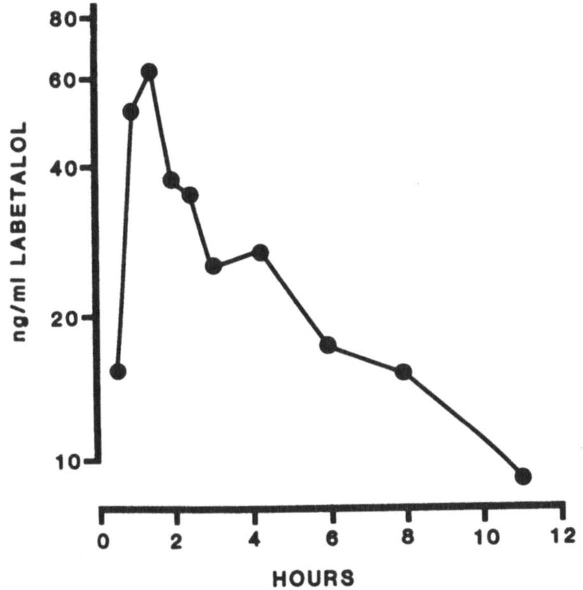

Fig. 2
Plasma concentrations of labetalol after oral administration of 200 mg. Typical results from one subject (Ref. [30]).

A typical graph of plasma concentrations of labelatol at the various times after administration of 200 mg orally to one subject is shown (Fig. 2). Typically, peak concentrations were observed at between 0.5 and 2.5 hours after oral administration of labetalol and this did not change with age. In the seven patients who received labetolol 200 mg, peak plasma concentrations varied from 63 ng/ml to 354 ng/ml and peak concentrations increased with age ($r = 0.87$, $p < 0.05$). Labetalol bioavailability varied from 8.9 % to 68.4 % and was also significantly related to age (see Fig. 3; % bioavailability $= 0.78 + 0.81$ age, $r = 0.7$, $p < 0.05$).

The mean volume of distribution of labetalol was 7.7 ± 1.1 1/kg s.e.m. (range 3.2—13.7 1/kg) and was not related to age. The mean clearance overall was 22.4 ± 3.5 ml/min/kg (range 8.8—41.8 ml/min/kg). Clearance tended to be lower in elderly people. The mean

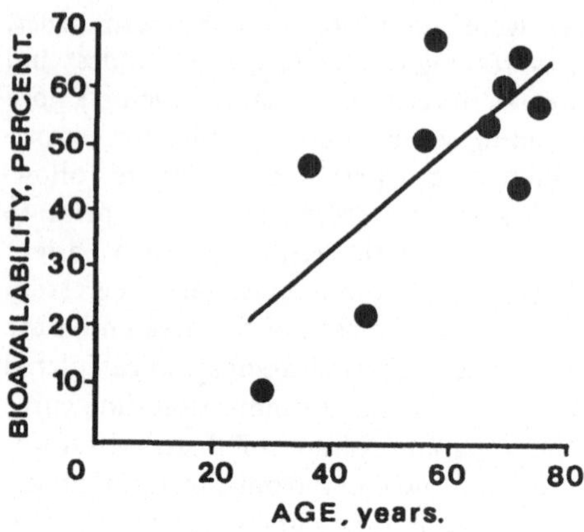

Fig. 3

Bioavailability of labetalol at various ages, showing the line of best fit (Ref. [30]).

clearance in younger subjects (aged less than 60 years) was 28.3 ± 5.5 ml/min/kg and in older subjects (aged greater than 60 years) was 16.4 ± 2.7 ml/min/kg. Elimination half life varied from 3.5 hours to 4.9 hours and increased with age (halflife = 2.62 + 0.026 age; r = 0.73, p. < 0.02).

Labetalol is a high 'first pass effect' drug demonstrating large variability in peak plasma concentrations and bioavailability after oral administration. Advancing age is associated with increases in peak plasma concentrations and bioavailability and a decrease in the rate of elimination of the drug.

For most metabolised drugs, age-related changes in elimination rates show no consistency. There are clear age associated effects for some but not for others [7]. Drugs subject to a high first pass effect, however, tend to show a fairly consistent age-related pattern. For these substances, the ability of he liver to extract the drug from blood is so high that the kinetics are determined by how quickly the drug is delivered to the liver [8]. Age related decreases in portal blood flow [9] together with possible decreases in rates of hepatic metabolism may contribute to a decreased first pass efficiency in the elderly. This is commonly seen as an increased bioavailability, previously reported for chlormethiazole [10], propranolol [11] and lignocaine. Labetolol then is no exception in that we have shown a pronounced age-related increase in its bioavailability. This is accompanied by decreased elimination of the drug. Changes of the magnitude found by us could result in greatly altered plasma concentrations of labetolol in the elderly. It would seem prudent then to administer labetalol in smaller doses to older people.

Hypertension in the Elderly

There are few data on which to base therapeutic decisions in hypertension in the elderly. Thiazide diuretics are effective in lowering blood pressure in the older hypertensive patient but long term use may be associated with a significant decrease in glucose tolerance, a rise in serum uric acid levels and serum creatinine, and a fall in serum potassium [13]. The blood pressure lowering effect of beta adrenoceptor blocking drugs in the elderly has not been well studied, and the possibility that they might have an adverse effect on the renal circulation is of concern. In young adult hypertensives a reduction in renal blood flow and/or glomerular filtration rate has been described following non-selective beta-adrenoceptor blocking drugs such as propranolol [14] and pindolol [15], when given intravenously, and following oral propranolol [16, 17]. Wilkinson et al. [18] have demonstrated a reduction in creatinine clearance with propranolol while they observed no change in patients taking the cardioselective agent atenolol. The situation is further complicated by the findings of Hollenberg and colleagues [19] who showed an increase in renal blood flow after intravenous administration of nadolol — a non-selective beta-adrenoceptor blocking drug. Recently Textor and collegues found that in chronic use nadolol did not change renal blood flow [20].

In order to assess the possible role of beta-adrenoceptor blocking drugs in the management of hypertension in the elderly we undertook to study the effects of labetalol — a non-selective beta-adrenoceptor blocking agent with alpha-blocking activity — both for it's blood pressure lowering effect and for any action it might have on renal circulation in elderly hypertensives.

Patients and Methods

Nine elderly and nine young outpatients with untreated essential hypertension were studied. Hypertension was defined as a diastolic blood pressure greater than 95 mmHg (phase 5) on each of three successive outpatient visits. Elderly was defined as 65 years of age or older and the young were 55 years of age or less. The age of the elderly group ranged from 65 to 85 years (mean 78); the younger patients ranged from 22 to 55 years (mean 40). Patients were excluded if they had the usual contraindications to beta-adrenoceptor blocking drugs, a recent myocardial infarction or liver disease. Those with raised blood urea nitrogen or serum creatinine were also excluded. Baseline blood urea nitrogen, serum creatinine and serum electrolytes were carried out in each patient prior to entry into the study and at the end of each treatment phase. Blood pressure was measured using a standard sphygmomanometer and heart rate was measured from the pulse rate for 30 seconds. Mean arterial blood pressure was calculated as one third of pulse pressure plus diastolic pressure.

All patients were started on labetolol 50 mg orally twice daily. The dose was doubled at weekly intervals until the diastolic pressure was lowered to or less than 90 mmHg or was reduced by 15 mmHg, or until a maximum daily dose of 1 g labetalol was reached. In all cases the appropriate blood pressure response was observed at doses below the maximum dose. Following this dose finding phase patients were entered into a randomised double-blind placebo-controlled trial, each phase lasting for 12 weeks.

Patients received the pre-determined dose of labetalol or appropriate placebo tablets. At the end of each 12 week period glomerular filtration rate and effective renal plasma flow were estimated using plasma clearance of intravenously injected ^{51}Cr EDTA and ^{125}I hippuran respectively. A single injection technique was employed, using $30\,\mu\text{Ci}$ of each isotope in 8 ml of normal saline. Venous blood samples were taken at intervals after the injection (5, 10, 15, 20, 30, 40, 50, 60, 80, 100, 120, 140, 160 and 180 minutes). Clearance values were calculated using an open two-compartment model [21]. The values obtained for GFR and effective renal blood flow were then corrected to 1.73 m^2 body surface area. Effective renal plasma flow was corrected for a simultaneous haemacrit to give effective renal blood flow. Data are presented as mean ± the standard error of the mean. Statistical comparison is by Student t-test, paired or unpaired as appropriate.

Results

Data for both supine and standing blood pressure are given in Table 1. Baseline data in the two age groups were different; in the elderly group supine mean arterial pressure was higher, the mean systolic pressure being 31.5 higher and diastolic 6.4 mmHg higher in the elderly.

Labetalol lowered supine blood pressure in all patients. In the elderly group supine mean arterial pressure fell by 17.1 ± 2.1 mmHg (P $<$ 0.001), the systolic pressure falling by 21.8 ± 7.4 mmHg (P $<$ 0.001), and the diastolic pressure by 14.8 ± 2.1 mmHg (P $<$ 0.001). In the young group supine mean arterial pressure was reduced 13.7 ± 2.5 mmHg (P $<$ 0.001), the systolic pressure falling by 17.4 ± 3.9 mmHg (P $<$ 0.001) and the diastolic pressure by 12.0 ± 2.1 mmHg (P $<$ 0.001). There was considerable variability in daily dose of labetalol required to get the desired blood pressure effect, but there was no significant difference in the daily mean dose for the elderly group (388.8 ± 58.8 mg) and the young group (266.7 ± 33.3 mg).

Heart rates for each age group were significantly lowered. The elderly group heart rate on placebo was 75.0 ± 4.3 compared to 70.7 ± 4.0 per minute on labetalol (P $<$ 0.02). In the young heart rate fell from 74.1 ± 2.2 to 68.5 ± 2.5 beats per minute (P $<$ 0.01).

Average glomerular filtration rate (Table 2) on placebo was 87.9 ± 8.2 in the young and 62.6 ± 6.3 ml/min/1.73 m^2 in the elderly (P $<$ 0.001). The average effective renal blood flow on placebo was 652.9 ± 68.0 in the young group and 469.0 ± 53.3 ml/min/1.73 m^2 in the elderly (P $<$ 0.001).

There was no significant change in either effective renal blood flow or glomerular filtration rate with labetalol. Following the 12 week course of labetalol mean glomerular filtration rate was 97.6 ± 7.1 in the young group and 60.2 ± 4.2 ml/min/1.73 m^2 in the

Table 1: Blood Pressure, Supine and Standing, on Placebo and Labetalol

Supine			
Blood Pressure mmHg		*Young*	*Elderly*
Mean arterial	Placebo	113.4 ± 3.1	128.2 ± 4.0
	Labetalol	99.7 ± 2.5	111.1 ± 3.7
Systolic	Placebo	149.2 ± 5.6	180.7 ± 9.0
	Labetalol	131.8 ± 5.0	158.9 ± 8.9
Diastolic	Placebo	95.6 ± 2.1	102.0 ± 2.4
	Labetalol	83.6 ± 1.5	87.2 ± 1.8
Standing			
Mean arterial	Placebo	113.7 ± 3.2	126.6 ± 8.1
	Labetalol	100.2 ± 2.1	108.0 ± 12.3
Systolic	Placebo	146.9 ± 5.5	176.4 ± 7.9
	Labetalol	132.6 ± 4.6	152.3 ± 8.0
Diastolic	Placebo	97.2 ± 2.4	101.7 ± 2.4
	Labetalol	83.7 ± 1.7	85.9 ± 3.1

Values are mean ± SEM

Table 2: Renal Haemodynamics on Placebo and Labetalol

		Young	*Elderly*	
GFR	Placebo	87.9 ± 8.2	62.6 ± 6.3	P < 0.001
ml/min/1.73 m^2	Labetalol	97.6 ± 7.1	60.2 ± 4.2	−
ERBF	Placebo	652.9 ± 68.0	469.0 ± 53.3	P < 0.001
ml/min/1.73 m^2	Labetalol	656.1 ± 35.9	385.4 ± 42.6	−

Values are mean ± SEM

elderly group, while effective renal blood flow was 656.1 ± 35.9 in the young group and 385.4 ± 42.6 ml/min/1.73 m^2 in the elderly group.

Neither serum creatinine or blood urea nitrogen were significantly altered in either group during labetalol therapy. Mean creatinine values on placebo were 88.9 ± 7.1 μmol/litre in the elderly and 78.6 ± 6.7 in the young. Corresponding values on labetalol were 90.2 ± 6.2 and 74.1 ± 5.8. Mean blood urea nitrogen was 6.3 ± 0.6 mmol/l in the elderly group while on placebo compared to 6.6 ± 0.5 during labetalol therapy. Corresponding values in the young group were 5.6 ± 0.3 and 5.5 ± 0.2 respectively.

A postural fall in blood pressure was seen in one elderly patient who was on a daily dose of 400 mg. His supine blood pressure on placebo was 170/105 mmHg and standing 150/100 mmHg. After three months on labetalol the corresponding figure were 130/80 and 105/68 mmHg.

Discussion

Doubts have been expressed about the efficacy of beta-adrenoceptor blocking drugs in the management of hypertension in the elderly [22]. The present results show that labetalol decreased blood pressure in the supine and erect positions in young and elderly hypertensives. The differences in baseline blood pressure values in the two groups make a comparison of blood pressure responsiveness in the two groups difficult. However, in both groups the fall in blood pressure was similar; 17.4/12.0 mmHg in the young, compared to 21.8/14.8 mmHg in the elderly hypertensives.

Most [2, 23, 24] but not all [25] reports indicate that in young hypertensives labetalol does not dramatically alter renal circulation or function. The lack of an effect of labetalol on effective renal blood flow or glomerular filtration rate may be due to two factors — the tendency of non-selective beta-adrenoceptor-blocking drugs to decrease effective renal blood flow [15, 18] on the one hand and the effect of vasodilators to increase it on the other [26]. Our findings of unaltered serum creatinine and blood urea nitrogen are in agreement with the flow data. Significantly, the elderly had a similar fall in blood pressure to the young hypertensives and in common with them demonstrated no adverse renal effects.

It is perhaps surprising that the pharmacodynamics of labetalol were similar in our old and young patients. Older people have been shown to be resistant to a number of effects of beta-adrenoceptor agonists and blocking drugs [27, 29]. On the other hand, and as described in this paper labetalol bioavailability increases with age [30]. It is likely therefore that the similarity of blood pressure and heart rate response in the young and elderly represent the balance between opposing pharmacokinetics and pharmacodynamic changes that occur with ageing, the former tending to increase effect with the latter decreasing responsiveness in the elderly.

Renal blood flow decreases with age [31], and as would be expected we found that baseline effective renal blood flow and glomerular filtration rate were reduced in elderly compared with younger hypertensive patients. It is important in such patients that antihypertensive therapy does not compromise renal function further. Therefore, the absence of a deleterious effect of labetalol on effective renal blood flow and glomerular filtration rate in such patients is particularly pertinent. While we cannot make general recommendations on the basis of these results in a small number of patients, it would seem that larger studies on efficacy and unwanted effects of beta adrenoceptor blocking drugs in elderly patients are worthwhile.

Conclusion

Like other beta adrenoceptor blocking drugs, it is possible to assay labetalol using a radio receptor technique. There is a marked increase in bioavailability of labetalol in the elderly. Labetalol is an effective blood pressure lowering drug in the elderly.

Acknowledgements

This work was supported by grants from the Medical Research Council of Ireland, the Royal College of Surgeons in Ireland and by Glaxo Ltd.

References

[1]   Richards, D. A., Maconochie, J. G., Bland, R. E., Hopkins, R., Woodings, E. P., Martin, L. E.: Relationship between plasma concentrations and pharmacological effects of labetalol. *Europ. J. Clin. Pharmacol.* **11**, 85–90 (1977).

[2]   Wood, A. J., Ferry, D. G., Bailey, R. R.: Elimination kinetics of labetalol in severe renal failure. *Br. J. Clin. Pharmac.* **13**, Suppl., 81–86 (1982).

[3]   Martin, L. E., Hopkins, R., Bland, R.: Metabolism of labetalol by animals and man. *Br. J. Clin. Pharmac.* **3**, Suppl., 695–710 (1976).

[4]   Breckenridge, A. M., Macnee, C. M., Orme, M. L'E., Richards, D. A., Sterlin, M. J.: Rate of onset of hypotensive response with oral labetalol. *Br. J. Clin. Pharmac.* **4**, 338P (1977).

[5]   Louis, W. J., Christophidis, N., Brignell, M., Vijayasekaran, V., McNeill, J., Vajda, F. J. E.: Labetalol, bioavailability, drug plasma levels, plasma renin and catecholamines in acute and chronic treatment of resistant hypertension. *Austr. N. Zeal. J. Med.* **8**, 602–609 (1978).

[6]   McNeill, J. J., Anderson, A. E., Louis, W. J., Morgan, D. J.: Pharmacokinetic and pharmacodynamic studies of labetalol in hypertensive patients. *Br. J. Clin. Pharmac.* **8**, Suppl., 157–161 (1979).

[7]   O'Malley, K., Laher, M., Cusack, B., Kelly, J. G.: Clinical Pharmacology and the elderly patient. In: M. J. Denham: *The treatment of medical problems in the elderly.* MTP Press 1–33 (1980).

[8]   Nies, A. S., Shand, D. G., Wilkinson, G. R.: Altered hepatic blood flow and drug metabolism. *Clin. Pharmacokin.* **1**, 135–155 (1976).

[9]   Sherlock, S., Bearn, A. G., Billing, B. H., Paterson, J. C. S.: Splanchnic blood flow in man by the bromsulphalein method: The relation of peripheral plasma bromsulphalein level to the calculated flow. *J. Lab. Clin. Med.* **35**, 923–932 (1950).

[10] Nation, R. L., Vine, I., Triggs, E. J., Learoyd, B.: Plasma levels of chlormethiazole and two

metabolites after oral administration to young and aged human subjects. *Eur. J. Clin. Pharmac.* **12**, 137–145 (1977).

[11] Castledon, C. M., George, C. F.: The effect of ageing on the hepatic clearance of propranolol. *Br. J. Clin. Pharmac.* **7**, 49–54 (1979).

[12] O'Malley, K., O'Brien, E.: Management of hypertension in the elderly. *N. Engl. J. Med.* **302**, 1397–1401 (1980).

[13] Amery, A., Berthaux, P., Birkenhager, W. et al.: Antihypertensive therapy in patients above age 60: third interim report of the European Working Party on High Blood Pressure in the Elderly (EWPHE). *Acta Cardiol.* **33**, 113–134 (1978).

[14] Sullivan, J. M., Adams, D. F., Hollenberg, N. K.: Beta adrenergic blockade in essential hypertension: Reduced renin release despite renal vasoconstriction. *Circ. Res.* 532–536 (1976).

[15] Heierli, C., Thoelen, H., Radielovic, P.: Renal function following a single dose of pindolol in hypertensive patients with varying degrees of impairment of renal function. *Int. J. Clin. Pharmac. Biopharm.* **15**, 67–71 (1977).

[16] Ibsen, H., Sederberg-Olsen, P.: Changes in glomerular filtration rate during long term treatment with propranolol in patients with arterial hypertension. *Clin. Sci.* **44**, 129–134 (1972).

[17] Falch, D. K., Odegaard, A. E., Norman, N.: Renal plasma flow and cardiac output during hydralazine and propranolol treatment in essential hypertension. *Scand. J. Clin. Lab. Invest.* **38**, 143–146 (1978).

[18] Wilkinson, R., Stevens, I., Pickering, M., Robson, V., Hawkins, T., Kerr, D., Harry, J.: A study of the effects of atenolol and propranolol on renal function in patients with essential hypertension. *Br. J. Clin. Pharmacol.* **10**, 51–59 (1980).

[19] Hollenberg, N. K., Adams, D. F., McKinstry, D., Williams, G. H., Borucki, L., Sullivan, J. M.: Beta adrenoceptor blocking agents and the kidney: effects of nadolol and propranolol on the renal circulation. *Br. J. Clin. Pharmacol.* **7**, (Suppl. 2) 219S–225S (1979).

[20] Textor, S. C., Fouad, F. M., Bravo, E. L., Tarazi, R. C., Vidt, D. G., Gifford, R. W.: Distribution of cardiac output to the kidneys during oral nadolol administration. *N. Engl. J. Med.* **307**, 601–605 (1982).

[21] Sapirstein, L. A., Vidt, D. G., Mandel, M. J., Hanhsek, G.: Volumes of distribution and clearances of intravenously injected creatinine. *Am. J. Physiol.* **181**, 330–336 (1955).

[22] Buhler, F. R., Burkart, F., Lutold, B. E., Kung, M., Marbet, G., Pfisterer, M.: Antihypertensive beta blocking action as related to renin and age: a pharmacologic tool to identify pathogenic mechanisms in essential hypertension. *Am. J. Cardiol.* **36**, 653–669 (1975).

[23] Rasmussen, S., Nielsen, P. E.: Blood pressure, body fluid volumes and glomerular filtration rate during treatment with labetalol in essential hypertension. *Br. J. Clin. Pharmacol.* **12**, 349–353 (1981).

[24] Cruz, F., O'Neill, M., Clifton, C., Wallin, J. D.: Effects of labetalol and methyldopa on renal function. *Clin. Pharmacol. Ther.* **30**, 57–63 (1981).

[25] Keusch, G., Weidmann, P., Ziegler, W. H., de Chatel, R., Reubi, F. C.: Effects of chronic alpha and beta adrenoceptor blockade with labetalol on plasma catecholamines and renal function in hypertension. *Klin. Wochenschr.* **58**, 25–29 (1980).

[26] Reubi, F. C.: Role of physical factors in the acute changes in renal function elicited by antihypertensive drugs. *Eur. J. Clin. Pharmacol.* **13**, 185–193 (1978).

[27] Vestal, R. E., Wood, A. J. J., Shand, D. G.: Reduced beta-adrenoceptor sensitivity in the elderly. *Clin. Pharmacol. Ther.* **26**, 181–186 (1976).

[28] Dillon, N., Chung, S., Kelly, J., O'Malley, K.: Age and beta-adrenoceptor mediated function. *Clin. Pharmacol. Ther.* **27**, 769–772 (1980).

[29] Conway, J., Wheeler, R., Sannerstedt, R.: Sympathetic nervous activity during exercise in relation to age: Effect of age on response to propranolol. *Cardiovasc. Res.* **5**, 577–581 (1971).

[30] Kelly, J., McGarry, K., O'Malley, K., O'Brien, E. T.: Bioavailability of labetalol increases with age. *Br. J. Clin. Pharmacol.* **14**, 304–305 (1982).

[31] Davies, D. F., Shock, N. W.: Age changes in glomerular filtration rate, effective renal plasma flow and tubular excretory capacity in adult males. *J. Clin. Invest.* **29**, 496–507 (1950).

Discussion

Borchard
You measured your pharmacokinetics after acute application. As we know from drugs with high bioavailability, after chronic administration the data could be different. Have you measured this?

O'Malley
What you say is absolutely true. There are very significant differences but we didn't get that information, I'm afraid.

N. N.
Könnten Sie bitte noch etwas zur Erklärung sagen, ob die Bioverfügbarkeit bei den älteren Patienten so stark zugenommen hatte? Der zweite Punkt ist, wie ist die Eliminationshalbwertzeit der Substanz?

O'Malley
There must be a decrease in the extraction of the drug as it goes to the liver, perhaps due to the shunting of blood; I don't know the answer. The half-lives in our study were about 3 hours to 4.5 hours. There was a positive correlation with age, but I don't think that it has any clinical significance.

Haim
Your renal function studies showed, at least a tendency to a decrease in effective renal plasma flow with an unchanged glomerular filtration rate. This would indicate or would be consistent with an increase in the filtration fraction. Did any of your elderly patients gain weight?

O'Malley
No, they didn't. We see this pattern also with atenolol, and I really cannot explain why that happend. There must be re-distribution.

Rietbrock, N.
Die Leberdurchblutung bei älteren Patienten kann sich doch nicht so total verändern, daß die Bioverfügbarkeit um etwa das Doppelte ansteigt. Haben Sie die über 4 Halbwertzeiten gemessen? Resultieren daraus Unterschiede?

O'Malley
It's possible. We measured for about 3 halflives, about 12 hours. The question of liver blood flow, I think, would probably explain differences in clearance, as systemic clearance does fall as a function of age. This wasn't very dramatic in the case of labetalol. When one refers to the first pass metabolism we are really concerned with portal blood flow and extraction by the liver. I think, there is some strange thing happening with extraction in aging. It may have to do with the distribution of the portal blood flow in the liver.

Heusinger
How is labetalol metabolised and which enzymes must be affected for the first-pass effect to be reduced?

O'Malley
I'm not sure. Hydroxylation and glucuronidation. Hydroxylation as such tends not to change with age, or doesn't change much with age, whereas glucuronidation tends not to change with the age. I feel that blood flow effects rather than enzyme activity are more important with age. For those drugs with a very long halflife and whose rate of elimination does not depend on liver blood flow, it is difficult to show much change in systemic clearance. The really dramatic changes occur in those drugs whose elimination depends on liver blood flow. That seems to be a flow phenomenon rather than a drug metabolising phenomenon.

Rietbrock, I.
Haben Sie die Verfügbarkeit von Sauerstoff gemessen? Wir haben gesehen, daß, wenn die Verfügbarkeit von Sauerstoff nicht hoch genug ist, die Extraktion abnimmt. Und damit könnte die Bioverfügbarkeit ansteigen.

O'Malley
No, we did not measure oxygen. Could you explain this study to me?

Rietbrock, I.
Wir haben einen Katheter in eine Lebervene geschoben und haben die Sauerstoffextraktion zwischen arteriellem und venösem Blut gemessen, und wir haben diese in Beziehung gesetzt zu der Extraktion. Wir haben nicht Labetalol, sondern andere Substanzen genommen. Es besteht eine enge Beziehung zwischen der Extraktion und der Verfügbarkeit von Sauerstoff. Ist nicht genügend Sauerstoff vorhanden, so sinkt die Metabolisierung bei älteren Patienten ab.

O'Malley
Could both of these problems be linked by shunting, i.e., if the liver blood flow was shunted, so that oxygen was not available for extraction, the drug is also not available for extraction? That may not explain everything, but it may contribute.

Koch
I propose a very simple explanation. Was there a high proportion of heavy drinkers in your material? Alcohol in geriatrics is the most common reason for raising the bioavailability.

O'Malley
I think that is unlikely in the older people. Alcohol is usually consumned before they become old. I would expect that would be a potential problem perhaps in the younger patients but not in the old patients. These are relatively healthy old patients with normal liver function tests.

Koch
We did a similar renal study in younger people and we saw a reduction of both glomerular filtration rate and renal blood flow by about 8 to 10 %.

O'Malley
Was that chronic treatment?

Koch
No, that was acute. Single doses.

O'Malley
I think one has to be very careful about extrapolation from single dose to chronic dose.

Heinicke
Are we discussing a problem which really does not exist? You only had three young persons, and you concluded that all young persons have a low bioavailability.

O'Malley
There were in fact five young people, but I take your point, the group was very small. We do the cut-off below 55. I'm not depending only on this study. It has been well demonstrated that propranolol, chlormethiazol, lignocaine, and many other drugs with high first-pass-metabolism are affected in this way. I'm leaning as much on that evidence as on these small numbers. .

On the Rationale of Combined Alpha/Beta Blockade (Labetalol) in the Treatment of Hypertension in Pregnancy and the Maintenance of Intra-Uterine Fetal Growth

H. Lardoux[1], J. Gerard[2], G. Blasquez[2], F. Chouty[1], B. G. Woodcock[3]

Department of Cardiology[1] and Obstetrics and Gynaecology[2], Centre Hospitalier, 91108 Corbeil-Essonnes, France
and
Abteilung für Klinische Pharmakologie, Universitätsklinik Frankfurt, Theodor-Stern-Kai 7, D-6000 Frankfurt/Main, F.R.G.[3]

Summary

Even if the broader question of the value of antihypertensive therapy during pregnancy remains to be answered, alpha-beta blockade therapy with labetalol appears to be of particular interest. Oral labetalol is a safe and effective compound during pregnancy and seems responsible for higher birth-weights. The intravenous application remains to be carefully evaluated in hypertensive emergencies (pre-eclampsia) but could be an important therapeutic approach. However, careful monitoring of neonatal blood glucose is needed during the first three days of life.

Hypertension in pregnancy may be responsible for eclampsia in the mother and deleterious complications in the fetus leading to repeated abortions, fetal death, intrauterine growth retardation of the fetus and prematurity.
Antihypertensive treatment is still controversial in mild to moderate hypertension associated with pregnancy and thus therapy is usually confined to those cases where hypertension is significant and implies some pathology. Antihypertensive treatment should be effective in not only reducing the blood pressure, but also in ensuring an adequate placental perfusion without harmful side effects.
The application of beta-blocking drugs in pregnant hypertensive women has frequently been associated with adverse effects, notably intrauterine growth retardation of the fetus [1]. In a recent randomised double-blind prospective study of 120 pregnant women with mild to moderate hypertension, atenolol was effective in controlling blood pressure in the majority of mothers but intrauterine growth retardation was the same as in the placebo group and neonatal bradycardia was more common during atenolol application [2].
These disadvantages of beta-blocking therapy do not appear to be present under combined alpha/beta blockade with labetalol. In a randomised trial involving 56 cases of hypertension in pregnancy, atenolol (mean daily dose 145 ± 48 mg) and labetalol (mean daily dose 614 ± 260 mg) produced equal blood pressure reduction but birth-weights were significantly higher in the labetalol treated group (mean difference in weight was 630 gm,

"/>

Table 1: Effects of Atenolol and Labetalol on Maternal Blood Pressure and Infant Birth-weight, and Maternal (M) and Infant (Umbilical Cord, UB) Drug Levels

	Atenolol	Labetalol
Blood pressure (mmHg)	128 ± 10/77 ± 8	131 ± 11/80 ± 9
Birth-weight (g)	2750 ± 630	3380 ± 550
Plasma drug levels (μg/l)	M 236 ± 268*	74 ± 63†
	UB 240 ± 215*	61 ± 42†

* n = 16; †n = 15.

Table 2: Relationship between maximal uricemia during pregnancy and neonatal birth-weight

	Birth-weight (g)	
Level of uricemia (μmol/l)	Atenolol treatment	Labetalol treatment
above 360	2600 ± 1207	3000 ± 1159
240 – 360	2700 ± 653	3300 ± 620
less than 240	3175 ± 480	3550 ± 463
	n = 28	n = 28

+ 22 %), Table 1 [3]. The birth-weights in both groups tended to be higher in those patients with the lowest levels of uricemia but birth-weights under labetalol were always higher than those for atenolol for any given level of uricemia (Table 2). Both labetalol and atenolol cross the placental barrier [3] as shown by the drug concentration in maternal blood and umbilical cord blood (Atenolol r = 0.90, p $<$ 0.001; and Labetalol r = 0.78, p $<$ 0.01). No deleterious effect on the Apgar score, neonatal heart rate or bronchospasm is seen. On the other hand, hypoglycemia ($\leqslant$ 1.4 μmol/l) is rather frequent (11 %) in the first day of life, but is easily controlled by force-feeding of the neonate. These adverse effects, even moderate, need careful monitoring of the neonate, during the first days of life. There were 2 still-births in the atenolol treated group and none in the labetalol treated group. However, in a recent study [4] including 70 consecutive hypertensive pregnant women treated with oral labetalol alone, five still-births were recorded. Four of them were directly related to the severity of the hypertension, complicated by pre-eclampsia. This underlines the limits of oral antihypertensive treatment in the severe pre-eclamptic patient.

Riley and Symonds (1982) [5] have documented investigations on the use of labetalol in the management of approximately 390 pregnancies. Their report contains evidence that lowering the blood pressure by the infusion of labetalol does not reduce uterine blood flow and this could be the basis for the higher birth-weights with labetalol in comparison with atenolol.

It is also of interest that labetalol has been reported to promote renal perfusion and reduce renal vascular resistance during maintenance treatment, whereas beta-blockade alone reduces renal perfusion. There are at least two studies which show that labetalol delays the onset of development of proteinuria [6]. According to renal histological investigations by Dame (1984) [7] pre-eclampsia could correspond to a latent renal disease and made manifest by the pregnancy condition. Thus irrespective of whether renal tissue changes are associated with the cause of, or result from, the hypertension, a drug with apparent beneficial effects on renal vasculature may alleviate the renal dysfunction or retard its development and thereby prevent the accompanying proteinuria. Preliminary results showing satisfactory responses with prolonged intravenous treatment with labetalol in 2 pre-eclamptic patients over 6 and 15 days support this view (unpublished observations).

We thank Martine Picaud for her secretarial help.

Literature

[1] Pruyn, S. C., Phelan, J. P., Buchanan, G. C.: Long term propranolol in pregnancy: maternal and fetal outcome. *Am. J. Obset. Gynecol.* **135**, 485–89 (1979).

[2] Rubin, P. C., Butters, L., Clark, D. M., Reynolds, B., Sumner, D. J., Steedman, D., Low, R. A., Reid, J. L.: Placebo-controlled trial of atenolol in treatment of pregnancy-associated hypertension. *Lancet* **1**, 431–34 (1983).

[3] Lardoux, H., Gerard, J., Blasquez, G., Chouty, F., Flouvat, B.: Hypertension in pregnancy evaluation on two beta-blockers atenolol and labetalol. *Europ. Ht. J.* **4** (Suppl. G), 35–40 (1983).

[4] Lardoux, H., Blasquez, G., Giraud, J., Jeuffroy, A., Touboul, A., Chouty, F., Gerard, J.: Experience with labetalol, an alpha-beta blocker in 70 pregnancies. 4th World Congress of the International Society for the study of hypertension in pregnancy. Amsterdam 18–21 June 1984.

[5] Riley, A., Symonds, E. M.: The investigation of labetalol in the management of hypertension in pregnancy. (editors). Excerpta Medica (International Congress series 591), Amsterdam, Oxford, Princeton (1982).

[6] Symonds, E. M.: In: The investigation of labetalol in the management of hypertension in pregnancy (Riley, A., Symonds, E. M., Eds.) International Congress Series 591, Excerpta Medica, Amsterdam, Oxford, Princeton (1982) pp. 165–166.

[7] Dame, W. R.: Die Präeklampsie – ein Syndrom, eine hypertensive Diathese? *Med. Welt* **35**, 651–4 (1984).

[8] MacGillivray, I., Campbell, D. M.: Antihypertensive therapy in pregnancy. In: The investigation of labetalol in the management of hypertension in pregnancy (Riley, A., Symonds, E. M., Eds.). Excerpta Medica (International Congress Series 591), Amsterdam, Oxford, Princeton (1982) pp. 5–9.

Discussion

Jähnchen
I would like to know at which gestational age did your treatment start because many conclusions depend on this?

Lardoux
Some patients were hypertensive before pregnancy others became hypertensive during pregnancy. We did not distinguish between different types of hypertension in these patients.

Jähnchen
Was the treatment for hypertension necessary in the last trimester or in the first trimester?

Lardoux
For some patients it was necessary during the whole of the pregnancy, for others during the later part of pregnancy.

Koch

Placental blood flow has been measured by a group in Stockholm and has been found to be unchanged under labetalol but lowered under the action of beta-blockers. This is a finding that can be expected on theoretical grounds.

N. N.

Are both of your groups comparable with regard to smoking habits and to the prevalence of diabetes?

Lardoux

They were equivalent on this point, but they were two consecutive groups and so we are now going to do a randomized trial because of such problems.

General Discussion

Taylor (to Prichard)
We heard this morning that there was pharmacological evidence to show that after some time the alpha-blocking effect of labetalol may be diminished yet, we know from work of yourself, of Lund-Johansen and of Koch, that the blood pressure effects are maintained over many years, with still what apparently are alpha-blocking vasodilator effects. How do you make these two quite different pharmacological and pragmatic clinical results compatible?

Prichard
When you give an alpha-blocker you are likely to see a relatively dramatic and immediate response due to alpha-blockade on the cardio-vascular system. You produce a sudden reduction in vascular resistence coincident with the administration of your alpha-blocker. Subsequent to that, in most cases, you are likely get fluid shifts and some compensatory increase in blood volume. This is seen particularly with prazosin in the first-dose phenomenon, and that is why one has to be a little careful with the initial administration of prazosin. Many physicians would tell the patients to go to bed after the first dose. I think, this probably applies to labetalol.
There is some evidence with chronic administration of labetalol that there is a modest increase in blood volume. Labetalol, acutely, lowers the blood pressure. This is primarily an alpha-effect, and is in marked contrast to that seen under beta-blockade. Whereas a beta-blocking-drug chronically lowers the blood pressure, acutely it has little effect. This does not mean that under chronic administration there is no significant alpha-blockade contributing to the blood pressure lowering action. I'm a little surprised about the results indicating that the antagonism to phenylephrine, though seen acutely, disappeared after 6 days to 1 month of administration. I must maintain an open mind on these results because firstly the investigators used small doses of labetalol and it is thus difficult to show much of a shift in the phenylephrine dose-response curve. The other feature about the results is by using relatively low doses they were not really getting up the dose response curve. It might be worth repeating these studies.
There is no doubt that during long-term labetalol treatment alpha-blockade is contributing substantianally to the anti-hypertensive effect. I would not wish to say anything different. I only want to say that acutely the alpha-component of the action of labetalol is relatively more predominant over its beta-effect. For these various reasons, I think, the principal factor is a fluid shift phenomenon.

N. N.
Beeinflußt Labetalol den Blutzuckerspiegel bei eingestellten Diabetikern? Gibt es z.B. eine Hypoglykämie bei Betablockern?

Koch
We have looked at the effect of labetalol, nifedipine, pindolol and metoprolol on blood-sugar changes in normal subjects during work. Whereas pindolol induced a decrease in blood sugar, the other substances did not. I do not know anything about the situation in the diabetic.

Feldschreiber
There is a published work by Parsons in London who has looked at diabetic patients with nephropathy and has used labetalol to control the hypertension. There has been no labetalol induced changes in the blood sugar responses.

Palm
You showed this morning, that there is partial tolerance against the alpha-blocking effect of labetalol. This is shown using phenylephrine and noradrenaline. Dr. Lund-Johansen had shown that after 6 years there is still a decreased total peripheral resistence. If there is tolerance, I think we should not talk about an alpha-1-antagonistic effect of labetalol, but may be of a direct vasodilating effect, since in pharmacological experiments it has been shown that besides having alpha-blocking activity labetalol also is a direct vasodilating drug.

Prichard
There is some pharmacological evidence for a modest direct vasodilator effect. I think it is probably true to say that the major part of the effects of labetalol is mediated through the alpha-receptor in

terms of its reduction in peripheral resistence. I think one has to be very careful about reference to this tolerance with labetalol in terms of antihypertensive effects. You know that here there is no tolerance. With regard to the evidence for tolerance against the alpha effect, it depends on what you mean by tolerance. I have just outlined a number of caveats about these studies showing tolerance, which I do not want to repeat. Before I am convinced there is some receptor tolerance, I would like to see more confirmative data. I think, if you like, it is a physiological tolerance — in so far that there is tolerance — which comes on acutely with the fluid shift but there is still significant and continuing alpha-blockade. If you wish to have more alpha-blockade you increase the dose and you can do this within a few days of commencing treatment.

Prichard (Summing-up)

I do not propose to repeat everything you have heard, but just exceedingly briefly; we started off with Prof. Lund-Johansen and Prof. Koch, and they were very much in accord with each other. Their remarks pointed out that hypertension involved particularly an increased peripheral resistence, associated with a reduction in cardiac output and stroke volume. They felt therefore that giving a drug, which as far as possible corrected these abnormalities, was a sound therapeutic approach. They pointed out that labetalol and the combination of beta- and alpha-blockade in different drugs, i.e., prazosin and tolamolol, did exactly this, reducing peripheral resistence without any concomitant reduction in cardiac output (beta-blockers are reducing cardiac output with a reduction in blood pressure with the exception of those beta-blockers which have intrinsic sympathomimetic activity, seen particularly with pindolol and perhaps penbutolol). These haemodynamic changes; the reduction in peripheral resistence, improved responses of the heart, cardiac-output etc. are maintained.

Dr. Bahlmann then talked about the response to stress, pointing out that the combination of alpha- and beta-blockade blunted the responses.

Prof. Franz made some interesting observations indicating that the rise in blood pressure on dynamic exercise, that is the systolic pressure, is functionally a response of the heart. In other words, of beta-mediated responses since he showed that the alpha-1-blocker prazosin did not affect this parameter very much at all, whereas beta-blockade with acebutolol did. Whereas both affected the rise in diastolic pressure the combination of two, overall, produced a greater anti-hypertensive effect.

We spent most of the afternoon discussion on the theoretical basis. It is of course a sound approach to therapeutics that we have a scientific basis, but we did not in fact spend very much time this afternoon talking about the practical use of labetalol although we did consider the use of labetalol in two particular areas. Prof. O'Malley making the point that labetalol was effective treatment in the elderly and disputing the dogma which is held is some quarters that the elderly do not respond to beta-blockers. He showed, at least in regard to labetalol, that there is a similar fall in blood pressure in the elderly, as in the young, and in passing, he also mentioned that he had seen good falls in blood pressure from nadolol and atenolol. He indicated that there was no reduction in glomerular filtration or effect on renal plasma flow in the elderly, and this was associated with chronic labetalol treatment, whereas in discussion Prof. Koch pointed out that he had found an effect associated with the acute use. I suspect that the explanation here is a fluid volume shift which has taken place by the time you measure the effect on renal plasma flow in a chronic situation as compared with the acute, and that this is the reason for the difference between acute and chronic treatment.

IV Balanced Alpha/Beta Blockade in the Therapy of Coronary Heart Disease

The Concept of Combined Alpha-Beta-Blockade in Coronary Heart Disease

S. H. Taylor

Department of Cardiovascular Studies, University of Leeds, England

Summary

The pathophysiological haemodynamic profile of coronary heart disease is dominated by the activities of the sympathetic nervous system. Attenuation of stimuli over a single sympathetic pathway allows unrestrained and enhanced acitivity of a potentially hazardous nature over the unblocked pathway. Controlled combined alpha-beta-adrenoceptor blockade appears to afford the most rational therapeutic approach to this common disease syndrome. Simultaneous blockade of both sympatho-adrenergic receptors does not appear to adversely alter the metabolic or other neuro-endocrine profiles, thus enhancing the therapeutic prospects for labetalol in the long-term treatment of this common chronic disease syndrome.

Coronary heart disease is now by far the most frequent cardiovascular illness in the adult population of the Western World and the greatest single cause of death [1]. Its deleterious economic impact on the community is equally large [2]. The intense therapeutic endeavours to ameliorate this threat by prevention are therefore understandable but so far have yielded poor returns [3]. Attention continues therefore to be directed to treatment of the established syndromes.

It has long been realised that the sympathoadrenal system plays a sinister, if illdefined, role in the evolution of the disease. However, clarification of the pathophysiological mechanisms involved was greatly accelerated with the development of clinically acceptable drugs with the ability to selectively and reversibly block the sympathoadrenal receptors in the heart and circulation [4]. The final therapeutic chapter has been the development of drugs that competitively block both adrenoceptors simultaneously [5, 6].

The sympathetic nervous system is responsible and essential for regulation of output of the heart and its distribution to the regional vascular territories. In normal man the sympathoadrenal system accomplishes these complex reflex tasks with ease and without excessive cost or detriment to the cardiovascular system. However, when the heart is afflicted by disease, this no longer holds true; the majority of circulatory reflexes are forced to operate with increasing intensity to maintain blood flow to the vital cerebral and coronary circulations as well as meet the metabolic demands of the peripheral tissues [7]. Ironically the increased activity of these vital circulatory reflexes further increases the hazard to the damaged heart and leading to its ultimate destruction. It is a necessary prerequisite, therefore, to examine not only the deranged morphology and physiology in coronary heart disease, but also the reflex circulatory mechanisms invoked so that their potentially deleterious activity may be sensibly attenuated.

Cardiac Morphology and Pathophysiology in Coronary Heart Disease

Pathology

Clinical attention has naturally been primarily concerned with the geography and nature of the easily defined occlusive lesions afflicting the coronary arteries. However, thickening of the walls of the coronary arteries has evaded clinical attention probably due to the difficulty of displaying such abnormalities of wall thickness except at operation or autopsy. However, the primary thickness of the coronary artery wall may play a vital role in the critical closure of the vessel during periods of vasomotricity, particularly if such constriction takes place over, or in the vicinity of, fixed atheromatous lesions.

Considerably more attention has also been directed to the pathology of the coronary arteries than to the resulting pathological changes in the myocardium they supply. Coronary heart disease is invariably associated with varying degrees of derangement of myocytic morphology [8]. Many of the contractile elements are replaced by fibrous tissue which aggravates their loss by impeding the normal contractile characteristics of those that remain. The growth of interstitial fibrosis also distorts the normal laminar arrangement of the myocytes; further impeding their contractile efficiency. These morphological changes in the ventricular myocardium grossly aggravate the functional embarrassment resulting from impairment of coronary blood flow (Fig 1). Further acute myocardial loss due to coronary occlusion invariably aggravates this functional impairment; this accounts for the frequency of left ventricular failure following infarction.

Pathology and function in coronary heart disease

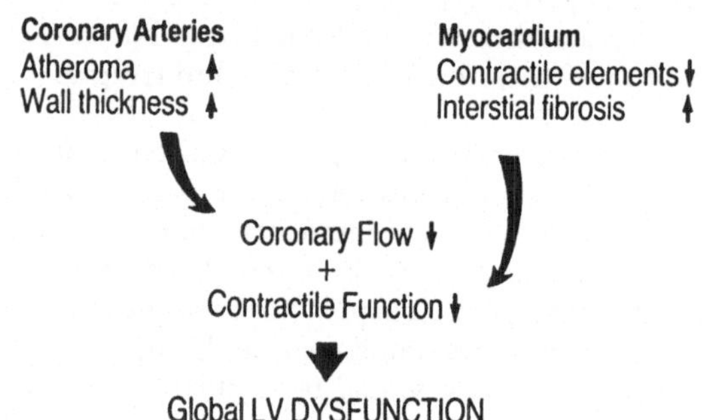

Fig. 1
Illustration of the pathological factors impeding left ventricular function in patients with coronary heart disease.

Pathophysiology

Considering these gross pathological changes in the coronary arteries and myocardium, it is not surprising that ischaemic heart disease is accompanied by significant changes in pumping function of the heart (Fig. 2). In stable coronary heart disease, without myocardial necrosis, increased work demand such as is occasioned by exercise, results in a haemodynamic pattern of acute reversible left ventricular failure [9, 10]. This is characterised by increase in left ventricular end-diastolic pressure and volume, together with a

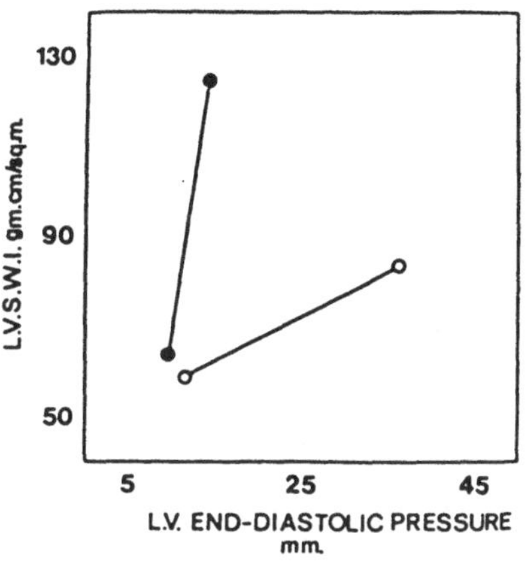

Fig. 2
Depression of left ventricular function exposed by exercise in patients with angina pectoris due to coronary artery obstructive disease (open circles of) compared to the response in normal subjects at the same external workload (from ref. [12]).

reduction in the ejection fraction [11] and depression of the Frank-Starling relationship [12]. The steep increase in end-diastolic pressure arises from a number of sources. Increased venous return due to sympathetically-induced venoconstriction, failure to expel the venous return, sympathetically-induced reduction in compliance of the left ventricular wall [13] and an unyielding pericardial sac all contribute to the excessive rise in left ventricular end-diastolic pressure. The increase in left ventricular end-diastolic and end-systolic volume is due not only to 'global' failure of left ventricular pumping activity, but also by areas of dyskensia and dilatation (pseudoaneurysm) in the regions most afflicted by impairment of coronary blood flow [14]. The pathophysiological censequences which follow from these primary haemodynamic changes add further detriment to the function of the ischaemic failing left ventricle [15]. The global derangement of the normal contraction geometry aggravates the pumping disadvantage and through the operation of the La Place theorem vastly increases left ventricular wall stress, work and oxygen consumption [16]. The large increase in intracavity pressure also impedes subendocardial blood flow during diastole. The intrinsic autonomic reflexes which these pathophysiological changes induce are quite incapable of spontaneously reversing the distorted haemodynamic profile of severe coronary heart disease. Similar haemodynamic changes occur following acute myocardial loss accompanying coronary occlusion, but the absence of a substantial increase in venous return (due to relative immobility of the patient in this situation) tends to hide the depressed left ventricular performance.

Circulatory Reflexes

The circulatory reflexes which occur following coronary heart disease are a caricature of the normal [15] (Fig. 3). They predominantly arise from two sources. First, and perhaps the predominating reflex, is that which arises from the substantial increase in left ventricular end-diastolic pressure. This is immediately reflected in an increase in the left atrial and pulmonary venous pressure which, through stretch of mechano-receptors in the atria and pulmonary veins results in afferent discharges to the vasomotor centres in the central

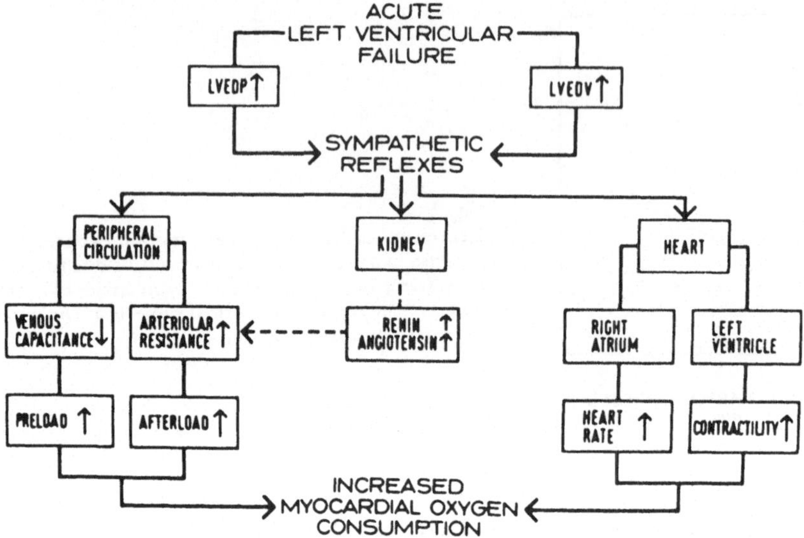

Fig. 3

Schema of the circulatory reflexes initiated by left ventricular dysfunction in patients with coronary heart disease (from ref. [15]).

nervous system [17]. Second, any failure to maintain the blood pressure also activates mechano-receptors in the aortic arch and carotid sinus which augment the afferent stimuli from the intra-cardiac receptors. The efferent outflow from the hind-brain vasomotor centres is directed over four main sympathetic pathways. Increased activity of sympathetic nerves to the heart, terminating on beta-adrenoceptors in the right atrium and left ventricle result in increased heart rate and increased left ventricular contractility respectively. Increased sympathetic nerve traffic to the periphery terminating on alpha-adrenoceptors in the arteriolar resistance and venous capacitance vessels results in vasoconstriction and increase in the systemic vascular resistance. Increased nerve traffic to beta-adrenoceptors in the juxtaglomerular apparatus of the kidney results in increased secretion of renin with subsequent activation of angiotensin and ultimately the salt-retaining aldosterone. Angiotensin directly augments the vasoconstrictive influence of sympathetic stimulation of alpha-adrenoceptors in the circulation and also heightens the activity of the central nervous system vasomotor centre, thus enhancing sympathetic efferent nerve traffic. Finally, increased sympathetic outflow over pre-ganglionic nerves to the adrenal medulla results in the secretion of catecholamines with further augmentation of all these primary sympathetic reflex responses. The enhanced profile of these circulatory reflexes are an integral part of the functional cardiovascular disturbance in coronary heart disease.

Deleterious Consequences of Excessive Sympathetic Activity in Coronary Heart Disease

These cardiovascular reflexes, so essential in normal man to facilitate the wide range of physiological responses that occur during normal daily life, are potentially deleterious in the presence of coronary heart disease. The increased sympathetic stimulation of the heart results in an immediate and direct increase in its oxygen consumption by increasing heart rate and left ventricular contractility [16]. These direct effects are augmented by the sympathetically induced loss of ventricular compliance [13]; this results in excessive elevation of the left ventricular end-diastolic pressure thus augmenting the intensity of the reflexes arising from intracardiac receptors. Peripheral vasoconstriction arising primarily from sympathetic stimulation of alpha-1 adrenoceptors in arteriolar resistance and venous capacitance vessels, and augmented by circulating catecholamines and angiotensin, increases the systemic vascular resistance and venous preload. These changes increase left ventricular afterload and wall stress and further increase myocardial oxygen consumption. Thus left ventricular myocardial oxygen consumption is progressively increased by the excessive heart rate, increased speed of left ventricular contraction and increased left ventricular afterload, particularly in the dilated and geometrically incompetent heart.

Moreover, the substantial increase in left ventricular myocardial oxygen consumption is accompanied by impeded subendocardial blood flow due to the increased pericapillary pressure. The resulting ischaemia leads to increased automaticity, reduced refractory period and reduction in fibrillation threshold of the subendocardial myocytes, thus opening the way to the initiation of sinister ventricular arrhythmias. This is the pathophysiological scenario which must be taken into account when treatment of coronary heart disease is contemplated. However, the obviously crucial and deleterious role of *both* sympathetic pathways in the pathophysiological progression of the syndrome immediately implicates combined sympathoadrenal blockade as the most rational pharmacological intervention.

Therapeutic Potential of Combined Alpha-Beta-Blockade in Coronary Heart Disease

Haemodynamic Aspects

Consideration of these pathophysiological mechanisms indicates that it is irrational to expect that blockade of one sympathetic pathway alone will achieve ultimate therapeutic benefit. Blockade of beta-adrenoceptors alone will reduce heart rate and left ventricular contractility, but only at the expense of an increase in left ventricular end-diastolic pressure and volume and a reduction in cardiac output and pulse pressure. These changes augment the reflex increase in sympathetic activity over the alpha-adrenoceptor pathway with the result that left ventricular afterload is increased by the subsequent vasoconstriction in arteries and veins. Conversely, blockade of the alpha-adrenoceptor pathway alone reduces arteriolar and venous constriction, blood pressure and work of the heart but only at the price of a reflex increase in sympathetic activity over the beta-adrenoceptor pathway; the associated increase in heart rate and contractility offsets the primary saving in left ventricular myocardial oxygen consumption [18]. Simultaneous blockade of both receptor pathways suffers from none of these disadvantages resulting from unbalanced sympathetic blockade (Table 1).

It is only in the presence of coronary heart disease that vasomotricity of the coronary vessels appears to achieve a substantial pathogenetic role. Vasomotor changes in the region of atherogenic lesions of the coronary vessels appear to be quite common and in some instances may be the final factor precipitating infarction [19]. The exact mechanisms responsible for such vasomotor changes are unclear, but it is likely that sympathoadrenal stimulation of alpha-adrenoceptors in these vessels may play a role. It would be attenuated by alpha-adrenoceptor blocking drugs but aggravated by beta-blockers.

These conceptual considerations clearly indicate a role for combined alpha-beta-adrenoceptor blockade in patients with stable coronary heart disease, particularly if angina is complicated by hypertension. It is equally reasonable to expect that combined attenuation of sympathetic stimuli will have advantages in the patient with the more acute syndrome of myocardial infarction. Alpha-adrenoceptor blockade of peripheral vessels can be expected to reduce pressure work of the heart [20] and thus counter any increase in left ventricular end-diastolic pressure and volume due to beta-blockade. In the coronary vessels, alpha-adrenoceptor blockade can also be expected to counter periinfarct vasomotor changes and thus prevent any further decrease in coronary blood flow [21]. Beta-blockade can be expected to exert a major myocardial oxygen-sparing benefit by reduction in heart rate and left ventricular contractility, particularly if the increase in left ventricular volume is offset by concomitant alpha-adrenoceptor blockade. This hypothesis is supported by recent experimental work demonstrating that labetalol had a substantially greater effect in sparing myocardial cell necrosis after acute coronary occlusion in the experimental animal than placebo or propranolol [22]. In many patients, myocardial infarction is complicated by co-existent hypertension. This may be the end result of chronic essential hypertension, but in many instances it is an acute response to the pain and physiological reflexes associated with the acute cardiac ischaemia. The increase in blood pressure in such circumstances is particularly deleterious to the infarcted left ventricle. It is reasonable to expect, therefore, that combined alpha-beta-adrenoceptor blockade will be highly effective in this condition and more effective than blockade of either sympathetic pathway alone. This supposition has now received ample support from haemodynamic studies in this emergency clinical situation [23–25]. The concept has received further support in patients with uncomplicated acute myocardial infarction. Although the overall clinical and haemodynamic response can be expected to be crucially dose-dependent [26], there are clear-cut haemodynamic benefits with combined alpha-beta-adrenoceptor blockade than beta-blockade alone in these patients.

Arrhythmia Aspects

Until recently it had been widely supposed that arrhythmias arising from the myocardium afflicted by coronary heart disease were largely engendered by sympathetic stimulation of beta-adrenoceptors in the subendocardium. However, the exciting possibility now exists that acutely ischaemic myocardium may also be the transient seat of receptors which are pharmacologically identical to alpha-adrenoceptors [5, 27]; this affords a potential role for alpha-adrenoceptor blockade in the occlusion and reperfusion phases of myocardial infarction. Experimental evidence now exists which clearly demonstrates the beneficial anti-arrhythmic effects of combined alpha-beta-adrenoceptor blockade in this emergency situation [27].

Labetalol exerts only weak membrane stabilising activity but possesses substantial Class I and perhaps Class III anti-arrhythmic activity [28]. The drug has also been demonstrated to increase the functional refractory period in the atrio-ventricular node and ventricles and to eliminate both catecholmine and ouabain-induced arrhythmias in the experimental animal. It also appears to enhance the maintenance of levels of high energy phosphate with the consequence that lactate and adenosine concentrations are significantly lower in ischaemic myocardium when compared to hearts not treated by the drug [29]. These findings indicate that labetalol may prove to be an effective agent in the prevention and treatment of ventricular arrhythmias associated with acute myocardial ischaemia [30]. The proportionate role of alpha- and beta-adrenoceptor stimulation in the genesis of arrhythmias arising in patients with stable coronary heart disease (angina pectoris) is at present unknown but unlikely to be substantially different from that observed in the more acute syndrome of myocardial infarction.

Non-cardiovascular Aspects

Combined alpha-beta-adrenoceptor blockade with labetalol does not appear to induce any deleterious changes in the lipoprotein cholesterol profile during either short-term or long-term administration [31, 32]. Combined alpha-beta-adrenoceptor blockade likewise does not appear to have any clinically consistent effects on fasting blood glucose concentration, basal insulin activity or its response to oral glucose load, either in normal or non-insulin requiring diabetics [33].

Chronic oral treatment with labetalol also does not appear to increase plasma or urinary adrenaline or noradrenaline concentrations [34]. Chronic alpha-beta-adrenoceptor blockade with labetalol also appears to reduce basal plasma renin activity and attenuate its increase during exercise [35]. Prevention in the release of renin is associated with significant reductions in angiotensin II concentration and in plasma aldosterone.

Alpha-adrenoceptor blocking drugs appear to have some bronchodilating activity which could be expected to offset the bronchoconstriction resulting from blockade of beta-2 adrenoceptors in the bronchii [36]. A number of investigative studies in man support this concept, but due to the potent beta-blocking activity of labetalol it should be avoided in patients with frank bronchial asthma.

In concept, combined alpha-beta-adrenoceptor blockade could also be expected to have a balanced effect on renal function. Beta-blockade alone usually diminishes renal plasma flow and glomerular filtration rate, whereas alpha-adrenoceptor activity usually increases renal blood flow and excretory function. Labetalol has no depressive effect on renal haemodynamics or excretory function [37]. It appears, therefore, that the concomitant alpha-blocking activity of the drug offsets the potentially deleterious effects of beta-blockade alone on renal excretory function.

References

[1]   Final Mortality Statistics, 1978. National Centre for Health Statistics: DHSS Publication (PHS) 80–1120, **29**, No. 6, Suppl. 2, 1980

[2]   Hjort, P. F. and Waaler, H. T. (1984): What is the economic impact of secondary prevention to society? *Eur Heart J.* **5**: (Suppl A) (In press)

[3]   Taylor, S. H.: Secondary prevention after myocardial infarction: facts and fallacies. *J. Cardiovasc. Pharmacol.* (In press)

[4]   Majid, P.A., Meeran, M.K., Benaim, M.E., Sharma, G. and Taylor, S.H. (1974): Alpha and beta-adrenergic receptor blockade in the treatment of hypertension. *Br. Heart J.* **36**, 588

[5]   Farmer, J.B., Kennedy, I., Levy, G.P. and Marshall, R.J. (1972): Pharmacology of AH 5158, a drug which blocks both alpha- and beta-adrenoceptors. *Br. J. Clin. Pharmacol.* **45**, 660

[6]   Richards, D.A. (1976): Pharmacologic effects of labetalol in man. *Br. J. Clin. Pharmacol.* **3**: (Suppl. 3), 721

[7]   Taylor, S.H.: The circulatory consequences of heart failure and shock. In: *Recent Advances in Cardiology* — 6th Edition. Ed: Hamer, J., Churchill Livingston, Edinburgh/London, 1974

[8]   Guthrie, R.B., Vlodaver, Z., Nicoloff, D.M. and Edwards, J.E. (1975): Pathology of stable and unstable angina pectoris. *Circulation* **53**: 823

[9]   Parker, J.O., Digiorgi, S., West, R.O. (1966): A haemodynamic study of acute coronary insufficiency precipitated by exercise. *Am. J. Cardiol.* **17**, 470

[10] Sharma, B. and Taylor, S.H. (1970): Reversible left ventricular failure in angina pectoris. *Lancet* ii, 902

[11] Sharma, B., Goodwin, J.F., Raphael, M.J., Steiner, R.E., Rainbow, R.G. and Taylor, S.H. (1976): Left ventricular angiography on exercise: a new method of assessing left ventricular function in ischaemic heart disease. *Br. Heart. J.* **38**, 59

[12] Sharma, B., Majid, P.A., Meeran, M.K., Whitaker, W. and Taylor, S.H. (1972): Clinical, electrocardiographic and haemodynamic effects of digitalis (ouabain) in angina pectoris. *Br. Heart. J.* **34**, 631

[13] Barry, W.H., Brooker, J.Z., Alderman, E.L. and Harrison, D.C. (1974): Changes in diastolic stiffness and tone of the left ventricle during angina pectoris. *Circulation* **49**, 255

[14] Sharma, B. and Taylor, S.H. (1975): Localisation of left ventricular ischaemia in angina pectoris by cineangiography during exercise. *Br. Heart. J.* **37**, 963

[15] Taylor, S.H.: Pathophysiological approach to the treatment of angina pectoris. In: *Recent Developments in Cardiovascular Drugs*, Ed: J. Coltart and D. Jewitt. Churchill Livingstone, Edinburgh/London/Melbourne/New York, 1982

[16] Braunwald, E. (1969): Thirteenth Bowditch Lecture. The determinants of myocardial oxygen consumption. *Physiologist* **12**, 65

[17] Linden, R.J. (1975): Reflexes from the heart. *Prog. Cardiovasc. Dis.* **18**, 201

[18] Taylor, S.H., Silke, B. and Nelson, G.I.C. (1982): Haemodynamic advantages of combined alpha-blockade and beta-blockade over beta-blockade alone in patients with coronary heart disease. *Br. Med. J.* **285**, 325

[19] Braunwald, E. (1978): Coronary artery spasm and acute myocardial infarction — a new possibility for treatment and prevention. *N. Eng. J. Med.* **299**, 1301

[20] Majid, P.A., Sharma, B., Taylor, S H. (1971): Phentolamine for vasodilator treatment of severe heart failure. *Lancet* ii, 719

[21] Maxwell, G.M. (1973): Effects of alpha- and beta-adrenoceptor antagonist (AH 5158) upon general and coronary haemodynamics of intact dogs. *Br. J. Pharmacol,* **44**, 370

[22] Chiariello, M., Brevitti, G., De Rosa, G. et al (1980): Protective effects of simultaneous alpha- and beta-adrenoceptor receptor blockade on myocardial cell necrosis after coronary occlusion in rats. *Am. J. Cardiol.* **46**, 249

[23] Marx, P. G. and Reid, D. S. (1979): Labetalol infusion in acute myocardial infarction with systemic hypertension. *Br. J. Clin. Pharmacol.* **8** (Suppl. 2), 233

[24] Timmis, A.D., Fowler, M.B., Jaggaro, N.S.V. (1982): Role of labetalol in acute myocardial infarction. *Br. J. Clin. Pharmacol.* **13** (Suppl. 1), 111

[25] Nelson, G.I.C., Silke, B., Ahuja, R.C., Hussain, M. and Taylor, S.H. (1983): Haemodynamic dose-response effects of intravenous labetalol in acute myocardial infarction. *Postgrad. Med. J.* **59** (Suppl. 3), 98

[26] Silke, B., Nelson, G.I.C., Ahuja, R.C., Choudhury, S. and Taylor, S.H. (1983): Pharmacokinetic and haemodynamic studies with labetalol in acute myocardial infarction. *Ir. J. Med. Sci.* **152**, 179

[27] Pogwizd, S.M., Sharma, A.D. and Corr, P.D. (1982): Influence of labetalol, a combined alpha- and beta-adrenergic blocking agent on the dysrhythmias induced by coronary occlusion and reperfusion. *Cardiovasc. Res.* **16**, 398

[28] Vaughan Williams, E.M., Millar, J.S. and Campbell, T.J. (1982): Electrophysiological effects of labetalol on rabbit atrial ventricular and Purkinje cells in normoxia and hypoxia. *Carciovasc. Res.* **16**, 233

[29] Lubke, W.F., Nguyen, T., Edward, M.F. (1983): Anti-arrhythmic action of labetalol and its effect on adenosine metabolism in the isolated rat heart. *J. Am. Coll. Cardiol.* **1**, 1296

[30] Mazzola, C., Ferrario, N. Calzavara, M.P. (1981): Acute antihypertensive and antiarrhythmic effects of labetalol. *Curr. Ther. Res.* **29**, 613

[31] Sommers, D.E.K., DeVilliers, L.S., Van Wyk, M., Schoeman, H.S. (1981): The effects of labetalol and oxprenolol on blood lipids. *S. Afr. Med. J.* **60**, 379

[32] Frishman, W., Michelson, E., Johnson, B. (1983): Effects of beta-adrenergic blockade on plasma lipids. *Am. J. Cardiol.* **49**, 984 (Abst)

[33] Andersson, O., Berglund, G., Hannson, L. (1976): Antihypertensive action, time of onset and effects on carbohydrate metabolism of labetalol. *Br. J. Clin. Pharmacol.* **3** (Suppl. 3), 757

[34] Keusch, G., Weidmann, P., Zugler, W.H. (1980): Effects of chronic alpha- and beta-adrenoceptor blockade with labetalol on plasma catecholamines and renal function in hypertension. *Klin. Wochenschr.* **58**, 25

[35] Lijnen, P. J., Amery, A. K., and Fagard, R. H. (1979): Effects of labetalol on plasma renin aldosterone and catecholamines in hypertensive patients. *J. Cardiovasc. Pharmacol.* **1**, 625

[36] Patel, K.R., and Kerr, J.W. (1975): Alpha-receptor blocking drugs in bronchial asthma. *Lancet* i, 348

[37] Rasmussen, S., Nielsen, P.E. (1981): Blood pressure, body fluid volumes and glomerular filtration rate during treatment with labetalol in essential hypertension. *Br. J. Clin. Pharmacol.* **12**, 349

Discussion

Borchard
Haben Sie Hinweise, daß die Kombination von Alpha- und Betablockern durch die alphaadrenale Blockade in der Lage ist, das Labetalol bei Patienten mit „Variant angine" einzusetzen?

Taylor
The answer to that is not known. The evidence for the usefulness of a variety of drugs in this condition, particularly alpha-blockers and beta-blockers, either is unsatisfactory or no benefit was seen. With regards to labetalol, I know of no study which has been specifically designed to look into that problem. Perhaps we should ask the speakers who are going to talk to us later in this field.

Pathophysiological Mechanisms of Alpha-Adrenoceptor Stimulation in the Ischemic Heart

P. B. Corr, K. A. Yamada
Cardiovascular Division, Washington University School of Medicine, 660 South Euclid Avenue, St. Louis, Missouri 63110, U.S.A.

Data derived from both multicenter clinical trials and experimental animals indicate that β-adrenergic stimulation of the myocardium can increase the propensity to malignant arrhythmias and that β-adrenergic blockade significantly reduces the incidence of sudden cardiac death [4, 19, 32, 34]. Despite these important findings, a very large number of patients taking β-adrenergic blocking agents post-myocardial infarction die, presumably of sudden death secondary to abnormalities in cardiac rhythm [4, 19, 32, 34]. In this brief review, we will consider recent experimental evidence from our laboratory and others indicating that in the ischemic heart, the effects of catecholamines may be mediated through stimulation of α-, as well as β-adrenergic receptors. These findings may be relevant not only to arrhythmogenesis but, to the development of irreversible injury in the ischemic and reperfused heart, due to the recently recognized effect of α-adrenergic stimulation on myocardial calcium.

Experimental animal studies have reported increased plasma catecholamines [37], increased catecholamine release from the heart [24] and increased efferent sympathetic nerve activity during acute myocardial ischemia and infarction [16]. The role of this sympathetic activation in the genesis of fatal ventricular arrhythmias is currently under active investigation.

Adrenergic Receptor Blockade and Arrhythmogenesis

Since the release of catecholamines in the ischemic and reperfused heart occurs through a number of different mechanisms, adrenergic receptor blockade would appear to be the most promising approach. During myocardial ischemia, β-adrenergic blockade reduces the incidence of arrhythmias in most experimental studies, but appears to be less effective in reducing the incidence of ventricular fibrillation [8]. In contrast, blockade of β-adrenergic receptors without direct membrane effects is uniformly ineffective in altering the arrhythmias associated with reperfusion in a number of different animal species [5, 40, 43].

Research from the authors' laboratory was supported by National Institutes of Health Grants HL-17646, SCOR in Ischemic Heart Disease, grant HL-28995 and by RR00396 from the Division of Research Resources. This work was done during the tenure of an Established Investigatorship (Dr. Corr), of the American Heart Association and with funds contributed in part by the Missouri Heart Affiliate.

In contrast to the variable effectiveness of β-adrenergic blockade, recent results from our laboratory and others suggest that the electrophysiological effects of catecholamines in the ischemic and reperfused heart can be mediated in part through stimulation of α-adrenergic receptors. This conclusion is derived from data obtained in a number of different species both *in vivo* and *in vitro*. For example, either non-specific α_1- and α_2-adrenergic blockade with phentolamine, specific α_1-adrenergic blockade with prazosin, and myocardial catecholamine depletion, all markedly reduced the incidence of ventricular fibrillation associated with coronary occlusion and reperfusion in the cat [40]. Similar antiarrhythmic effects have also been demonstrated in our laboratory using labetalol, a combined α- and β-adrenergic blocking agent [35] and BE2254, a specific water soluble α_1-adrenergic blocking agent. The beneficial antiarrhythmic effects of α-adrenergic blockade were independent of hemodynamic alterations including differences in heart rate, mean arterial pressure, left ventricular end diastolic pressure, cardiac output, peak dP/dt and stroke work [35, 40], as well as independent of changes in regional coronary blood flow assessed using radiolabeled microspheres in the ischemic and reperfused heart [40]. The antiarrhythmic effects of prazosin in the cat during ischemia have been reported by others, using lower doses [11] and in the dog, intravenous [41] or intracoronary [45] phentolamine also attenuates the incidence of ventricular arrhythmias associated with reperfusion of the ischemic region. The effects obtained with phentolamine alone need to be viewed with caution since this agent can also result in cholinergic blockade, inhibit the action of tyramine and potentiate the action of norepinephrine on isolated guinea pig atrium and in higher doses, induce direct membrane effects independent of any interaction with the adrenergic receptor [38].

Opie and colleagues have recently assessed the effects of adrenergic blockade in the isolated perfused rat heart with a 15 minute ligation of the left anterior descending coronary artery followed by reperfusion [43]. Although this isolated perfused heart preparation was non-working and not directly innvervated, one major advantage includes the 100 % incidence of ventricular fibrillation during reperfusion. In this preparation, α_2-adrenergic blockade with yohimbine exhibited the greatest antiarrhythmic efficacy, with phentolamine and prazosin producing comparable antiarrhythmic effects at higher doses, and β-adrenergic blockade producing antiarrhythmic effects only at doeses far in excess of those required for adequate β-adrenergic blockade [43].

Thus, the antiarrhythmic effects of α-adrenergic blockade has now been confirmed by several groups of investigators using different species. Subsequent work in our laboratory has centered on elucidating the electrophysiological effects of α-adrenergic stimulation in the ischemic heart as well as the mechanisms responsible for the recently recognized effects of α-adrenergic blockade on calcium movement in the reperfused heart.

Potential Mechanisms Responsible for Enhanced α-Adrenergic Responsivity

Myocardial α-adrenergic effects were first demonstrated by a prolongation of atrial refractory period [18]. Subsequently, it has been demonstrated *in vitro* that α-adrenergic stimulation decreases Purkinje fiber automaticity [38] and *in vivo* decreases idioventricular [20] and sinus node rate [21]. There is also a prolongation of Purkinje fiber action potential duration *in vitro* [17]. In depressed tissue, there is evidence to suggest that α-adrenergic mediated effects are very different. For example, in rabbit papillary muscle depolarized by elevated $(K^+)_0$, α-adrenergic stimulation augments the slow inward current (I_{si}) [28]. Analogous findings are seen in bovine ventricular muscle [6]. *In vivo*, the augmentation of contractility produced by stellate nerve stimulation is mediated by α-adrenergic receptors in the ischemic region but by β-adrenergic receptors in the normal zone [22]. Both of these α-adrenergic mediated effects may involve modulation of intracellular calcium. In the cat, reperfusion after coronary occlusion results in an increased idioventricular rate, which can be prevented by α-adrenergic blockade or catecholamine depletion with 6-hydroxy-dopamine [40]. Likewise, in animals depleted of myocardial catecholamines, the idioventricular rate can be increased on reperfusion by methoxamine, an α-agonist [40]. In contrast, in normal cats the idioventricular rate may only be increased by β-adrenergic stimulation. Thus, there is evidence to suggest that α-adrenergic stimulation may result in electrophysiologcial derangements peculiar to myocardial ischemia and reperfusion but not readily apparent in normal tissue. This may, in part, be secondary to the increase in number of α_1-adrenergic receptors in ischemic tissue [10] and may explain the potent antiarrhythmic efficacy of α-adrenergic blocking agents in the setting of acute myocardial ischemia and subsequent reperfusion.

The mechanisms responsible for the apparent increased sensitivity of the myocardium to α-adrenergic stimulation may be related to alterations in adrenergic receptors. In the cat, 30 min of myocardial ischemia is associated with a two-fold increase in the density of α_1-adrenergic receptors confined to the ischemic region, with no alteration in receptor affinity [10]. This increased α-adrenergic receptor number is present when reperfusion occurs at 35 min after occlusion and is associated with increased α-adrenergic responsivity of the tissue assessed electrophysiologically which appears to contribute to the onset of malignant arrhythmias [40]. The increase in α_1-adrenergic receptors returns to control levels with sustained reperfusion with a time course which corresponds to the decrease in α-adrenergic responsivity [10, 40]. In the dog, both α_1-adrenergic [30] and β-adrenergic receptor number [31] increases in ischemic myocardium, although the increase in β-receptor number does not occur until 1 hour after occlusion. At this time, the increase in β-receptor number was associated with an increase in the tissue production of cyclic AMP and phosphorylase kinase activity in response to isoproterenol [31]. Thus, adrenergic receptor alterations during ischemia suggest that augmented tissue responsivity to both α- and β-adrenergic receptor stimulation may occur during ischemia. The effect of ischemia on the coupling of α-receptors to intracellular mediators remains to be determined.

α-Adrenergic Stimulation and Calcium Accumulation

Several lines of evidence suggest that the effects of α-adrenergic stimulation of the myocardium during ischemia and reperfusion may be mediated through an increase in calcium movement into the cell. First, in partially depolarized myocardium *in vivo*, α-adrenergic stimulation potentiates the calcium mediated I_{si} (6,28). Second, in the ischemic dog heart *in vivo*, the positive inotropic effect of catecholamines is mediated through α-adrenergic stimulation in the ischemic region and β-adrenergic stimulation in the adjacent normal myocardium [22]. Third, several studies have demonstrated an interaction between α-adrenergic receptors and calcium antagonists which appears to parallel their antiarrhythmic potency [9, 29, 33]. Fourth, there is substantial evidence that α-adrenergic stimulation increases cytosolic calcium in a number of other tissues including vascular smooth muscle [12], liver [15], nerve [1] and parotid gland [36]. Fifth, a recent study demonstrated that a catecholamine induced cardiomyopathy was mediated through stimulation of α-

adrenergic receptors, associated with increased calcium uptake [13]. Sixth, recent preliminary findings indicate that lowering the perfusate calcium in isolated hearts result in an antifibrillatory effect during reperfusion [44].

In a recently completed series of studies, we demonstrated an important role for α-adrenergic stimulation in the movement of calcium into reversibly injured tissue during reperfusion [39]. After 35 minutes of ischemia, reperfusion resulted in a two-fold increase in total tissue calcium. Pretreatment with either phentolamine or prazosin completely prevented the increase in total tissue calcium [39]. In contrast, propranolol reduced but did not prevent the rise in total tissue calcium. Calculated intracellular calcium was determined by measurements of the extracellular space (^{3}H-inulin) and blood volume (^{51}-Cr-RBC). Although 35 minutes of ischemia and 10 minutes reperfusion increased the apparent extracellular space by 10 % of total tissue volume, the calculated intracellular calcium increased by 160 % accounting for most of the observed increase in total tissue calcium. Phentolamine and prazosin administered prior to ischemia prevented both the increase in extracellular space and intracellular calcium [39].

Since the α-adrenergic blocking agents were administered prior to ischemia, the treatment may have reduced the severity of ischemia and thereby contributed to the beneficial effect. However, administration of either phentolamine or the water soluble α_1-specific agent BE2254 after 33 minutes of ischemia, just two minutes prior to reperfusion also completely prevented the increase in intracellular calcium associated with reperfusion [39]. To assess the subcellular localization of calcium, tissue was fixed with osmium tetroxide and calcium precipitated by potassium pyroantimonate, and sections taken for electron microscopy. Reperfused tissue showed numerous precipitates of calcium antimonate in mitochondria and the presence of calcium was verified by x-ray microprobe analysis of these precipitates and by prevention of granule formation by perfusion with EGTA during fixation. Although the tissue did not demonstrate evidence of irreversible injury, there was evidence of antecedant ischemia in the form of glycogen depletion. Animals pretreated with phentolamine and rendered ischemic did not demonstrate any mitochondrial calcium precipitates although there was evidence of glycogen depletion. Thus, based on several lines of evidence, α-adrenergic blockade specifically prevented uptake of calcium by the reversibly injured myocyte during reperfusion. In contrast, when the ischemic period was lengthened to 70 minutes, α-adrenergic blockade only partially prevented the increase in total tissue calcium. Light microscopy of the tissue revealed patchy evidence of irreversible damage, suggesting that α-adrenergic blockade was effective in reversibly ischemic but not irreversibly damaged tissue [39].

Mechanism of α-Adrenergic Mediated Calcium Uptake During Reperfusion

Sarcolemmal calcium influx may occur via the slow inward current (I_{si}), sodium-calcium exchange, passive diffusion, via endogenous calcium ionophores and possibly through potassium-calcium exchange. In contrast, calcium efflux may occur via sodium calcium exchange and the active transport of calcium.

Influx

The I_{si} has been studied using voltage-clamp techniques and ion substitution. The I_{si} is characterized as both voltage and time-dependent with a threshold of approximately -50 mV [27]. The channels show selectivity for Ca^{+2} over the cations Na^+, K^+ or Mg^{+2}

and the extent to which it contributes to calcium transport is estimated to be 1 pmol/ beat/cm^2 [3]. The magnitude of the I_{si} increases with increases in $(Ca^{+2})_0$ and decreases with increases in $(Ca^{+2})_i$. Under physiological conditions, epinephrine augments the I_{si} via stimulation of β-adrenergic receptors, as similar results are produced by isoproterenol, a relatively pure β-adrenergic agonist, and β-adrenergic blockade reduces the magnitude of the I_{si} [27]. The channel mediating the I_{si} may be blocked both by the inorganic compounds Cd^{2+} Co^{+2}, Mn^{+2}, La^{+3}, and Ni^{+3} as well as by several organic calcium antagonists. Studies using ^{3}H-nitrendipine binding to cardiac membranes indicates that the relative affinity of these organic compounds for the voltage dependent calcium channel is greatest for nifedipine with lower affinities for verapamil and diltiazem [14]. The order of affinity of these compounds for the α_1-receptor is opposite, with verapamil exhibiting the greatest potency [9, 29, 33]. This suggests that the α_1-adrenergic receptor is probably not interacting with the voltage dependent calcium channel.

Evidence indicates that sodium-calcium exchange may be a major mechanism responsible for the influx of calcium in the myocardial cell [2]. Cellular uptake of $^{45}Ca^{2+}$ has been measured in isolated myocytes in culture and found to increase with decreases in $(Na)_0$ or increases in $(Na)_i$. Consistent with Na-Ca exchange, the slow channel blocking agent verapamil failed to significantly modulate this $^{45}Ca^{2+}$ uptake [2]. Sodium-calcium exchange has also been examined using ion sensitive intracellular microelectrodes [23]. Simultaneous measurements of the activity of sodium (aNa_i) and calcium (aCa_i) have demonstrated that Na-Ca exchange is coupled in a ratio of 2.5 [23]. Thus, Na-Ca exchange appears to be electrogenic with a net transfer of current into the cell, and if the carrier system is reversible it would be expected to be variable with the level of the transmembrane potential.

Since the free calcium concentration in the interstitial space is approximately 10,000 fold higher than that found in the intracellular compartment assessed by either microelectrodes, Arzenazo III or aqueorin [25], the potential exists for passive diffusion of calcium into the cell. Fortunately, passive diffusion across the sarcolemma is small, but following irreversible myocardial necrosis, loss of sarcolemmal integrity may allow passive accumulation of calcium. Similarly, during ischemia or evolving infarction, calcium influx may be augmented by the presence of agents such as prostaglandins which can experimentally act as endogenous calcium ionophores [42]. This may be particularly important since recent observations indicate that infarcted myocardium possesses a greatly increased capacity to metabolize arachidonic acid to prostaglandin products [26]. Finally, evidence suggests that potassium-calcium exchange may also contribute to the influx of calcium, although the precise role in maintenance of intracellular calcium has not been defined.

Efflux

One major mechanism responsible for efflux is sodium-calcium exchange [25]. This mechanism results in calcium efflux during diastole when $(Na)_i$ is relatively low and the membrane potential is negative. There is also evidence, though indirect, for active transport of calcium out of the cell. In support of this mechanism, binding within sarcolemmal vesicles occurs coincident with Mg^{2+}-dependent-ATP hydrolysis, and as a result, calcium is actively taken up by the vesicle [7]. Both mechanisms of calcium efflux would be expected to be depressed during myocardial ischemia, sodium-calcium exchange by the increased intracellular sodium and loss of membrane potential and active calcium transport out of the cell due to the fall in cellular ATP. Therefore, sodium-calcium exchange is likely to play a major role in calcium uptake that occurs on reperfusion and the effect of α-adrenergic blockade in modulating calcium by this mechanism will require investigation.

Conclusion

Clinical and experimental evidence demonstrates an important role of adrenergic stimulation in the genesis of fatal arrhythmias secondary to ischemia and reperfusion. There is experimental evidence to show that β-adrenergic blockade reduces the incidence of arrhythmias associated with ischemia but not reperfusion. α-adrenergic blockade has demonstrated considerable efficacy in the prevention of arrhythmias associated with both ischemia and reperfusion. The potent arrhythmogenic effects of α-adrenergic stimulation may be due to the recently recognized reversible increase in α_1-adrenergic receptors during ischemia and early reperfusion. One of the major manifestations of α-adrenergic stimulation during reperfusion appears to be enhanced myocardial calcium uptake, potentially contributing to both malignant arrhythmias and myocardial cell damage.

References

[1]   Atlas, D., Adler, M.: α-adrenergic antagonists as possible calcium channel inhibitors. *Proc. Nat'l. Acad. Sci. (USA)* **78**, 1237–1242 (1981).

[2]   Barry, W.H., Smith, T.W.: Mechanisms of transmembrane calcium movements in cultured chick embryo ventricular cells. *J. Physiol. (Lond.)* **325**, 243–260 (1982).

[3]   Beeler, G.W., Reuter, H.: Membrane calcium current in ventricular myocardial fibers. *J. Physiol. (Lond.)* **207**, 191–209 (1970).

[4]   Beta-Blocker Heart Attack Study Group. The beta-blocker heart attack trial. *J. Am. Med. Assoc.* **246**, 2073–2074 (1981).

[5]   Brooks, W.W., Verrier, R.L., Lown, B.: Protective effect of verapamil on vulnerability to ventricular fibrillation during myocardial ischemia and reperfusion. *Cardiovasc. Res.* **14**, 295–302 (1980).

[6]   Bruchner, R., Scholz, H.: Effects of phenylephrine in the presence of propranolol on slow potentials in mammalian ventricular fibers. *Naunyn Schmied. Arch. Pharmacol.* **311**, R37 (1980) (abstract).

[7]   Caroni, P., Carafoli, E.: An ATP-dependent Ca^{2+}-pumping system in dog heart sarcolemma. *Nature* **283**, 765–767 (1980).

[8]   Corr, P.B., Gillis, R.A.: Autonomic neural influences on the dysrhythmias resulting from myocardial infarction. *Circ. Res.* **43**, 1–9 (1978).

[9]   Corr, P.B., Sharma, A.D.: Alpha-adrenergic mediated effects on myocardial calcium. In: *Calcium Antagonists and Cardiovascular Disease*. Edited by L.H. Opie, Raven Press, New York, pp 193–204 (1984).

[10] Corr, P.B., Shayman, J.A., Kramer, J.B., Kipnis, R.J.: Increased α-adrenergic receptors in ischemic cat myocardium: a potential mediator of electrophysiological derangements. *J. Clin. Invest.* **67**, 1232–1236 (1981).

[11] Davey, M.J.: Relevant features of the pharmacology of prazosin. *J. Cardiovasc. Pharm.* **2**, S287–S301 (1980).

[12] Deth, R., van Breeman, C.: Relative contributions of Ca^{2+} influx and cellular Ca^{2+} release during drug induced activation of the rabbit aorta. *Pflugers Arch.* **348**, 13–22 (1974).

[13] Downing, S.E., Lee, J.C.: Contribution of α-adrenergic activation to the pathogenesis of norepinephrine cardiomyopathy. *Circulation Res.* **52**, 471–478 (1983).

[14] Ehlert, E.J., Roeske, W.R., Hoga, E., Yamamura, H.I.: The binding of ^{3}H Nitrendipine to receptors for calcium channel antagonists in the heart, cerebral cortex, and ileum of rats. *Life Sciences* **30**, 2191–2202 (1982).

[15] Exton, J.H.: Molecular mechanisms involved in α-adrenergic responses. *Mol. Cell. Endocrinol.* **23**, 233–264 (1981).

[16] Gillis, R.A.: Role of the nervous system in the arrhythmias produced by coronary occlusion in the cat. *Am. Heart J.* **81**, 677–684 (1971).

[17] Giotti, A., Ledda, F., Mannaioni, P.F.: Effects of noradrenaline and isoprenaline, in combination with α- und β-receptor blocking substances, on the action potential of cardiac Purkinje fibers. *J. Physiol. (Lond.)* **229**, 99–113 (1973).

[18] Govier, W.C.: Prolongation of myocardial functional refractory period by phenylephrine. *Life Sci.* **6**, 1367–1371 (1967).

[19] Herlitz, J., Malek, I., Ryden, L. Effect on mortality of metroprolol in acute myocardial infarction: a double-blind randomized trial. *Lancet.* **II**, 823–827 (1981).

[20] Hordof, A.J., Rose, E., Danilo, P., Jr., Rosen, M.R.: α- and β-adrenergic effects of epinephrine on ventricular pacemakers in dogs. *Am. J. Physiol.* **242**, 677–682 (1982).

[21] James, T.N., Bear, E.S., Lang, K.F., Green, E.W.: Evidence for adrenergic alpha-receptor depressant activity in the heart. *Am. J. Physiol.* **215**, 1366–1375 (1968).

[22] Juhasz-Nagy, A., Aviado, D.M.: Increased role of alpha-adrenoceptors in ischemic myocardial zones. *Physiologist* **19**, 245 (1976) (abstract).

[23] Lado, M.G., Sheu, S-S., Fozzard, H.A.: Changes in intracellular Ca^{2+} activity with stimulation in sheep cardiac Purkinje strands. *Am. J. Physiol.* **243**, H133–H137 (1982).

[24] Lammerant, J., DeHerdt, P., DeSchryner, C.: Direct release of myocardial catecholamines into left heart chambers: The enhancing effect of acute coronary occlusion. *Arch. Int. Pharmacodyn.* **163**, 219–226 (1966).

[25] Langer, G.A.: Sodium-calcium exchange in the heart. *Ann Rev. Physiol.* **44**, 435–449 (1982).

[26] McClusky, E.R., Corr, P.B., Lee, B.I., Saffitz, J.E., Needleman, P.: The arachidonic acid metabolic capacity of canine myocardium is increased during healing of acute myocardial infarction. *Circulation Res.* **51**, 743–750 (1982).

[27] McDonald, T.R.: The slow inward current in the heart. *Ann. Rev. Physiol.* **44**, 425–434 (1982).

[28] Miura, Y., Inui, J., Imamura, H.: Alpha-adrenoceptor-mediated restoration of calcium dependent potentials in the partially depolarized rabbit papillary muscle. *Naunyn Schmied. Arch. Pharmacol.* **301**, 201–205 (1978).

[29] Motulsky, H.J., Snavely, M.D., Hughes, R.J., Insel, P.A.: Interaction of verapamil and other calcium channel blockers with α_1- and α_2-adrenergic receptors. *Circulation Res.* **52**, 226–231 (1983).

[30] Mukherjee, A., Hogan, M., Mc Coy, K., Buja, I-M., Willerson, J.T.: Influence of experimental myocardial ischemia on alpha$_1$-adrenergic receptors. *Circulation* **64** (Suppl. III), 149 (1980), abstract.

[31] Mukherjee, A., Bush, L.R., McCoy, K.E., Duke, R.J., Hagler, H., Buja, L.M., Willerson, J.T.: Relationship between β-adrenergic receptor numbers and physiological responses during experimental canine myocardial ischemia. *Circ. Res.* **50**, 735–741 (1982).

[32] Multicenter International Study: Improvement in prognosis of myocardial infarction by long-term beta-adrenoreceptor blockade using practolol. *Br. Med. J.* **3**, 735–740 (1975).

[33] Nayler, W.G., Thompson, J.E., Jarrott, B.: The interaction of calcium antagonists (slow channel blockers) with myocardial alpha-adrenoceptors. *J. Mol. Cell. Cardiol.* **14**, 185–188 (1982).

[34] Norwegian Multicenter Study Group.: Timolol-induced reduction in mortality and reinfarction. *N. Engl. J. Med.* **304**, 801–807 (1981).

[35] Pogwizd, S.M., Sharma, A.D., Corr, P.B.: The influences of labetalol, a combined α- and β-adrenergic blocking agent on the dysrhythmias induced by coronary occlusion and reperfusion. *Cardiovasc. Res.* **16**, 398–407 (1982).

[36] Putney, J.W.: Stimulus-permeability coupling: Role of calcium in the regulation of membrane permeability. *Pharmacol. Rev.* **30**, 209–245 (1979).

[37] Richardson, J.A., Woods, E.F., Bagwell, E.E.: Circulating epinephrine and norepinephrine in coronary occlusion. *Am. J. Cardiol.* **5**, 613–618 (1960).

[38] Rosen, M.R., Hordof, A.J., Ilvento, J.P., Danilo, P., Jr.: Effects of adrenergic amines on electrophysiological properties and automaticity of neonatal and adult Purkinje fibers. *Circ. Res.* **40**, 390–400 (1977).

[39] Sharma, A.D., Saffitz, J.E., Lee, B.I., Sobel, B.E., Corr, P.B.: α-adrenergic mediated accumulation of calcium in reperfused myocardium. *J. Clin. Invest.* **72**, 802–818 (1983).

[40] Sheridan, D. J., Penkoske, P. A., Sobel, B. E., Corr, P. B.: Alpha-adrenergic contributions to dysrhythmia during myocardial ischemia and reperfusion in cats. *J. Clin. Invest.* **65**, 161–171 (1980).

[41] Stewart, J. R., Burmeister, W. E., Burmeister, J., Lucchesi, B. R.: Electrophysiologic and anti-arrhythmic effects of phentolamine in experimental coronary artery occlusion and reperfusion in the dog. *J. Cardiovasc. Pharmacol.* **2**, 77–91 (1980).

[42] Sugiyama, S., Norimatsu, I., Takayuki, O.: Possible roles of prostaglandins and calcium in ventricular vulnerability during coronary reperfusion. *J. Appl. Biochem.* **1**, 402–409 (1979).

[43] Thandroyen, F. T., Worthington, M. G., Higginson, L. M., Opie, L. H.: The effect of alpha- and beta-adrenoceptor antagonist agents on reperfusion ventricular fibrillation and metabolic status in the isolated perfused rat heart. *J. Am. Coll. Cardiol.* **1**, 1056–1066 (1983).

[44] Thandroyen, F. T., Opie, L. H.: Reduction in extracellular calcium ion concentration prevents reperfusion ventricular fibrillation. *J. Amer. Coll. Cardiol.* **3**, 586 (1984), (abstract).

[45] Williams, L. T., Guerrero, J. L., Leinbach, R. C. Prevention of reperfusion dysrhythmia by selective coronary alpha-adrenergic blockade. *Am. J. Cardiol.* **49**, 1046 (1982) (abstract).

Discussion

Scholz
Manche Tiere bzw. einige Spezies haben nicht gut ausgebildete Alpharezeptoren. Z. B. Hund, Meerschweinchen. Offen ist dabei die Zahl oder die Funktion der Rezeptoren. In ihrer Abb. nimmt innerhalb von 30 Minuten nach Reperfusion die Zahl der Alpha-Adrenozeptoren ungefähr um den Faktor 2 zu. Um welche Spezies handelt es sich— Ist das nicht unvorstellbar, daß innerhalb von 30 Minuten ein neuer Rezeptor entsteht, oder kann es sein, daß Bindungsstellen für vorhandene Rezeptoren durch die Ischämie geschaffen werden?

Corr
The slide did show a change in alpha-1-adrenoceptors within 30 minutes. I might point out that the changes in the receptors actually occur earlier than that. We now know, using techniques where we can freeze the tissue instantly and look radiographically at the receptors, that the increase is much earlier. The slide that I showed here was the very early work, where in the isolation of the tissue, you produce some reversibility of the receptors and they go back to the control levels.
Your second question; How can the receptor simply be exposed so quickly? In the slide that I showed with the isolated myosides, all receptors are exposed within minutes. Presumeably there are latent receptors in the membrane. They are certainly not being synthesized and transported to the membrane. They are simply being exposed. There are many precedents for that happening. We know from studies in human beings, for example giving catecholamines and looking at peripheral lympocytes, that the receptors can be exposed in 15 or 20 minutes. Whether these are functionally important receptors in the heart needs to be determined. That is what we are doing now. I have not proven that these exposed receptors are functionally coupled, but they appear to have the same characteristics as the normal receptors on the cell. I might point out that during ischemia alpha-1-adrenergic receptors go up in the dog as well. Wilson and collegues have shown that. I agree with you that they are very low in the normal dog heart; they are very low in the normal cat heart; very low in many species, but the point is that ischemia apparently can expose the receptor sites.

Woodcock
I have a comment to make which is relevant to this question of activation of the alpha-adrenoceptors. About 14 years ago I published results of experimental work on rats treated for about 6 weeks with a protein deficient diet. At the end of this period we found that there was an increase in the activity of membrane-bound enzymes isolated from the liver microsomes. The cause of this increase in activity was due to the large increase in lysophosphatides which had occured during the treatment period. Of course, a protein deficient liver is not an ischemic heart, but both are abnormal tissues, and in both there are changes occuring in metabolism. One can produce this increase in liver enzyme activities by simply adding the lysophosphatides to the enzyme *in vitro*. The stimulation in activity is something like 5-fold, and this occurs immediately. One can concieve of a similar sort of effect occuring in the cardiac tissue, providing that the lysophosphatides can be liberated at the time of ischemia.

Jahrmärker
I have two questions. First, your data on calcium seems to be a plea for calcium antagonists. Can you give a statement on which events can be prevented by calcium antagonists and which not? Secondly, you had an increase in irritability and idio-ventricular rate following vagal stimulation and stellate ganglion stimulation. This is in contrast to many findings which show lowering of irritability and an increase in fibrillation-threshold following vagal stimulation under these conditions because the balance between sympathetic and vagal stimulation is changed.

Corr
During vagal stimulation the idio-ventricular rate was only about 60 beats per minute. That was our way to measure the idio-ventricular rate. It was very low and then it went up in response to sympathetic stimulation. So vagal stimulation was used to enable us look at the instrinsic idio-ventricular rate. The literature would suggest that calcium antagonists, particularly nifedipine, given at the time of reperfusion, will not influence the calcium movement that occurs into the reperfused irreversibly injured tissue. Nifedipine however, given prior to ischemia, will protect against the movement of calcium during subsequent reperfusion. Those two points suggest that the protective influence is because it delayed the development of tissue ischemia during the ischemia interval. We have assessed the effects of specific calcium antagonists in this model. I might point out that several calcium antagonists are also alpha-adrenergic-blocking agents. The best known is probably verapamil. Verapamil at a concentration of 10^{-7} M, which is certainly comparable with what would occur in the myocardium, is a relatively potent alpha-adrenergic blocker. My answer would be that the movement of calcium through these cells is not simply movement through the voltage dependent calcium channel but is probably Ca^{++} movement through some other calcium channel that is controlled in some way by receptor stimulation, and I would suggest that may be that was the alpha-1-adrenergic receptor and that calcium antagonist likely to be effective in this sort of arena would be those that were also alpha-1-adrenergic blocking agents.

Palm
Could you please comment on the drug concentrations used to inhibit calcium uptake where you used labetalol, prazosin, propranolol and phentolamine.

Corr
Although we used higher and lower levels, the lowest level of prazosin that will work is 50 micrograms per kg. The concentration of phentolamine that will work at the lowest end is 0.7 mg, or 750 micrograms per kg because it is a relatively weaker alpha-blocker. What we attempt to do in each case is to go 3 times the dose ratio 10. So the drugs are comparable in terms of their relative alpha-adrenergic blocking level. The doses of the drugs vary, but the grade of alpha-blockade is similar across for each one. The dose of Ba 2254 is 0.2 mg per kg. These doses are in experimental animals and you can not obviously take a mg per kg basis and apply that to human beings.

Bahlmann
I would like to come back to the vagal stimulation. You know of the work using morphine before applying this kind of cardiac ischemia. The preventive effect on the sinister arrhythmias you mentioned was postulated to be due to vagal stimulation. How could this agree with the scheme you draw?

Corr
The vagal stimulation, I must point out again, was only used as a pulse stimulation of the vagus in order to find out what the intrinsic idio-ventricular rate was. We published studies nearly 12 years ago that showed also that vagal stimulation could be protective in the ischemia heart, but these that we used were only pulses to look at the intrinsic idio-ventricular rate. The other approach to measure the idio-ventricular rate would be the use of formalin injection into the vein and the problem with that is that you destroy the sympathetic fibres that cross through that area and you change the results of the stimulation, i.e., what you are trying to measure. That is the reason why we had to use vagal stimulation in the form of pulse-stimulation.

Bahlmann
The question still remains, how could you explain the beneficial effect of morphine in a system where you postulate that you must block alpha-1-receptors to get a beneficial result?

Corr

The easiest answer to that question would be that the acetylcholine release was affecting, and has been shown to affect, the release of catecholamines in the nerve endings. That may be one mechanism that is involved. There are obviously effects in several systems. Acetylcholine can affect calcium movement into cells, probably via the voltage sensitive calcium channel. Those would be two potential mechanisms.

N. N.

I think it is generally accepted that the beta-adrenoceptor is located on the outside of the cell membrane. Do we have any idea where the alpha-adrenoceptor is located? Is it within the cell membrane, is it on the inside of the cell membrane?

Corr

In the normal tissue it is on the outside of the membrane. We know that from autoradiographic studies. That is definitive. They are on the outside.

N. N.
Is it published?

Corr
Almost.

Beta-Adrenoceptor Blockers, Calcium Antagonists and Combined Alpha-Beta-Receptor Blockade in Coronary Heart Disease: Haemodynamic Profiles

G. Koch

Department of Clinical Physiology, Centrallasarettet, Karlskrona, Sweden, and Department of Physiology, Free University of Berlin, West-Berlin, FRG

Summary

Both beta-receptor blockers and calcium antagonists reduce angina and increase exercise tolerance in ischemic heart disease. Similar beneficial effects can be achieved a balanced blockade of both beta- and alpha-1-adrenoceptors. However, the underlying mechanisms differ profoundly. The hemodynamic responses at rest and during exercise elicited by the three regimens was evaluated in 3 matched groups of men with ischemic heart disease, mean age for the groups 55, 56 and 58 years. They were studied invasively at rest and during exercise, before and after single oral doses of metoprolol (100 mg), labetalol (200 mg) and nifedipine (10 mg). Metoprolol reduced mean arterial pressures, heart rate and cardiac output. Systemic vascular resistance and left ventricular filling pressure increased. Nifedipine treatment resulted under all conditions in a distinct decrease of systemic vascular resistance and arterial pressures, and a slight increase of heart rate and cardiac output. Left ventricular filling pressure was significantly reduced, the more the higher the initial level. The effect of labetalol was similar to that of nifedipine; however, cardiac output was unchanged, heart rate was slightly reduced. Left ventricular filling pressure was significantly lower.
Suppression of adrenergic stimulation by beta-receptor blockade alone may have adverse hemodynamic effects in ischemic heart disease with further functional deterioration. Converserly, both calcium and combined alpha-beta receptor blockade tend to improve left ventricular function mainly due to their vasodilator action on the precapillary resistance vessels. The results strongly suggest that in patients in whom beta-receptor blockers appear indicated, their adverse hemodynamic effects can be offset by concomitant alpha-1-receptor blockade or vasodilation without losing but rather enhancing symptomatic efficacy. Combined alpha-beta receptor blockade has the advantage over calcium antagonists alone of preventing any increase in adrenergic activity and related hyperkinetic responses.

Zusammenfassung

Beta-Rezeptoren-Blocker, Calcium-Antagonisten sowie eine gleichzeitige Blockade von Beta- und Alpha-Rezeptoren haben alle einen etwa gleich günstigen Einfluß auf Angina pectoris und Arbeitskapazität bei der koronaren Herzkrankheit. Die dieser günstigen Wirkung zugrunde liegenden Mechanismen unterscheiden sich jedoch stark. In drei vergleichbaren Gruppen von Patienten mit ischämischer Herzkrankheit (mittleres Alter 55, 56 und 58 Jahre) wurde untersucht, wie die Ruhe- und Belastungshämodynamik durch diese drei verschiedenen Behandlungsformen beeinflußt wird und in welchem Maße die jeweilige Wirkung den pathophysiologischen Veränderungen gerecht wird. Die Untersuchungen erfolgten invasiv im Liegen und bei Fahrradergometer-Arbeit im Sitzen jeweils vor und nach oraler Verabreichung von 100 mg Metoprolol (Beta-1-Rezeptoren-Blocker), 10 mg (Nifedipin Ca-Antagonist) bzw. 200 mg Labetalol (Alpha-1-Beta-Rezeptoren-Blocker).

Unter Metoprolol kam es zu einem Abfall von arteriellem Blutdruck, Herzfrequenz und Herzminutenvolumen; der totale periphere Widerstand und der linksventrikuläre Füllungsdruck stiegen. Nifedipin führte unter allen Bedingungen zu einer deutlichen Erniedrigung des peripheren Widerstandes, des linksventrikulären Füllungsdruckes und zu einem leichten Abfall des arteriellen Druckes; Herzfrequenz und Herzminutenvolumen waren höher nach Nifedipin. Die Wirkung von Labetalol war der von Nifedipin ähnlich, jedoch war das Herzminutenvolumen unverändert, die Herzfrequenz niedriger. Wie nach Nifedipin war auch nach Labetalol der linksventrikuläre Füllungsdruck bedeutend niedriger, insbesondere nach Belastung.

Eine Unterdrückung der sympathischen Stimulierung durch eine alleinige Beta-Rezeptoren-Blockade kann bei Patienten mit koronarer Herzkrankheit ungünstige hämodynamische Folgen mit weiterer Verschlechterung der linksventrikulären Dynamik haben. Dagegen führen eine Behandlung mit Ca-Antagonisten oder eine Kombination von Beta- und Alpha-Blockade im allgemeinen zu einer Verbesserung der Funktion der linken Kammer, hauptsächlich aufgrund der dabei erfolgenden Vasodilatation im Bereich der präkapillären Widerstandsgefäße. Die Ergebnisse lassen den Schluß zu, daß eine gleichzeitige Alpha-1-Rezeptoren-Blockade oder geeignete Vasodilatation in Fällen, in denen eine Behandlung mit Beta-Rezeptoren-Blockern indiziert erscheint, deren ungünstige hämodynamischen Wirkungen ausgleichen kann, ohne daß es zu einer Abschwächung des symptomatischen Effektes kommt. Eine kombinierte Alpha-Beta-Rezeptoren-Blockade hat den Vorteil gegenüber den Ca-Antagonisten, daß eine Erhöhung der sympathischen Aktivität und damit verbundene hyperkinetische hämodynamische Reaktionen unterdrückt werden.

Both beta-adrenoceptor blockers and calcium antagonists are widely used in the management of ischemic heart disease. In the clinical setting both have similar beneficial effects on angina threshold and incidence, and on exercise tolerance. However, beta-receptor blockers tend to depress cardiac function and thus carry the risk of precipitating functional deterioration particularly in cases with severe left ventricular dyskinesia [5].
Conversely, calcium antagonists, and in particular nifedipine, tend to improve ventricular dynamics [5, 6], but enhance adrenergic activity and tend to elicit hyperkinetic responses [5]. Combining the vasodilator action of nifedipine with the beta-adrenoceptor blocking effects of the beta-1-selective antagonist metoprolol has been shown to minimize the adverse hemodynamic effects of the beta-receptor blockade whilst preventing hyperkinetic responses [5]. On theoretical grounds, the combination of an alpha-1-receptor antagonist with a beta-receptor-blocker can be expected to yield at least similar advan-

tages as those obtained with the combination of nifedipine and metoprolol. The present study summarizes and compares the hemodynamic effects of the three different regimens: combined alpha-beta-blockade, beta-blockade alone and slow channel calcium inhibition.

Since labetalol combines alpha-and beta-receptor blocking properties in the same molecule [10] and has been shown to have favourable hemodynamic effects in hypertension [3, 4], the drug was chosen for combined alpha-beta blockade. Beta-blockade was achieved with metoprolol, slow channel calcium blockade with nifedipine.

Patients and Methods

All patients were men with established ischemic heart disease, low angina threshold and greatly restricted exercise tolerance. Roughly one fourth had a history of previous myocardial infarction. They were subjected to hemodynamic evaluation including analysis of the effect of pharmacological intervention because of poor control of angina. The allocation to the different intervention groups was randomised; in some of the patients different therapeutic regimens were assessed. 22 patients were studied before and 60 minutes after 100 mg metoprolol. 16 patients before and 30 minutes after 10 mg nifedipine, 15 patients before and 60 minutes after 200 mg labetalol. All drugs were orally administered. The groups were fairly well matched with respect to age, functional restriction, heart volume and pre-treatment hemodynamic function (Table 1). The control and post-treatment studies were done in a strictly identical manner. The pressures in the brachial artery and in the pulmonary circulation were measured by means of polyethylene catheters percutaneously inserted into the respective vessels. Cardiac-output was determined according to the Fick principle. Measurements at rest were done with the patient in the supine position, exercise was performed for 3 minutes at a low and for 6 minutes at a high submaximal load in the seated position on an electrodynamically braked bicycle ergometer. The work loads were selected according to the individual functional capacity, exercise at the highest work inducing typical angina during control conditions. Details concerning the general investigation procedure, analyses, calculations including the reproducibility of the methods and the statistical evaluation, are given elsewhere [3].

Table 1: Some anthropometric and pre-treatment function data (means and standard deviations). LVFP: left ventricular filling pressure.

Groups	Metoprolol n = 22	Nifedipine n = 16	Labetalol n = 15
Age, ys	55 ± 7	56 ± 6	58 ± 5
Height, cm	175 ± 7	177 ± 7	176 ± 6
Weight, kg	74 ± 11	77 ± 8	76 ± 10
Heart volume, ml/m^2	589 ± 238	568 ± 173	545 ± 83
Work load, Watt	90 ± 24	95 ± 28	95 ± 19
Heart rate, rest	74 ± 12	70 ± 9	76 ± 12
Cardiac output, L/min, rest	5.7 ± 1.1	6.4 ± 1.6	6.6 ± 1.1
LVFP, mmHg, rest	7 ± 4	6 ± 4	8 ± 2
Heart rate, exercise	129 ± 18	126 ± 17	133 ± 20
Cardiac output, L/min, exercise	11.2 ± 2.5	12.2 ± 2.6	10.5 ± 1.5
LVFP, mmHg, exercise	17 ± 5	13 ± 7	21 ± 6

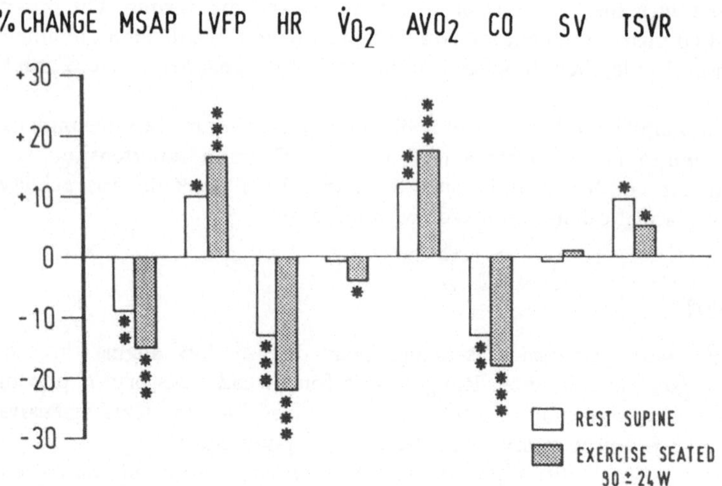

Fig. 1

Percentage changes from pre-treatment values of some hemodynamic variables after 100 mg of oral metoprolol (MSAP: mean systemic arterial pressures, LVFP: left ventricular filling pressure, HR: heart rate, $\dot{V}_{O_2}$: oxygen uptake, AV_{O_2}: arterio-mixed venous oxygen difference, CO: cardiac output, SV: stroke volume, TSVR: total systemic vascular resistance).

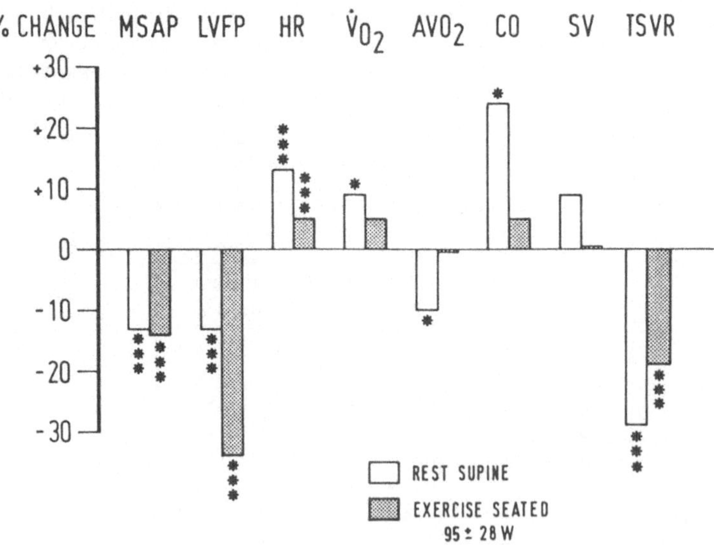

Fig. 2

Percentage changes from pre-treatment values of some hemodynamic variables after 10 mg of oral nifedipine. For abbreviations see Fig. 1.

174

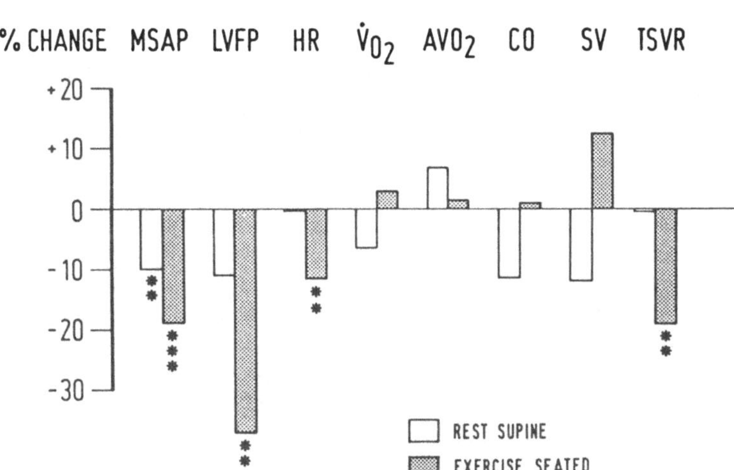

Fig. 3

Percentage changes from pre-treatment values of some hemodynamic variables after 200 mg of oral labetalol. For abbreviations see Fig. 1.

Results

Metoprolol (Fig. 1) induced a slight decrease of systemic arterial pressure mainly due to a reduction of cardiac-output; systemic vascular resistance increased. The reduction of cardiac-output was entirely due to lower heart rates. Left ventricular filling pressures increased by 1 ± 3 (standard deviation) mmHg at rest, and by 4 ± 5 mmHg during exercise. Nifedipine (Fig. 2) resulted under all circumstances in a considerable reduction of systemic vascular resistance and left ventricular filling pressure, and slightly lower systemic arterial pressures, while heart rate and cardiac-output were higher, in particular at rest. The effect of labetalol (Fig. 3) was similar to that of nifedipine with respect to left ventricular dynamics: afterload in terms of systemic arterial pressure and systemic vascular resistance was significantly reduced, in particular during exercise, preload in terms of left ventricular filling pressure was lowered by 1 ± 3 mmHg at rest and by 8 ± 5 mmHg during exercise. Heart rate was lower and stroke volume was higher during work; cardiac-output and the arterio-venous oxygen difference were not significantly affected either at rest or during work. The effect of metoprolol and labetalol on the product of systolic pressure and heart rate were similar whereas left ventricular stroke work during work appeared to be more affected by labetalol.

Discussion

Quite evidently the hemodynamic effects of the three regimens studied differ profoundly: beta-receptor blockers lower myocardial oxygen demand by decreasing pulse rate and contractility, and hence cardiac work for a given oxygen uptake. Calcium antagonists lower predominantly the systolic load on the left ventricle by reducing precapillary vascular resistance; however, nifedipine not only lowers afterload but also preload in terms of left ventricular end-diastolic pressure, apparently by reducing capacitance vessel tone in some vascular beds. Concomitantly however, pulse rates and cardiac output tend to rise, obviously due to enhanced adrenergic activity judging from plasma catecholamines [5]. Combined alpha-beta receptor blockade by labetalol exerts a similar action as nifedipine with respect to afterload and preload, but without eliciting a hyperkinetic response.

Despite the differences in the hemodynamic profiles all regimens had similar beneficial effects with respect to onset and duration of angina and to exercise tolerance. Also in a subgroup in which the effects of metoprolol and labetalol were compared in the same patient no significant difference between the two agents could be demonstrated though there was a tendency for labetalol to be more efficacious (Koch, unpublished observations). One of the oldest and most widely used antianginal drugs, nitroglycerine, has a hemodynamic profile still different from that of the three agents studied, lowering pre- and afterload, but in particular, postcapillary capacitance vessel tone, and reducing cardiac output [2]. Again, the antianginal efficacy in coronary heart disease appears similar to that of the agents studied, judging from the results of a comparative placebo controlled double blind study of the effects of nifedipine and isosorbide-mononitrate on exercise capacity, angina perception and ST-segment displacement (Koch, unpublished data). From all these observations it would appear that the mechanism by which myocardial oxygen requirement is reduced is not crucial for a specific drug's symptomatic efficacy in the majority of cases.

However, in individual patients the response to different treatment regimens may vary considerably and require careful adjustment of treatment according to the specific condition.

According to La Place's law wall tension (T) and thus myocardial oxygen demand during a single contraction is directly proportional to intraventricular systolic pressure (P) and radius (r) and reciprocally related to wall thickness (n): $T = P \cdot r/n$. This would imply that reduction of afterload (P) and of preload (r) are equally important, as is prevention of (further) dilatation of the cardiac chamber. Furthermore, it has been shown that coronary vascular resistance is closely correlated to left ventricular enddiastolic pressure [9]. Accordingly, a regimen tending to raise enddiastolic volume and pressure as occurring with beta-receptor blockade [1], appears less appropriate in this context than interventions that do not prompt further increases of preload such as calcium antagonists, nitrates or combined alpha-beta blockade.

However, there is no doubt that beta-receptor blocking drugs offer a clinically effective treatment in many patients with exercise induced angina pectoris. Furthermore, recent epidemiological studies suggest their usefulness in the secondary prevention of myocardial infarction [7, 8]. The present results strongly suggest that in patients in whom beta-receptor blockade appears indicated, the adverse hemodynamic effects of the beta-receptor blocker alone can be offset by concomitant alpha-1-receptor blockade or vasodilation without losing but rather enhancing symptomatic efficacy. These results are in complete accordance with those obtained by Taylor et al. who compared labetalol with propranolol in a similar group of patients [11] and in our own study comparing the effects of the combination of metoprolol and nifedipine with those of metoprolol alone [5]. An additional advantage of combined alpha-beta receptor blockade is the absence of the increases in adrenergic activity and related hyperkinetic hemodynamic responses which frequently accompany treatment with calcium antagonists, particularly nifedipine.

References

[1] Dehmer, G. J., Falkoff, M., Lewis, S. E., Hillis, L. D., Parkey, R. W., Willerson, J. T.: Effect of oral propranolol on rest and exercise left ventricular ejection fraction, volumes, and segmental wall motion in patients with angina pectoris. Assessment with equilibrium gated blood pool imaging. *British Heart Journal* **45**, 656–666 (1981).

[2] Kasparian, H., Wiener, L., Duca, P. R., Gottlieb, R. S., Brest, A. N.: Comparative hemodynamic effects of placebo and oral isosorbide dinitrate in patients with significant coronary artery disease. *American Heart Journal* **90**, 68–74 (1975).

[3] Koch, G.: Acute hemodynamic effects of an alpha- and beta-receptor blocking agent (AH 5158) on the systemic and plumonary circulation at rest and during exercise in hypertensive patients. *American Heart Journal* **93**, 585–591 (1977).

[4] Koch, G.: Haemodynamic adaption at rest and during exercise to long-term antihypertensive treatment with combined alpha- and beta-adrenoceptor blockade by labetalol. *British Heart Journal* **41**, 192–198 (1979).

[5] Koch, G.: Beta-receptor and calcium blockade in ischemic heart disease: effects on systemic and pulmonary hemodynamics and on plasma catecholamines at rest and during exercise. In: *4th International Adalat Symposium. New Therapy of Ischemic Heart Disease* (P. Puech and R. Krebs, eds.) pp. 131–142, Amsterdam, Oxford, Princeton: Excerpta Medica, 1980.

[6] Lydtin, H., Schierl, W., Lohmöller, G.: Exercise pulmonary wedge pressure after acute and chronic administration of nifedipine in ischemic heart disease. In: *4th International Adalat Symposium. New Therapy of Ischemic Heart Disease* (P. Puech and R. Krebs, eds.) pp. 249–254, Amsterdam, Oxford, Princeton: Excerpta Medica, 1980.

[7] Multicentre International Study. Reduction in mortality after myocardial infarction with long-term beta-adrenoceptor blockade. *British Medical Journal* **280**, 419–421 (1977).

[8] Norwegian Multicentre Study Group. Timolol induced reduction in mortality and reinfarction in patients surviving acute myocardial infarction. *New England Journal of Medicine* **304**, 801–807 (1981).

[9] Opherk, D., Mall, G., Zebe, H., Schwarz, F., Weihe, E., Manthey, J., Kübler, W.: Reduction of coronary reserve: a mechanism for angina pectoris in patients with arterial hypertension and normal coronary arteries. *Circulation* **69**, 1–7 (1984).

[10] Richards, D. A., Prichard, B. N. C.: Clinical Pharmacology of labetalol. *British Journal of Clinical Pharmacology* **8**, 89 S-93 S (1979).

[11] Taylor, S. H., Silke, B., Nelson, G. I. C., Okoli, R. C., Ahuja, R. C.: Haemodynamic advantages of combined alpha-blockade and beta-blockade over beta-blockade alone in patients with coronary heart disease. *British Medical Journal* **285**, 325–327 (1982).

Oral Beta and Alpha Blockade (Labetalol) in the Management of Stable Angina Pectoris in Normotensive Patients – A Preliminary Report

J.W. Upward, F. Akhras, G. Jackson
Department of Cardiology, King's College Hospital, London, SE5 9RS, and Lewisham Hospital, London, SE13 6LH, U.K.

Summary

The efficacy of labetalol, an alpha and beta receptor antagonist, has been evaluated in nine normotensive patients with stable angina pectoris in a single blind dose ranging study. After a 2 week control placebo period labetalol was administered twice daily at dosages of 100, 150, 200 and 300 mg b.i.d. All patients had fewer anginal attacks and consumed fewer glyceryl trinitrate tablets than during the placebo period. Maximal symptom limited treadmill exercise tests performed 3 and 12 hours after dosage showed increased exercise time and decreased double products for all doses, but especially 200 and 300 mg b.i.d. Trough point exercise tolerance did not differ significantly from that at peak dosage. Thus, labetalol is an effective antianginal agent when given twice daily, especially at 200 mg and 300 mg b.i.d. dosage.

The value of beta receptor antagonists in the management of patients with stable angina pectoris is well established [1, 2]. The benefits of beta blockade are, however, achieved at the expense of a decrease in cardiac output and an increase in peripheral vascular resistance [3]. These haemodynamic effects may be important in the aetiology of the not infrequent side effects of beta blockade: cold hands and feet, and fatigue. Labetalol is an agent which possesses both alpha and beta adrenoceptor antagonist properties [4]. Acute studies have shown a reduction in peripheral vascular resistance following its intravenous administration [3, 5] and, compared with propranolol, less impairment of left ventricular haemodynamic performance [3]. In addition, in contrast to propranolol, labetalol produces a reduction in coronary vascular resistance [5].
Labetalol's main role has been in the treatment of hypertension [6, 7, 8] and in a preliminary report of labetalol therapy in patients with both hypertension and angina, amelioration of anginal symptoms has been described [9].
The object of this study was to assess the effects of labetalol in normotensive patients with stable angina pectoris, with reference to control of anginal symptoms and effect on exercise tolerance.

Patients and Methods

Patients

Twelve patients, nine men and three women, with a mean age of 59 years (range 41–66 years) participated in the study. All had had clinically stable exercise induced angina pectoris for three months or longer. Patient details are summarised in Table 1. No patient had valvular heart disease, cardiac failure, obstructive airways disease, hypertension (resting diastolic > 100 mmHg), diabetes, or renal or thyroid disease. All patients were limited on treadmill exercise testing by angina pectoris accompanied by horizontal or down sloping depression of the ST-segment of 1.0 mm or more, persisting to 80 msec beyond the 'J' point. Eleven patients had angiographically proven coronary disease, defined as greater than 70 % stenosis of at least one major vessel. The remaining patient who declined angiography, had typical angina and 4 mm ST depression inferolaterally at peak exercise. Suitable patients were entered into the study after informed written consent had been obtained.

Table 1: Patient Profiles

Patient Number	Age	Sex	Exercise limited by	Coronary arteriogram
1	58	M	Angina	3 vessel CAD
2	51	F	Angina	2 vessel CAD
3	66	M	Angina	2 vessel CAD
4	61	F	Angina	2 vessel CAD
5	63	M	Angina	not done
6	62	M	Angina	2 vessel CAD
7	64	M	Angina	Single vessel CAD
8	64	M	Angina	2 vessel CAD
9	60	M	Angina	3 vessel CAD
10	41	F	Angina	3 vessel CAD
11	54	M	Angina	2 vessel CAD
12	64	M	Angina	2 vessel CAD

Drug Dosage and Administration

The study was divided into five two week periods. After a single blind placebo control period, labetalol was administered in twice daily dosage for the following eight weeks. The labetalol dosage was increased at two weekly intervals. The total daily labetalol dosage for the four treatment periods was 200 mg, 300 mg, 400 mg and 600 mg respectively.

Antianginal Assessment

Patients kept diaries to record frequency of angina attacks and glyceryl trinitrate consumption. At each visit, supine and standing blood pressures were measured using a standard sphygmomanometer. Patients were asked if they had experienced any side effects, but were not questioned about specific symptoms.

Exercise Testing

Maximal symptom limited treadmill exercise tests were performed, using the Bruce protocol, before entry into the study and in the second week of the placebo period and each
treatment period. In each of the two week periods exercise tests were performed three
hours and twelve hours after dosage on separate days. The treadmill, the recording equip-
ment and the recording methods have been described previously [10].

Statistical Method

To assess drug efficacy, angina attack frequency and glyceryl trinitrate consumption in
the control period were compared to those on therapy with labetalol. Exercise tolerance
on therapy was compared with that on the second placebo exercise test to minimise any
learning or training effect. Statistical analysis was made using two way analysis of variance
and the Student's "t" test for paired data. The latter was corrected, when this was appropriate, using the Bonferroni correction for multiple comparisons [11].

Results

Full data was obtained in nine patients. One patient required dosage reduction because
of mild heart failure. Two patients were withdrawn from the study: one because of
"scalp tingling" while taking labetalol, and one because of progressive worsening of his
angina while taking placebo.

Angina attack frequency

Frequency of angina attacks decreased in all of the nine patients who completed the
study (Fig 1). There was a progressive reduction in anginal attack frequency as labetalol
dose was increased, the decrease was statistically significant at daily labetalol dosages of
300 mg, 400 mg and 600 mg daily. On these doses the reduction compared to placebo
was 40 % ($p < 0.05$) 56 % ($p < 0.01$) and 63 % ($p < 0.01$) respectively.

Glyceryl trinitrate consumption (Fig 1)

The reduction in nitrate consumption paralleled the reduction in angina attack frequency.
The reduction in consumption was statistically significant on the 400 mg and 600 mg
daily labetalol dosage. The percentage reduction compared to placebo was 60 % ($p < 0.01$)
at both dosage levels.

Exercise tolerance

Exercise time, expressed as seconds of the Bruce protocol, is shown in Figure 2 and Table 2
(a and b). The mean exercise times of the two exercise stress tests in the placebo period
differed by only 6 % (not significant). Exercise tolerance on labetalol therapy increased
with increasing dosage. The increase in exercise time became significant compared to the
placebo exercise test, on labetalol 300 mg daily. The mean exercise time on labetalol

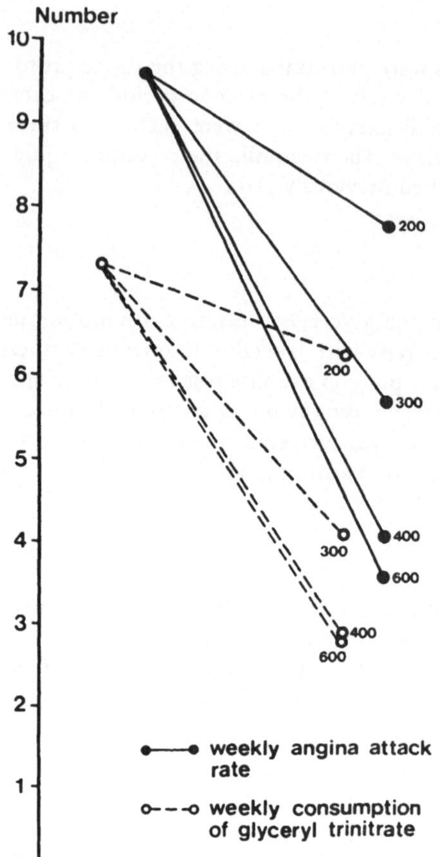

Fig. 1
The effect of labetalol therapy on angina attack frequency and glyceryl trinitrate consumption

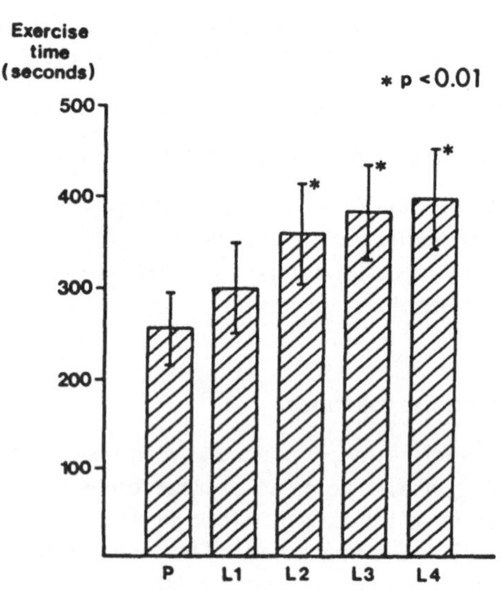

Fig. 2
The effect of labetalol therapy on exercise tolerance in patients with angina pectoris. P, L1, L2, L3, and L4 denote placebo therapy and therapy with labetalol in dosages of 100 mg, 150 mg, 200 mg and 300 mg b.i.d. respectively

Table 2a: Placebo Reproducability

	on no medication	Placebo visit 1	Placebo visit 2
Resting Blood Pressure (mmHg)			
Systolic	154 ± 8.0	152 ± 8.5	152 ± 8.3
Diastolic	91 ± 2.9	87 ± 4.0	86 ± 3.3
Resting Heart Rate (beats/minute)	76 ± 2.3	74 ± 2.9	74 ± 3.0
Peak Exercise Blood Pressure (mmHg)			
Systolic	178 ± 7.6	173 ± 8.6	178 ± 6.5
Diastolic	91 ± 2.9	87 ± 2	86 ± 3.3
Peak Exercise Heart Rate (beats/minute)	131 ± 8.7	127 ± 7.5	126 ± 7.1
Duration of Exercise (sec)	213 ± 35	243 ± 40	258 ± 39

Table 2b: Placebo and Labetalol — Rest and Exercise Data

| | Placebo visit 2 | Labetalol dose mg/daily | | | |
		200	300	400	600
Resting Blood Pressure (mmHg)					
Systolic	152 ± 8.3	137 ± 7.9**	128 ± 6.5**	128 ± 6.5**	121 ± 7.2**
Diastolic	86 ± 3.3	80 ± 4.7	78 ± 3.0	75 ± 3.8**	74 ± 2.6**
Resting Heart Rate (beats/min)	74 ± 230	69 ± 4.0	69 ± 2.8	67 ± 1.3	71 ± 2.3
Peak Exercise Blood Pressure (mmHg)					
Systolic	178 ± 6.5	160 ± 8.4**	152 ± 7.5**	152 ± 6.2**	144 ± 5.7**
Diastolic	86 ± 3.3	80 ± 4.7*	78 ± 3.0**	75 ± 3.8**	74 ± 2.6**
Peak Exercise Heart Rate (beats/min)	126 ± 7.1	112 ± 4.1	116 ± 6.0	116 ± 4.4	114 ± 4.7
Duration of Exercise (sec)	258 ± 39	300 ± 50	361 ± 54**	387 ± 52**	399 ± 54**

* p < 0.05 (paired "t" with Bonferroni correction)

** p < 0.01 (paired "t" with Bonferroni correction)

300 mg, 400 mg and 600 mg daily was respectively 40 % (p < 0.01) 50 % (p < 0.01) and 55 % (p < 0.01) greater than on placebo. Importantly at these dosage levels, the exercise tolerance three hours after dosage did not differ significantly from that at the end of the dosage interval (Table 3). The maximum ST segment change seen on the 12 lead electrocardiogram at peak exercise is shown in Table 4. There was a trend towards a reduction in degree of ST segment change at peak exercise, but this did not reach statistical significance.

Table 3: Peak and Trough Exercise Time (seconds)

Labetalol dose mg/day	3 hours post drug	12 hours post drug		
300	361 (± 54)	352 (± 54)	(n = 9)	NS
400	387 (± 52)	366 (± 58)	(n = 9)	NS
600	426 (± 54)	415 (± 52)	(n = 8)	NS

Table 4: Exercise Data

	2nd exercise test on placebo	Daily Labetalol Dose (mg)			
		200	300	400	600
Rate-pressure product at peak exercise (mmHg · min-1)	22564 (± 1863)	18068* (± 1259)	18317** (± 1435)	17578* (± 937)	16480** (± 870)
Exercise Tolerance (seconds of Bruce protocol)	258 (± 3!)	300 (± 50)	361 (± 54)**	387 (± 52)**	399 (± 54)**
Maximum ST segment depression (mm)	2.1 (± 0.3)	1.5 (± 0.2)	1.6 (± 0.4)	1.8 (± 0.2)	1.7 (± 0.3)
Heart rate at work load which was achieved on the 2nd placebo test (beats/min)	126 (± 7)	109 (± 4)**	109 (± 5)**	106 (± 5)**	107 (± 3)**

*   p < 0.05 (paired "t" test)
**   p < 0.01 (with Bonferroni correction)

The Effect on Blood Pressure and Heart Rate (Tables 2 and 4)

There was a significant reduction in resting systolic and diastolic blood pressure on labetalol therapy. On the highest dosage the percentage reduction in both parameters was 14 % (Table 2). There was a trend towards reduction in resting heart rate, but the change was small and when compared with the heart rate on placebo using the paired "t" test, not significant.

Peak exercise systolic and diastolic blood pressures were significantly lower on labetalol therapy than in the control period. On the highest labetalol dosage the percentage reduction in systolic and diastolic pressure was 19 % and 13 % respectively (Table 2).

Table 5: The Effect of Posture on Blood Pressure 3 Hours After Dosage on the Highest Labetalol Dose

	Measurement after 5 minutes in supine position	Measurement 2 minutes after standing	
Systolic (mmHg)	124 ± 4.4	125 ± 5.6	NS
Diastolic (mmHg)	72 ± 8.3	76 ± 7.8	p < 0.05

NS = not significant

The heart rate at peak exercise on labetalol therapy was not significantly different from that at peak exercise in the control period. It should be noted however, that peak exercise on therapy, was at a significantly higher workload than that in the placebo period. Heart rate on labetalol therapy, measured at the workload achieved in the placebo period is shown in Table 4. A significant reduction is seen at all dosage levels. (Table 4).
There was a significant reduction in peak exercise rate-pressure product on labetalol therapy. The percentage reduction on the highest dosage being 27 % (Table 4). On the highest labetalol dosage there was no significant postural drop in blood pressure (Table 5).

Side Effects and Withdrawals

Patient 3 was withdrawn after three days of therapy because of scalp tingling. Patient 6 developed dyspnoea on exertion while taking labetalol 200 mg daily. He did not have clinical signs of heart failure, but chest x-ray showed pulmonary venous congestion which was not previously present. Dosage reduction to 100 mg daily and the addition of a thiazide diuretic resulted in a marked symptomatic improvement. On placebo therapy he had experienced 14 attacks of angina per week and had consumed 4 GTN tablets per week. On his final labetalol dosage he only experienced one attack of angina in a 6 week period. His exercise tolerance increased from 160 seconds in the control period to 221 seconds on his final dosage regime and his symptomatic improvement has been maintained in a six month follow-up period.
Patient 8 experienced progressive worsening of his angina while taking placebo and was withdrawn from study before receiving labetalol. No patients complained of fatigue or cold peripheries and none had symptoms referrable to postural hypotension.

Discussion

Labetalol is the only agent, currently available, with combined alpha and beta adrenoceptor antagonist properties [4]. It is effective in the treatment of hypertension [6, 7, 8] and, in hypertensive patients has been shown to have an antianginal effect [9].
The main determinants of myocardial oxygen consumption are the systolic blood pressure and the heart rate [12]. The patient with angina may derive symptomatic benefit from agents which reduce one or both of these variables [1, 2, 9]. The administration of the alpha blocking agent phentolamine results in a fall in blood pressure, but any potential benefit is offset by the increased oxygen requirement from the resulting reflex tachycardia. In some patients this may actually precipitate an angina attack [13].

In this study of normotensive patients with angina, labetalol produced a significant increase in exercise tolerance accompanied by a significant reduction in frequency of angina attacks and in nitrate consumption. The resting heart rate was not significantly affected but the rate response to exercise was reduced, and there was a significant reduction in peak exercise rate − pressure product. Labetalol therapy was generally well tolerated; only one patient had to be withdrawn from study in the active treatment period. This patient had the uncommon but well documented side effect of scalp tingling [14]. Labetalol had less effect on resting heart rate than would be expected with agents such as propranolol or atenolol (1,2). This difference probably reflects the balance between the depressant effect of beta blockade on the sinus node, and the tendency to reflex tachycardia in response to the alpha blockade mediated vasodilatation [3, 4]. Importantly however, despite this effect, significant antianginal properties were evident.

The combination of alpha and beta blockade may have advantages over beta blockade alone in the management of patients with angina pectoris. It has been demonstrated in acute studies that labetalol produces less depression of left ventricular function than propranolol [3] and, unlike propranolol, it reduces [3, 5, 7] or has no effect on peripheral vascular resistance [8]. These properties may render labetalol acceptable to the patient who cannot tolerate other beta receptor antagonists because of side effects of fatigue and cold peripheries. Labetalol unlike propranolol, has a coronary vasodilator effect [5, 15]. This may be of little benefit to some angina sufferers, but in others, in whose symptomatology coronary spasm plays a role [16] labetalol may offer a significant advantage over other beta receptor antagonists.

In conclusion labetalol is an effective, well tolerated antianginal agent which can be administered twice daily. It was most effective in this study at dosage levels of 200 mg b.i.d. One patient developed mild heart failure on a lower dose and it would seem prudent therefore to start therapy on labetalol 200 mg daily, and titrate the dose to suit the individual patient's needs. Labetalol has some theoretical advantages over pure beta receptor antagonists but further studies are needed to determine their clinical significance.

References

[1]   Hamer, J., Sowton, E.: Effects of propranolol on exercise tolerance in angina pectoris. *Am. J. Cardiol.* **18**: 354−358 (1966).

[2]   Jackson, G., Harry, J.D., Robinson, C., Kitson, D., Jewitt, D.E.: Comparison of atenolol with propranolol in the treatment of angina pectoris with special reference to once daily administration of atenolol. *Br. Heart J.* **40**: 998−1004 (1978).

[3]   Silke, B., Nelson, G.I.C., Ahuja, R.C., Taylor, S.H.: Comparative haemodynamic dose response effects of propranolol and labetalol in coronary artery disease. *Br. Heart J.* **48**: 6 364−371 (1982).

[4]   Richards, D.A., Prichard, B.N.C., Boakes, A.J., Tuckman, J., Knight, E.J.: Pharmacological basis for antihypertensive effects of intravenous labetalol. *Br. Heart J.* **39**: 99 106 (1977).

[5]   Gagnon, R.M., Morisette, M., Presant, S., Savard, D., Lemire, J.: Haemodynamic and coronary effects of intravenous labetalol in coronary artery disease. *Am. J. Cardiol.* **49**: 1267−1269 (1982).

[6]   Frick, M.H., Porsti, P.: Combined alpha and beta adrenoceptor blockade with labetalol in hypertension. *Br. Med. J.* **1**: 1046−1048 (1976).

[7]   Joekes, A.M., Thompson, F.D.: Acute haemodynamic effects of labetalol and its subsequent use as an oral hypotensive agent. *Br. J. Clin. Pharmacol.* **3** (suppl 3) 789−793 (1976).

[8]   Timmis, A.D., Fowler, M.B., Jaggarao, N.S.V., Chamberlain, D.A.: Labetalol infusion for the treatment of hypertension in acute myocardial infarction. *Eur. Heart J.* **1**: 413−416 (1980).

[9] Halprin, S., Frishman, W., Kirschner, M., Strom, J.: Clinical pharmacology of the new beta adrenergic blocking drugs. Part II. Effects of oral labetalol in patients with both angina pectoris and hypertension: a preliminary experience. *Am. Heart J.* **99**: 388—396 (1980).

[10] Akhras, F., Upward, J., Stott, R., Jackson, G.: Early exercise testing and coronary angiography after uncomplicated myocardial infarction. *Br. Med. J.* **284**: 1293—1294 (1982).

[11] Wallenstein, S., Zucker, C.L., Fleiss, J.L.: Some statistical methods useful in circulation research. *Circ. Res.* **47**: 1—9 (1980).

[12] Robinson, B.F.: Relation of heart rate and systolic blood pressure to the onset of pain in angina pectoris. *Circulation* **35**: 1073—1083 (1967).

[13] Kelly, D. T., Delgado, C. E., Taylor, D. R., Pitt B., Ross, R. S.: Use of phentolamine in acute myocardial infarction associated with hypertension and left ventricular failure. *Circulation* **47**: 729—735 (1973).

[14] Hua, A. S. P., Thomas, G. W., Kincaid-Smith, P.: Scalp tingling in patients on labetalol. *Lancet* **2**: 295 (1977).

[15] Kern, M.J., Ganz, P., Horowitz, J.D., Gaspar, J., Barry, W.H., Lorell, B.H., Grossman, W., Mudge, G.H.: Potentiation of coronary vasoconstriction by beta-adrenergic blockade in patients with coronary artery disease. *Circulation* **6**: 1178—1185 (1983).

[16] Leading article. Coronary artery spasm *Br. Med. J.* **1**: 969—970 (1979).

Discussion

Borchard
Sie stellten eingangs die Frage, ob eine kombinierte Alpha-, Betarezeptorenblockade Vorteile gegen-über einer einfachen Betarezeptorenblockade aufweisen würde. Können Sie die Vorzüge der kombi-nierten Alpha- plus Betarezeptorenblockade aufzeigen?

Jackson
The principal benefits in addition to less adverse effects, should theoretically be the beneficial haemo-dynamic response. There are theoretical advantages with regard to the lower negative inotropic action of the beta- and alpha-combination with labetalol in comparison with a conventional beta-blocker. Whether labetalol has a similar metabolic profile in terms of, for example, pacing induced lactate metabolism, needs to be determined.

Heinicke
Are you surprised that you did not find any changes in spite of the fact that you ameliorate angina pectoris? Normally under beta-blockade we find quite definite changes in the ST-segment.

Jackson
I found such observations also when looking at the beta-blocker timolol. There is a trend down-wards. It may be that we are short on numbers, but I think the important thing is that we have taken the criterion of maximum ST-depression and have not 'bent' our data to find a more favourable lead. I agree entirely that it is the total ST-depression that we should look at, although we don't have the facilities, with mapping, to look at that in our department.

N. N.
Is labetalol the only anti-angina medication during this period, or have your patients further medica-tion like nitrates of calcium-channel-blockers?

Jackson
They were only allowed to have sublingual nitrates to be used for anginal attacks.

Schulz
Gibt es vom gleichen Untersucher Befunde, in der ein reiner Betablocker mit Labetalol verglichen worden ist? Ich frage nach der Wirksamkeit von Labetalol und Betablockern.

Jackson
The important thing before starting any comparison is to find out if your drug works. The next, to ask; is this drug better than other drugs we have? Firstly in the whole population and then in the group for whom adverse effects of cold hands and feet and heavy legs are a problem, which is probably 15 % of the beta-blocker-group. Does that answer your question?

Schulz
No.

Jackson
There is no study going on at present. Those two areas, I agree, need work, but we could not start these studies unless we could show in this study that the drug worked.

N. N.
You have one patient who developed congestion. Did you look for the reason for this congestion? Had he a myocardial infarction?

Jackson
No, he had, according to our angiograms, acceptable left ventricular function, and it was a surprise to us when he developed heart failure at that dosage level.

Schmidt
Sie haben empfohlen, die Dosis zu titrieren. Dazu zwei Fragen. Nach welchen Kriterien soll man sich bei der Titration richten. Welches Intervall soll man wählen? Wir wissen aus anderen Untersuchungen, daß die anginöse Wirksamkeit des Betablockers sicher nicht nach 2 Wochen voll erreicht ist.

Jackson
I think that the conventional criterion must be a combination of the patient's angina attack rate and his well-being. We titrated patients at 2-weekly intervals. I take your point that a maximum benefit can come on with the beta-blocker over a 2 to 4 week period. In clinical practice I titrate the dose at monthly intervals.

Borchard
Unter Betarezeptorenblockade steigt der linksventrikuläre Füllungsdruck bei Belastung jeweils bei Normotonen an. Gibt es irgendwelche Untersuchungen, die diesen linksventrikulären diastolischen Füllungsdruck unter Labetalol bei Koronarpatienten unter Belastung untersucht haben?

Jackson
Could I ask you to comment on that Dr. Taylor?

Taylor
We carried out a study and it shows that during exercise, comparing equivalent degrees of beta-blockade as assessed by reduction in exercise heart rate, labetalol did not cause a rise in filling pressure, whereas propranolol did. It also maintained the cardiac output at rest and during exercise in contrast to the depression caused by propranolol. So it is just what you would expect. A decrease in afterload caused by vasodilation maintains the filling pressure during exercise better than beta-blockade alone.

The Use of Labetalol for Acute Myocardial Infarction in Normotensive Patients

D. A. Chamberlain, M. E. Heber, E. Rosenthal, N. B. Thomas,
R. D. Burwood, J. Lutkin, R. Vincent
Royal Sussex County Hospital, Brighton, England

Summary

Pharmacodynamic considerations raise the possibility that combined alpha- and beta-blockade may be safer and more efficacious as an acute intervention for patients with myocardial infarction than pure beta-blockade. Arteriolar dilatation and venodilatation should make failure less likely and reduce myocardial metabolic demands. Moreover, pure beta-blockers may constrict coronary arteries under some conditions, an effect which should be attenuated by alpha-blockade. Accordingly the policy of giving labetalol in the acute phase of myocardial infarction was tested, using immediate bolus doses, 6-hour infusions, and oral therapy for 5 days. A 3-level dose schedule was designed to reduce systolic pressure no further than 100 mmHg. 166 patients (age limit 75) were randomised to treatment or control groups, with exclusions including severe LVF, conduction disorders, and treatment with beta-blockers or vaso-active drugs. No benefit was seen in the group on active treatment in terms of ejection fraction, enzyme release, R-wave loss, or arrhythmias judged by aberrant counts on dynamic electrocardiography. Enzyme release and aberrant counts showed a tendency to be greater in the group on active therapy. These results were obtained with doses of labetalol constrained by blood pressure readings and relatively low doses were used. Adequate sympathetic blockade was unlikely to have been achieved in most cases.

The combination of alpha- and beta-blockade of adrenoceptors is widely accepted as appropriate for the treatment of hypertension, but evaluation is incomplete for the management of acute and chronic ischaemic heart disease. Preliminary studies of the use of labetalol in patients with acute myocardial infarction complicated by hypertension [1, 2, 3, 4] have been promising: the vasodilatation promoted by alpha-blockade can control the blood pressure and may aid the resolution of heart failure. Theoretical considerations suggest both beneficial and adverse effects from vasodilatation in normotensive subjects with acute infarction and only clinical trials can show whether or not the balance is favourable. In this paper we review the data available at present; they suggest that intervention with labetalol in the acute stage of infarction is unlikely to have more than a limited therapeutic role.

Historical Background and Theoretical Considerations

Adrenoceptor blockade in acute myocardial infarction has attracted wide interest since Snow [5] conducted a small non-randomized trial with propranolol, and claimed to have observed a protective effect. Many small negative trials of beta-blockers followed, but definitive information on the value of beta-adrenoceptor antagonists became available only when large-scale studies were conducted. These have been reviewed [6, 7]: the evidence suggests benefit from treatment with oral beta-blockers started late in the hospital phase, but adequate data on the value of intravenous beta blockers in the early hours of infarction are not yet available.

The response to beta-adrenoceptor blockade after infarction is complex, but the advantageous effects must − on balance − outweight those which are potentially harmful. In the convalescent phase, complex arrhythmias are suppressed [8], reinfarction is less likely [6, 7], and mortality is lessened by treatment [6, 7]. Regarding the intravenous use of beta-blockers in the acute phase of infarction, evidence exists for a reduction in the incidence of ventricular fibrillation [9], and for a favourable effect on indices of infarct size − namely CPK release and R-wave scores [10]. But beta-blockade will exacerbate any tendancy to heart failure, may worsen conduction disorders, and may increase any tendancy to coronary constriction. These adverse actions must curtail the benefits of treatment particularly in the acute phase, and also restrict the proportion of victims of infarction who can appropriately be treated.

Combined alpha- and beta-blockade should retain many of the benefits of beta-blockade alone, and mitigate some of the disadvantages. The venodilatation and arterioler dilatation ensure that any tendancy to heart failure is countered, and indeed studies with hypertensive patients during infarction confirm a reduction in left atrial pressure (measured indirectly as pulmonary capillary wedge pressure) [1, 2]. The coronary constriction believed to follow beta-blockade in some instances is thought to result from unopposed alpha-mediated tonus, a response which combined blockade would not induce. Moreover reperfusion arrhythmias are mediated in part by alpha-adrenoceptors [11] and labetalol may protect against these [12]. The plasma concentrations required are likely, however, to be outside any attainable therapeutic range.

The alpha component of combined alpha- and beta-receptor blockade introduces one additional problem. The greater fall in blood pressure, helpful in the treatment of hypertension, will reduce perfusion pressure of the coronary arterial tree. To a degree, compensation can be expected from the reduced coronary constricter effect and from autoregulation; but the impact on survival of jeopardized ischaemic myocardium cannot be predicted and the clinical relevance of induced hypotension in this situation is unknown.

Labetalol, with its balanced pharmacological profile, offers a useful means of testing the clinical efficacy of combined alpha- and beta-blockade in patients with acute infarction, but few data are available at present.

Review of Previous Studies of Labetalol in Acute Infarction

The early studies in acute infarction were in patients who had hypertension during the acute phase of the illness [1, 2, 3, 4] and the haemodynamic response has been well defined. Systolic and diastolic pressures can be lowered effectively whilst calculated peripheral resistance shows little change. The fall in cardiac index tends to parallel the decrease in heart rate. Raised left atrial pressure tends to fall on treatment, whilst normal left atrial pressure remains unchanged.

Nelson and colleagues in Leeds [13] were the first to report on the use of labetalol in normotensive patients in the early stage of acute infarction (4 to 18 hours after the onset of symptoms). Haemodynamic responses were measured in nine patients, with heart rate and blood pressure monitored in an additional six. Infusion of labetalol in a dose of 0.5 mg/Kg/hr was given for 90 minutes (total dose 48–66 mg). Average systolic pressure fell from 143 to 115 mmHg, heart rate from 70 to 64 beats per minute, cardiac index from 3.2 to 2.9 L/min/m^2, with little change in indirect left atrial pressure or stroke volume. The response was therefore similar to that in hypertensive patients. The reduction in major determinants of myocardial oxygen consumption suggested that the combination of alpha- and beta-blockade may be advantageous in normotensive patients with acute infarction and further exploration of the field was deemed important.

The Brighton Study of Labetalol in Acute Myocardial Infarction

A total of 166 patients were studied in a randomized open trial of the value of labetalol, with treatment started early after the onset of symptoms of infarction or suspected infarction. All were aged less than 75 and had a typical history. Subsequent categorization into those with and without definite infarction was based upon either characteristic evolution of ECG changes or diagnostic enzyme rises. Inclusion demanded that the onset of symptoms be within 6 hours. We excluded those with severe left ventricular failure, hypotension (less than 100 mmHg) or hypertension (more than 200 mmHg), conduction disorders and arrhythmias requiring treatment, valvular regurgitation, a history of bronchospasm, recent treatment with labetalol or verapamil, and those with hepatic or renal disease.

Labetalol was given as a bolus dose followed by an infusion for six hours. At five hours the first oral dose was given and continued eight hourly for five days. Doses were at three levels with the aim of maintaining systolic pressure near but not below 100 mmHg. The schedule is shown in Table 1, and the doses attained using this scheme are presented in Table 2.

Table 1 Treatment schedules

B.P. (Systolic)	Bolus dose (10 mins)	Maintenance (rate/min for 6 Hrs)	Oral dose 9 hrly for 5 days
100 – 129	0.25 mg/Kg	62.5 ug	50 mg
130 – 159	0.5 mg/Kg	125 ug	100 mg
160 +	1.0 mg/Kg	250 ug	200 mg

Table 2

Bolus dose	Maintenance I.V.	Oral dose
0 – 24 mg 29 pts	0 – 9 mg 17 pts	0 – 499 mg 27 pts
25 – 49 mg 40 pts	10 – 19 mg 22 pts	500 – 999 mg 41 pts
50 – 74 mg 10 pts	22 – 29 mg 19 pts	1000 – 1499 mg 12 pts
75 – 100 mg 4 pts	30 + 16 pts	1500 + mg 2 pts

The following measurements were made: blood pressure and heart rate response, R-wave score, ejection fraction acutely (single crystal scintigraphic counter) and at six weeks (Gamma camera), and arrhythmias as recorded over 10-hours of taped electrocardiogram. Blood pressure fell significantly more in the 83 patients treated with labetalol than in the equal number who acted as controls (Fig. 1). Heart rate was also reduced by labetalol (Fig. 2). No effect was observed on R-wave score or ejection fraction — either acutely (Fig. 3) or at six weeks — when the labetalol and control patients were compared.

CPK MB release was greater in those treated with labetalol, both for all patients who had observations successfully completed and for the subgroup subsequently shown to have infarction. No evidence was obtained that labetalol prevented the progression from threatened to completed infarction. A clear tendency emerged for patients treated with labetalol to have more aberrant beats, defined by abnormal QRS width and prematurity on Pathfinder (Reynolds Medical) analysis (Fig. 4).

The Brighton study of labetalol in normotensive patients with infarction was designed to test a *policy* of using combined alpha- and beta-blockade from the earliest possible time after the onset of symptoms and continuing treatment throughout the acute phase. We wished to know whether treatment could be controlled readily without hazard to the patients, whether effective doses of labetalol could be given — bearing in mind the constraints of induced hypotension, whether advantages accrued for the patient in terms of arrhythmia control and indices of infarct size, and whether a large-scale mortality study might be worthwhile.

Our experience showed the labetalol dosage was constrained by hypotension to an extent which would have limited the degree and protective value of beta-blockade. We

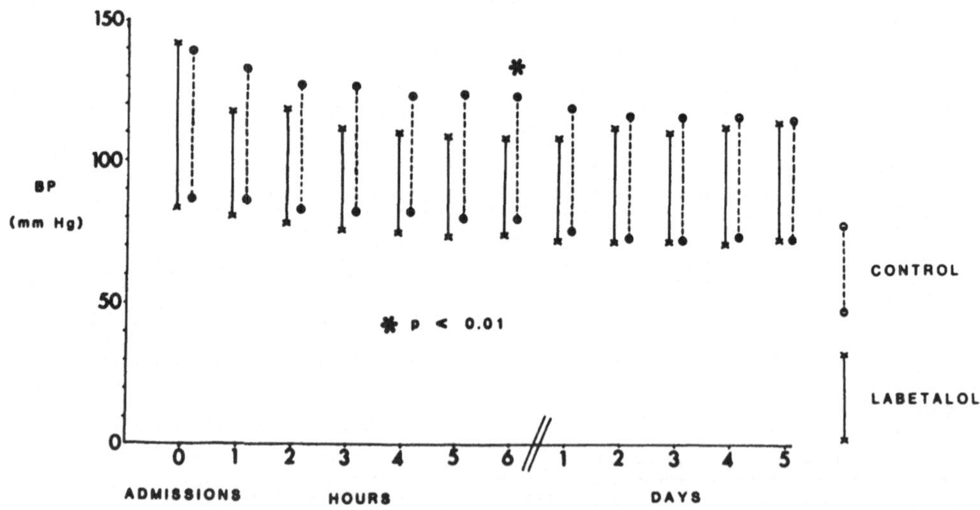

Fig. 1

Averaged blood pressure responses hourly for six hours and daily for five days for the patients treated with labetalol and those who served as controls.

192

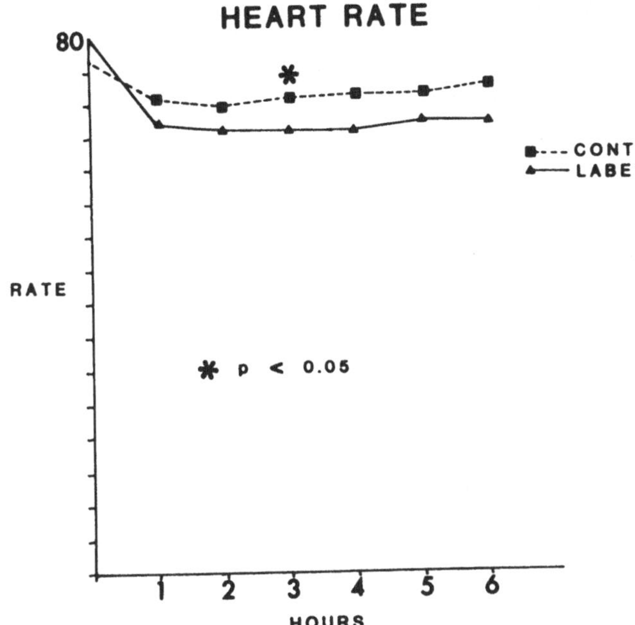

Fig. 2

Averaged heart rates over six hours for patients treated with labetalol and those who served as controls.

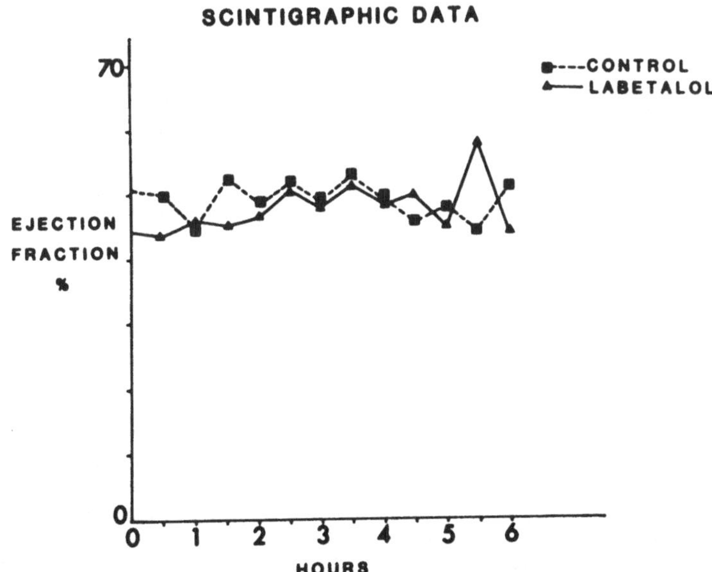

Fig. 3

Averaged ejection fraction measured by a single crystal probe over six hours for 46 patients treated with labetalol and 40 patients who served as controls. (Patients were selected for scintigraphic measurements on the basis of availability of isotope.)

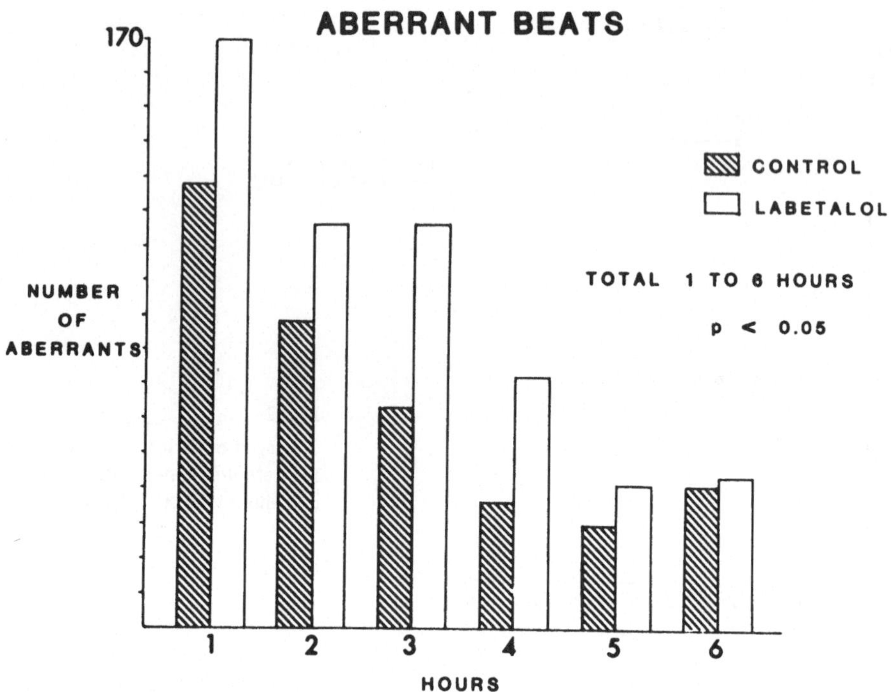

Fig. 4

The average counts of aberrant (widened premature) beats over six hours in patients treated with labetalol and in those who served as controls.

observed no effect of our treatment on left ventricular function as assessed by scintigraphy. The augmented enzyme release did not necessarily indicate a tendency for an increase in infarct size as a result of labetalol treatment. Only about 15 per cent of enzyme loss from infarcted myocardium is released into the circulation, whilst the remainder is destroyed *in-situ* [14]; if coronary vasodilation did occur from the alpha-blockade an increased washout may have occurred without there necessarily being an increase in cellular damage. Our data cannot distinguish between these two possible mechanisms.

The increase in arrhythmias indicated by a higher count of aberrant complexes is disturbing. The consistency of the effect over the monitored hours makes this unlikely to have been only the play of chance. Labetalol must have a proarrhythmic effect in this situation, but we do not know if this is because extrasystoles may be bradycardia-dependent, because of increased myocardial ischaemia following induced hypotension, or because of other known or unknown actions of the drug.

We do not believe there are grounds at present for planning a large-scale mortality study using labetalol in a manner similar to that adopted in our own protocol. Unless more favourable evidence is forthcoming we advise at present that the use of labetaolol in patients with acute myocardial infarction be restricted to those for whom control of hypertension is judged to be important.

References

[1] Marx, P. G., Reid, D. S.: Labetalol infusion in acute myocardial infarction with systemic hypertension. *Br. J. Clin. Pharmacol.* **8** (suppl. 2), 233s–238s (1979).

[2] Timmis, A. D., Fowler, M. B., Jaggarao, N. S. V., Chamberlain, D. A.: Labetalol infusion for the treatment of hypertension in acute myocardial infarction. *Europ. Heart J.* **1**, 413–416 (1980).

[3] Renard, M., Rivière, A., Jacobs, P., Bernard, R.: Treatment of hypertension in acute stage of myocardial infarction. *Brit. Heart J.* **49**, 522–527 (1983).

[4] Silke, B., Verma, S. P., Nelson, G. I. C., Taylor, S. H.: Effects of alpha/beta blockade on cardiac performance in hypertension complicating myocardial infarction. This volume, pp. 195–203.

[5] Snow, P. J. D.: Effect of propranolol in myocardial infarction. *Lancet* **II**, 551–553 (1965).

[6] Chamberlain, D. A.: Beta adrenoceptor antagonists after myocardial infarction — where are we now? *Brit. Heart J.* **49**, 105–110 (1983).

[7] Furberg, C. D., Friedewald, W. T., Eberlein, K. A. (Eds): Proceedings of the workshop on implications of recent beta-blocker trials for post-myocardial infarction patients. *Circulation* **67** (Suppl. I) (1983).

[8] Lemberg, L., Castellanos, A., Arcebal, A. G.: The use of propranolol in arrhythmias complicating acute myocardial infarction. *Amer. Heart J.* **80**, 479–487 (1970).

[9] Rydén, L., Ariniego, R., Arnman, K., Herlitz, J., Hjalmarson, Å., Holmberg, S., Reyes, C., Smedgåard, P., Svedberg, K., Vedin, A., Waagstein, F., Valdenström, A., Wilhelmsson, C., Wedel, H., Yamamoto, M.: A double-blind trial of metoprolol in acute myocardial infarction. Effects on ventricular tachycardias. *New Engl. J. Med.* **308**, 614–618 (1983).

[10] Yusuf, S., Sleight, P., Rossi, P., Ramsdale, D., Peto, R., Furze, L., Sterry, H., Pearson, M., Motwani, R., Parish, S., Gray, R., Bennett, D., Bray, C.: Reduction in infarct size, arrhythmias and chest pain by early intravenous beta-blockade in suspected myocardial infarction. *Circulation* **67** (Suppl. I), 32s–42s, 1983.

[11] Corr, P. B., Yamada, K. A.: Pathophysiological mechanism of alpha-adrenoceptor stimulation in the ischemic heart. This volume pp. 161–170.

[12] Sheridan, D. J., Penkoske, P. A., Sobel, B. E., Corr, P. B.: Alpha adrenergic contribution to dysrhythmia during myocardial infarction and reperfusion in cats. *J. Clin. Invest.* **65**, 161–171 (1980).

[13] Nelson, G. I. C., Ahuja, R. C., Hussain, M., Silke, B., Taylor, S. H.: α- and β-blockade with labetalol in acute myocardial infarction. *J. Cardiovasc. Pharmacol.* **4**, 921–924 (1982).

[14] Bleifeld, W., Mathey, D., Hanrath, P., Buss, H., Effert, S.: Infarct size estimated from serial creatine phosphokinase in relation to left ventricular hemodynamics. *Circulation* **55**, 303–311 (1977).

Discussion

Taylor
Would you comment on the dosage you were using within the first hour or two, compared to those used by Corr? He pointed out as you did, that the ectopic beat formation didn't really reflect mortality from ventricular arrhythmia, but I think he was using dosages which were different.

Chamberlain
Very different. We would like to reproduce these sort of dose levels, but it is very difficult to do that in a clinical situation. I think that we could have been a little bit bolder, because if you use a bigger dose of labetalol it may be that the blood pressure doesn't come down all that much, but slightly lower. I do not think that we could get to the dose levels used experimentally.

Taylor
Presumably we could get to larger doses if the patient was hypertensive.

Chamberlain
Yes, absolutely.

Rietbrock, N.

Wie war das Verhältnis von Erhaltungsdosis und Initialdosis? Bei der Wahl der Initialdosis geht man aus von der wirksamen Erhaltungsdosis, und legt dann die Initialdosis fest. Das ist nur optimal möglich, wenn die pharmakokinetischen Daten der Substanz bekannt sind.

Chamberlain

We certainly did not adjust our doses on pharmacokinetic data, it is true, but in a pilot study we explored how large a dose we could give without causing severe hypotension and our aim was to use the maximum dose. We looked at blood levels in earlier small subsets. The aim was to use the biggest dose possible, without causing the blood pressure to go below 100. The measurement was arranged on the basis of a study of 25 patients where we did dose titrations.

Corr

You have looked at your data, separated as to more malignant arrhythmias, rather than number of premature beats? Have you looked at runs of ventricular tachycardias? Did you have a higher incidence in one group than than the other?

Chamberlain

There are rather few episodes of ventricular tachycardia and from a quick look at the data there seems to be little difference in the two groups. It certainly doesn't stand out as being good news, but it may simply be that there were not enough of the sinister arrhythmias.

Prichard

I would like to comment on the value of pharmacokinetic data. I think it must be said that pharmacokinetics is very much the hand-maiden of pharmacodynamics. In other words, it is sometimes a useful servant to tell us how to understand the effect of drugs, but often it is rather irrelevant. I think the only relevance in this context is that when you give a bolus injection of labetalol, and even a bolus injection over 10 minutes (a cross between a bolus injection and infusion) you are going to get initially a very high level. What really matters is; what is the response of that patient to that particular drug? The drug levels are, within broad limits, irrelevant as to what effect you get, and particularly so in this sort of situation where there are many other factors, in terms of sympathetic tone, degree of damage to the myocardium, which will influence the final outcome, rather that the mere blood level.

Chamberlain

I think it is worth emphasizing too, that we were testing a policy, not looking at clinical pharmacology. We were looking at a policy in a clinical context and it may not tell us all there is to know about labetalol.

Taylor

I would like to support Prichard and Chamberlain. I think that to measure the plasma concentration of a drug with mixed action in a patient, where we do not quite know how much alpha-stimulation against beta-stimulation is present, is a useful exercise in pharmacology, but is of little use to the physicians. I think that it is extremely limited, particularly when you are using drugs in combination, in this instance with diametrically opposed pharmacological effects, in serious disease.

Effects of Alpha-Beta Blockade on Cardiac Performance in Hypertension Complicating Myocardial Infarction

B. Silke, S. P. Verma, G. I. C. Nelson, S. H. Taylor

University Department of Cardiovascular Studies,

and

Department of Medical Cardiology, The General Infirmary, Leeds, England.

Summary

The haemodynamic effects of α-β blockade with labetalol were evaluated in 36 male patients following acute myocardial infarction, within 18 hr of the onset of symptoms. Continuous intravenous labetalol infusion resulted in linear reductions in systemic arterial blood pressure and vascular resistance, the rate of pressure reductions being proportional to the initial control systolic blood pressure level. There was a small reduction in cardiac output and heart rate which was independent of the reduction in systemic arterial pressure. Slow calcium channel blockade (nifedipine) was compared with α-β blockade with labetalol in patients with systemic hypertension ($> 160/95$ mmHg) complicating myocardial infarction. At equivalent reductions in systemic blood pressure and left ventricular afterload, labetalol resulted in greater ($p < 0.05$) reduction in stroke work index than nifedipine, due to reflex sympathetic activation and tachycardia induced by the latter therapy. These data suggest that labetalol is an effective and safe intervention, when applied under haemodynamic monitoring control, both in normotensive and hypertensive myocardial infarction.

In recent years there has been intense interest in the pharmacological manipulation of the circulation, to reduce left ventricular afterload and limit infarct size [1]. Hypertension complicating myocardial infarction is not an uncommon problem; reduction of persistently raised blood pressure has been advocated to reduce oxygen consumption and limit the extent of muscle injury [2, 3].
Labetalol, a competitive antagonist at alpha and beta-adrenoceptors, is an effective antihypertensive agent [4, 5]; moreover, the addition of alpha to beta-blockade in pattients with stable coronary heart disease reduces the increase in left ventricular afterload induced by beta-blockade alone [6—8]. The haemodynamic disadvantages of beta-blockade alone in acute myocardial infarction [9, 10] may therefore be modified by concomitant vasodilatation. Laboratory animal studies with labetalol have also demonstrated theoretical advantages for alpha- and beta-blockade in the occlusion and reperfusion phases of acute myocardial infarction [11]. Combined alpha and beta-blockade reduced the incidence of ventricular fibrillation in a dose-response fashion [12]. Moreover, in such studies

labetalol also reduced myocardial cell necrosis and infarct size after acute coronary occlusion [13].

Recently the haemodynamic effects of such treatment in patients in the early stages of acute myocardial infarction have been described [14–17]. Our studies were designed to further explore the dose-response effect of intravenous therapy on cardiovascular dynamics in patients admitted within a few hours of the onset of symptoms of acute myocardial infarction.

Methods

Patients

Male patients, aged 44–64 yr. were studied in the Coronary Care Unit within 4–18 hours of the onset of symptoms of acute myocardial infarction. Serum cardiac enzymes were raised in all. On admission all patients were in sinus rhythm and without clinical or radiographic evidence of left ventricular failure. Hypertension was defined as persistent (> 4 hr), elevation of the systemic arterial blood pressure (systolic BP > 160 mmHg or diastolic BP > 95 mmHg). All patients with persisting pain had received a single dose of a narcotic analgesic but none required supplementary doses within 2 hours of the study's commencement. No other cardioactive drug was administered before or during these studies. Patients were informed of the object of the treatment and the study was agreed to by the hospital Ethics Committee.

Design (Study 1)

The first study was designed as an open dose-response evaluation of the haemodynamic effects of a continuous intravenous (i. v.) infusion of labetalol in 21 patients with different levels of systemic blood pressure. Control systolic arterial pressure was > 160 mmHg in 6, between 135–160 mmHg in 9 and between 100–134 mmHg in a further 6 patients. Control measurements were made at 20 min intervals for 60 min following which i. v. labetalol was infused, commencing at 0.5 mg/kg/hr for the first 60 min then 1.0 mg/kg/hr for 60 min and finally 2.0 mg/kg/hr for 60 min; the infusion was discontinued if the systolic blood pressure fell below 100 mmHg. Haemodynamic measurements were made every 30 min during the infusion period.

Design (Study 2)

The second study was designed as a randomised between-group comparison of the haemodynamic effects of nifedipine (20 mg sublingually) or labetalol (1 mg/kg i. v. over 15 min) in patients whose myocardial infarction was complicated by hypertension, with or without haemodynamic decompensation (PAOP > 18 mmHg). Following a 1 hour control period haemodynamic measurements were made at 15, 30, 60 and 120 min after each drug. 7 patients were studied in each of the 4 groups.

Haemodynamic Measurements

Electrocardiographic and haemodynamic monitoring was established in each patient immediately after admission. Heart rate was measured from the electrocardiogram and systemic arterial pressure through a brachial artery catheter. Pulmonary vascular pressures were measured through a balloon-tipped thermodilution catheter introduced via the cubital fossa and positioned by pressure monitoring so that inflation of the balloon resulted in replacement of the pulmonary artery pressure by a typical pulmonary wedge pressure tracing (pulmonary artery occluded pressure – PAOP). Pressures were externally transduced (Bell and Howell 4-327-I) with strain gauges recorded together with heart rate on a thermal recorder (MFE 1440). Zero reference point was taken at the mid-chest level.

Mean pressures were integrated electronically and heart rate and pressures were averaged over at least two respiratory cycles. Cardiac output was measured in triplicate by thermo-dilution and automatically computed (Edwards Laboratories Computer 9520/Recorder 9812). A gas-operated constant speed injector (OMP Model 3700) was used with 10 ml of dextrose saline at 0 °C as indicator. This system has been shown to be linear in vitro with a coefficient of variation of 6.2 % in similar patients.

Statistical analysis of difference between control and post-drug data was tested by analysis of variance of repeated measurements [18]. Tukey's studentised test was then used to generate the single value by which difference between drug and control values was tested. Variability of measurements during the control studies was determined by the coefficient of variation and expressed as a percentage of the mean. There was no trend to change in any variable during the period; for clarity of presentation the values during the control period are presented as averages.

Results

The labetalol infusion was not associated with untoward symptoms in any patient. No patient suffered ventricular tachycardia or fibrillation and none developed a conduction defect or died during their hospital admission.

Table 1: Effects of Labetalol infusion in patients with Myocardial Infarction related to pre-treatment Systolic Arterial Blood Pressure

Group	Total Dose (mg)	Duration of Infusion (min)	Plasma Concentration (ng/ml)[1]	Rate of SBP Reduction (mmHg/100 mg Labetalol)
I (> 160) (n = 6)	242 ± 27	165 ± 10	735 ± 147	31.8 ± 6.3
II (135–160) (n = 9)	179 ± 33	137 ± 13	571 ± 70	28.0 ± 5.5
III (100–134) (n = 6)	154 ± 23	128 ± 9	660 ± 10	11.0 ± 2.1

Data expressed as Mean ± S.E.M.
1 At end of Infusion.

Study 1 Intravenous dose plasma concentration and effects of labetalol (Table 1)

The average cumulative doses of labetalol and plasma concentrations achieved in the different entry blood pressure groups are shown. The critical end-point for stopping the infusion was a systolic blood pressure of 100 mmHg. All 21 patients tolerated the initial infusion of 0.5 mg/kg/hr for 30 min. In hypertensives, all but one patient tolerated all infusion levels including the final infusion dose of 2.0 mg/kg/hr. In normotensives the infusion was discontinued at 1.0 mg/kg/hr in five patients and at 2.0 mg/kg/hr in four. In patients with low blood pressure, three patients tolerated only 1.0 mg/kg/hr although three received 2.0 mg/kg/hr without reduction in systolic blood pressure below 100 mmHg. The rate of reduction in systolic blood pressure was quadratically related to its initial height (Table 1). The dose-related fall in blood pressure resulted in small reductions in cardiac output in each group (Fig. 1). Cardiac output was reduced equally in all patient groups at the first dose level (0.5 mg/kg/hr at 30 min) but continuation of the labetalol infusion produced no further change. There was a significant dose-related reduction in the systemic vascular resistance in the hypertensive patients but not in the other groups (Fig. 2). There were no significant changes in pulmonary artery occluded pressure in any patient group.

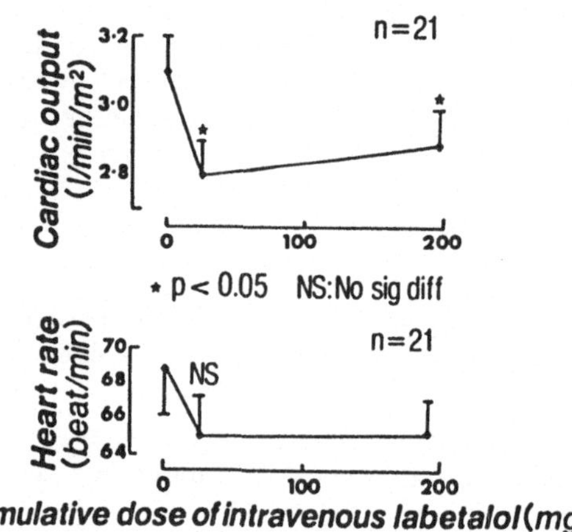

Fig. 1
Effect of continuous labetalol infusion on cardiac output and heart rate in 21 patients with acute myocardial infarction.
(Data expressed as Mean ± S.E.M. Statistics related to comparison with control * p < 0.05).

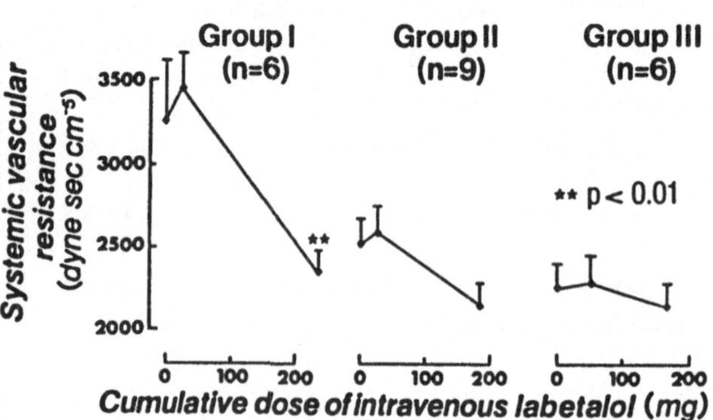

Fig. 2
Effect of labetalol infusion on systemic vascular resistance related to pre-entry systolic blood pressure.
(Data expressed as Mean ± S.E.M. Statistics related to comparison with control).

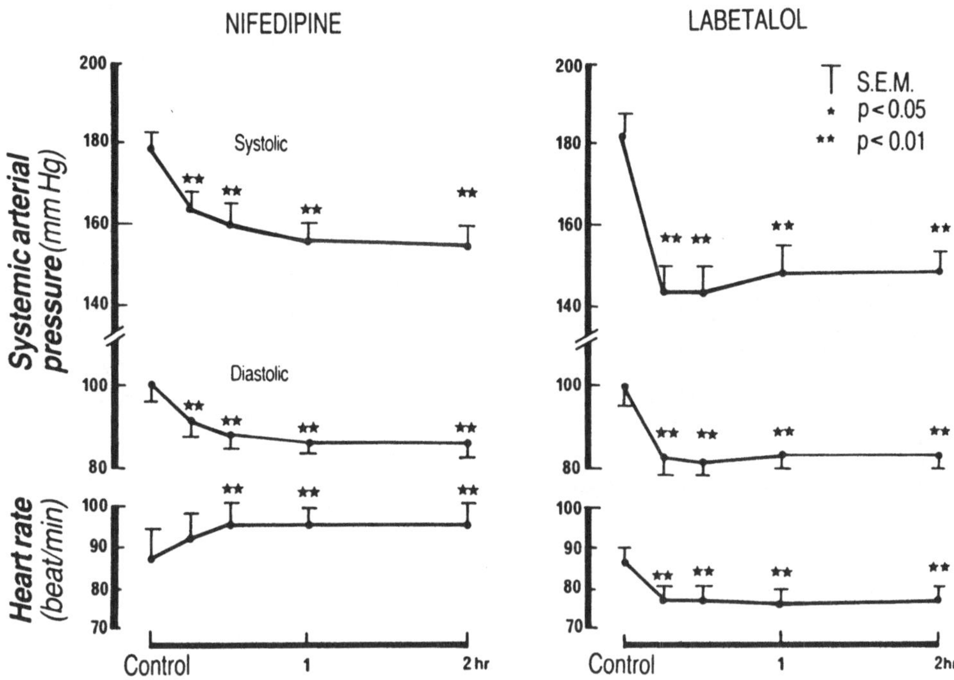

Fig. 3 Comparison of effects of labetalol and nifedipine in acute myocardial infarction. (Data expressed as Mean ± S.E.M. Statistics related to comparison with control).

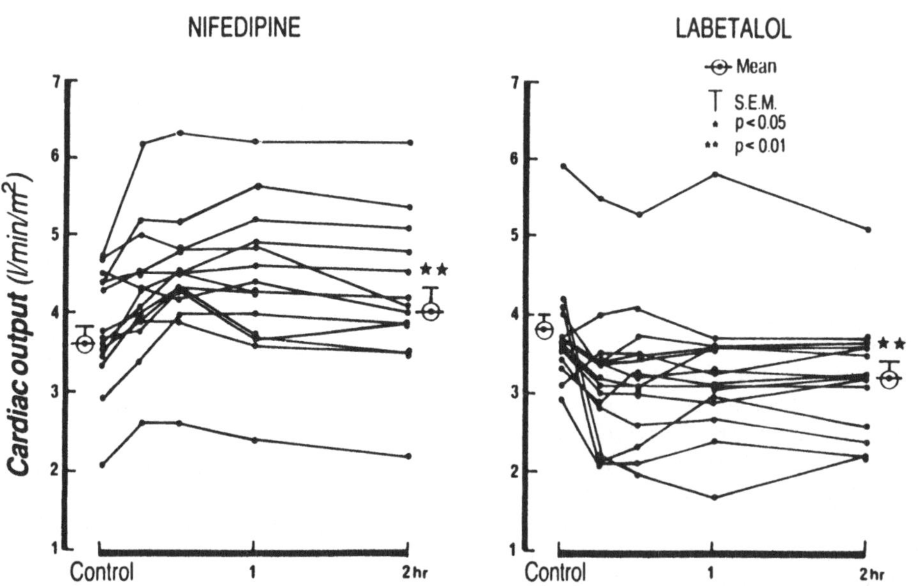

Fig. 4 Effects of nifedipine (20 mg sublingually) or labetalol (1 mg/kg i.v.) on cardiac output at rest following acute myocardial infarction.

201

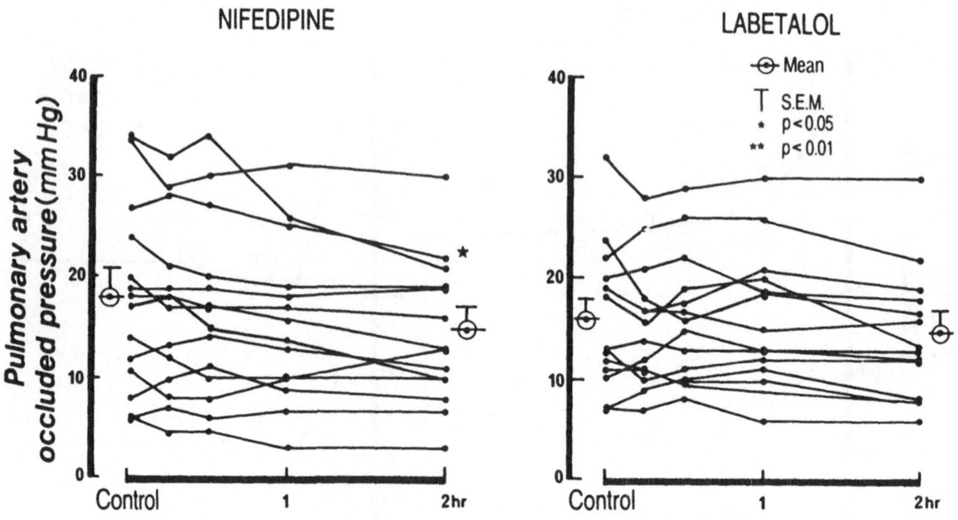

Fig. 5 Effects of nifedipine (20 mg sublingually) or labetalol (1 mg/kg i.v.) on PAOP at rest following acute myocardial infarction.

Study 2

Both nifedipine (20 mg) and labetalol (1 mg/kg i.v.) achieved similar reduction in diastolic blood pressure (Fig. 3) and presumably left ventricular afterload. The average labetalol dose was 78 mg (57—104 range). This was associated with significant falls in systemic blood pressure, and a reduction in heart rate ($p < 0.05$) and cardiac output (Fig. 4—5) without changes in PAOP. Nifedipine, in contrast, increased heart rate ($p < 0.01$) and cardiac output ($p < 0.01$) with a reduction in PAOP, which was confined to patients with an initial starting value > 18 mmHg. These effects were maintained for the 120 min of the observation period.

Discussion

These results suggest that intravenous labetalol is clinically efficacious in the therapy of hypertension complicating acute myocardial infarction. These data clearly showed that the sensitivity to the alpha-blocking component of the drug was related directly and in a dose-response fashion to the patient's initial systemic arterial pressure and vascular resistance. In contrast, the effects of the beta-adrenoceptor blocking component of the drug were maximum at the initiation to treatment and independent of the arterial pressure. Moreover, with subsequent dosage increments the potentially adverse haemodynamic consequences of beta-blockade were offset by concomitant alpha-adrenoceptor blockade mediated vasodilatation.

Our results with intravenous labetalol are similar to published reports [14—17]. Timmis et al. observed falls in systolic and diastolic arterial pressure of -59 and -19 mmHg respectively with small reductions in heart rate and cardiac output. These results are similar to those of Marx and Reid [15]. Renard et al. [17] showed a difference in response of pulmonary artery occluded pressure, relative to its initial pre-treatment value, following labetalol. These data, in agreement with those of Timmis et al., showed an unchanged PAOP when initial value was low; where initial PAOP was > 15 mmHg labetalol usually resulted in a fall. These results are similar to that following intravenous propranolol and may be related to an effect on ventricular compliance [19].

The observed effects of slow-calcium channel blockade were compatible with previous data on nifedipine in stable ischaemic heart disease [20, 21]. Nifedipine reduced blood pressure, left ventricular afterload and the cardiac output increased as the systemic vascular resistance was lowered. However, presumably as the result of the fall in mean blood pressure, and reflex sympathetic activation [22], the heart rate rose. Thus the reduction in stroke work index on nifedipine was less than at a similar reduction in left ventricular afterload on labetalol.

One of the prime objectives of this study was to compare the haemodynamic effects of labetalol and nifedipine in patients with sustained hypertension after acute myocardial infarction, with particular reference to those patients having concomitant left ventricular failure. Although both regimens effectively corrected the elevations in systemic arterial pressure, there were major haemodynamic differences in the mechanisms by which this was achieved. In patients with or without pulmonary congestion combined α and β blockade reduced afterload and was accompanied by falls in heart rate and cardiac output. Stroke volume was unchanged. In contrast, nifedipine by predominant arteriolar dilatation, but without sympathetic blockade, resulted in increase in heart rate, cardiac output and stroke volume. Nifedipine did not, however, alter PAOP when initial values were normal (< 18 mmHg) but the LV filling pressure (-5 mmHg; $p < 0.05$) fell when initially elevated. The data on nifedipine is in agreement with effects observed in patients with chronic ischaemia and heart failure [23, 24, 25].

In conclusion, these results suggest that labetalol is a useful therapy for the acute management of hypertension with or without heart failure. Slow calcium channel blockade would only seem indicated in patients whose hypertension is accompanied by LV dysfunction. The possible impact of acute alpha-beta blockade on the outcome of myocardial infarction complicated by hypertension in terms of attenuation of dysrhythmics, reduction in infarct size or improvement in prognosis must await more definitive and pragmatic studies.

Acknowledgements

We wish to thank Sister S. Winterburn and Nursing Staff of the Cardiac Care Unit for their help, and Mrs. A. Richmond, B. Sc., for assistance with the statistical programme. We also wish to acknowledge financial support for the study from the Yorkshire Regional Hospital Board, West Riding Medical Research Trust and Glaxo UK (Ltd.).

References

[1] Braunwald, E. and Moroko, P. R.: The reduction of infarct size — an idea whose time (for testing) has come. *Circulation* **50**, 206–209 (1974).

[2] Kelly, D. T., Delgado, C. E., Taylor, D. R., Pitt, B. and Ross, R. S.: Use of phentolamine in acute myocardial infarction associated with hypertension and left ventricular failure. *Circulation* **47**, 729–735 (1973).

[3] Shell, W. E. and Sobel, B. E.: Protection of jeopardised ischaemic myocardium by reduction of ventricular afterload. *New Eng. J. Med.* **291**, 481–486 (1974).

[4] Prichard, B. N. C. and Boakes, A. J.: Labetalol in long-term treatment of hypertension. *Brit. J. Clin. Pharmacol.*, Suppl. 743–750 (1976).

[5] Rǿnne-Rasmussen, J. O., Andersen, G. S., Bowal Jenson, N. and Andersson, E.: Acute effect of intravenous labetalol in the treatment of systemic arterial hypertension. *Brit. J. Clin. Pharmacol.*, *Suppl. 805–808* (1976).

[6] Gagnon, R. M., Morisette, M., Presant, S., Savard, D. and Lemire, J.: Haemodynamic and coronary effects of intravenous labetalol in coronary artery disease. *Am. J. Cardiol.* **49**, 1267–69 (1982).

[7] Taylor, S. H., Silke, B., Nelson, G. I. C., Okoli, R. C. and Ahuja, R. C.: Haemodynamic advantages of combined alpha-blockade and beta-blockade over beta-blockade alone in patients with coronary heart disease. *Br. Med. J.* **285**, 325–27 (1982).

[8] Silke, B., Nelson, G. I. C., Ahuja, R. C. and Taylor, S. H.: Comparative haemodynamic dose-response effects of propranolol and labetalol in coronary heart disease. *Br. Heart J.* **48**, 364–371 (1982).

[9] Bay, G., Lund Larson, P., Lorentsen, E. and Silvertsen, E.: Haemodynamic effect of propranolol in acute myocardial infarction. *Br. Med. J.* **1**, 141–143 (1967).

[10] Jewitt, D. E., Burgess, P. A. and Shillingford, J. P.: The circulatory effects of practolol in patients with acute myocardial infarction. *Cardiovasc. Res.* **4**, 188–193 (1970).

[11] Sheridan, D. J., Penkoske, P. A., Sobel, B. E. and Corr, P. B.: Alpha-adrenergic contributions to dysrhythmias during myocardial ischaemia and reperfusion in cats. *J. Clin. Invest.* **65**, 161–171 (1980).

[12] Pogwizd, S. M., Sharma, A. D. and Corr, P. B.: Influences of labetalol and combined alpha- and beta-adrenergic blocking agent on the dysrhythmias induced by coronary occlusion and reperfusion. *Cardiovasc. Res.* **16**, 398–407 (1982).

[13] Chiarello, M., Brevetti, G., de Rosa, G., Acunzo, R., Petillo, F., Rengo, F. and Condorelli, M.: Protective effects of simultaneous alpha- and beta-adrenergic receptor blockade on myocardial cell necroses after coronary arterial occlusion in rats. *Am. J. Cardiol.* **46**, 249–254 (1980).

[14] Marx, P. G. and Reid, D. S.: Labetalol infusion in acute myocardial infarction with systemic hypertension. *Br. J. Clin. Pharmacol* **8**, Suppl. 2, 233S–238S (1979).

[15] Timmis, A. D., Fowler, M. B., Jaggaroso, N. S. V. and Chamberlain, D. A.: Labetalol infusion for the treatment of hypertension in acute myocardial infarction. *Eur. Heart J.* **1**, 413–416 (1980).

[16] Nelson, G. I. C., Silke, B., Ahuja, R. C., Hussain, M., Taylor, S. H.: Haemodynamic dose-response effects of intravenous labetalol in acute myocardial infarction. *Postgrad. Med. J.* **59** (Suppl. 3) 98–103 (1983).

[17] Renard, M., Melot, R., Haardt, H., Vainsel, H. and Bernard, R.: Effect of labetalol on preload in acute myocardial infarction with systemic hypertension. *J. Cardiovasc. Pharmacol.* **6**, 90–93 (1984).

[18] *Biomedical Computer Programs* – 'P' Series. Eds. Dixon, W. J. and Brown, M. B., 1979. University of California Press, Berkeley, p. 540.

[19] Mueller, H. S., Ayres, S. M.: The role of propranolol in the treatment of acute myocardial infarction. *Prog. Cardiovasc. Dis.* **19**, 405–412 (1977).

[20] Henry, P. D.: Comparative pharmacology of calcium antagonists: nifedipine, verapamil and diltiazem. *Am. J. Cardiol.* **46**, 1047–1058 (1980).

[21] Winniford, M. D., Mark Lam, R. V., Firth, B. G., Nicod, P., Hillis, L. D.: Haemodynamic and electrophysiologic effects of verapamil and nifedipine in patients on propranolol. *Am. J. Cardiol.* **50**, 704–710 (1982).

[22] Amlie, J. P., Landmark, K.: The effects of nifedipine on the sinus and atrioventricular node of the dog heart after beta-adrenergic receptor blockade. *Acta Pharmacol. Toxicol. (Copenh)* **42**, 287–291 (1972).

[23] Zacca, N. M., Verani, M. S., Chahine, R. A., Miller, R. R.: Effect of nifedipine on exercise-induced left ventricular dysfunction and myocardial hypoperfusion in stable angina. *Am. J. Cardiol.* **50**, 689–695 (1982).

[24] Elkayam, U., Weber, L., Torkan, B., Berman, D. and Rahimtoola, S.: Acute haemodynamic effect of oral nifedipine in severe chronic congestive heart failure. *Am. J. Cardiol.* **52**, 1041–1045 (1983).

[25] Nelson, G. I. C., Silke, B., Ahuja, R. C., Hussain, M. and Taylor, S. H.: Haemodynamic effects of nifedipine during upright exercise in patients with stable angina pectoris and either normal of severely impaired left ventricular function. *Am. J. Cardiol.* **53**, 451–455, 1984.

Discussion

Borchard
Könnten Sie etwas zur Häufigkeit und zur Schwere von Rhythmusstörungen in den Gruppen, die Sie untersucht haben, sagen?

Silke
None of these patients had disrhythmias. We did not specifically subject them to 24-hour-monitoring and evaluate disrhythmias as such, but these patients would not have been entered into this study had there been clinically significant incidences of disrhythmias requiring therapy. There were no incidences of disrhythmias observed during monitoring over the course of these studies.

General Discussion

Taylor
There is one important question I would like to remind you of, and that is dose. There is no doubt that in hypertension where there is marginal, if any, increase in vasoconstriction sensitive to alpha-blockade, the dose of the drug required to lower the blood pressure is obviously greater than in patients who are vasoconstricted, either during exercise-angina or following myocardial infarction. The dosage regimen that seems tenable in hypertension, that is a starting dose of 200 mg twice a day, can be stepped up in many patients to 400 mg twice a day with increased effectiveness. There are obviously a few patients, particularly those of light weight, in which 200 mg twice a day probably is too much, and who therefore need only 100 mg twice a day. So we are having, in hypertension an optimal effect with probably between 400 and 800 mg a day. In angina pectoris, from the studies of Dr. Jackson and those of our own and other workers, the dose is at least half of this. That is a maximum dose of 400 mg per day with many patients responding to 200 mg a day. Dr. Chamberlain pointed out and Dr. Silke emphasized, that in acute myocardial infarction it may be even less than that. This emphasizes to us that we must adjust the dose of a sympatholytic combined agent like labetalol to the clinical condition, that is the physiological state which we are trying to correct. I think this is a very important aspect that hasn't been brought up until now.

Rietbrock, N.
Wo würden Sie denn, Dr. Taylor, die Substanz jetzt einordnen? Mehr auf Seite der Betablocker, oder mehr auf die Seite der Kalziumantagonisten? Könnten Sie das noch einmal umreißen? Welche Eigenschaften ähneln den Kalziumantagonisten und welche Eigenschaften den Betablockern?

Taylor
I suppose, one could deal with this from two aspects. One from the field of high blood pressure, and the other from coronary heart disease. I think that in hypertension there is no single agent that can invariably be advocated to lower the blood pressure in every patient. We do not know the cause of the hypertension we can only treat the physiological abnormality. There is no doubt that blockade of the sympathetic nervous system is now a favourite treatment, and at least it does lower the blood pressure. The beta-blockers do this but there is no doubt also that vasodilators, in particularly vasodilators with alpha-blocking properties, may also be important. I think we shall eventually find, for each patient, that drug which not only satisfactorily lowers blood pressure and is rational in its use but also produces less side-effects than other combinations. Beta-blockers are very good in some patients, without side-effects, in others they have intolerable side-effects. It may be that labetalol, as far as we can see from our experience, has a very definite place as one of these agents. It will not replace all beta-blocking drugs, or all calcium-antagonists. All these drugs have side-effects. We shall eventually find a small group of patients with essential hypertension in which alpha- and beta-blockade in combination is the most efficacious treatment for that patient. I think that was already alluded to by Dr. Jackson when he said that many patients with angina will respond very satisfactorily to a beta-blocker drug alone. Others will get relief of angina, but only at the price of intolerable side-effects. Those are the patients for whom alpha-, beta-blockade might well offer advantages. We are modifying the physiological derangement that results from the disease, we are not modifying the disease. This is the crucial issue.

Kuhlmann
Habe ich nicht therapeutische Vorteile, wenn ich eine Substanz mit nur alpha- oder betablockierender Wirkung anwende und diese individuell oder liegen größere Vorteile bei einer Substanz, die sowohl alpha- als auch betablockierende Wirkungen hat?

Taylor
I think that really is a matter of opinion. If I understand from the practice of German physicians, that is not their view-point. Their view-point is that they would like to give a single agent with a minimum of titration. I do not feel that the physician in general practice is in anyway able to titrate what he really requires. He can measure the blood pressure, but that is not all that is required in these people. I think it may be as Dr. Corr intimated earlier, we may not be able, the clinicians and physicians, to detect the alpha-blocking activity of a drug we give to our patients but it may be important in a hidden way. Just to quote one possible example, the hypertensive patient who develops an infarction.

Many of our hypertensive patients unfortunately will develop an infarction at some point. It might be a good thing to have both, alpha-, and beta-blocking drugs aboard. Dr. Corr was intimating or even going out of his way to say that some of the arrhythmias, particularly late one, may be due to activation of beta-receptors but there is no doubt that there is a patch in the evolution of myocardial infarction when the sinister killing arrhythmias are due to alpha-stimulation. The doctor can never determine this when he is treating a hypertensive. He just must go on what knowledges he has supplied to him.

Greeff

Ich möchte dann doch noch einmal auf die Pharmakokinetik eingehen. Ich bin nicht ganz Ihrer Meinung, Dr. Taylor, daß die Pharmakokinetik unnötig ist. Herr Rietbrock hat sicherlich auch nicht den Blutspiegel gemeint, sondern mehr den zeitlichen Verlauf des Effektes. Nun hat diese Substanz eine alpha- und betablockierende Wirkung. Es wäre z. B. interessant zu wissen, ob die Kinetik der Alpha- und Betarezeptoren identisch ist. Es ist in einigen klinischen Situationen wichtig zu wissen, wann man die zweite Dosis geben muß, und dafür müssen wir die pharmakodynamische Halbwertzeit kennen.

Taylor

I do not disagree, I think that we do need to have additional information, from whatever source in pharmacokinetics. I believe as physician, whatever the pharmacokinetic knowledge displayed to me, I need to know the effects of that drug on that patient. I was not particularly decrying pharmacokinetics, but explaining that with a mixed action drug like labetalol with both, alpha- and beta-blocking activitiy we are not measuring the pharmacokinetics of its alpha-blocking component or its beta-blocking component, we are measuring labetalol and that is where the difficulties must arise.

Rietbrock, N.

Labetalol hat einen First-Pass-Effekt und ähnliches gilt für Nifedipin. Wir wissen, wie groß die Variablität solcher Substanzen ist, etwa eine Abweichung von ± 50 %. Kann man dann überhaupt eine sublinguale Verabreichung vergleichen mit einer intravenösen Gabe? Das ist gerade beim Nifedipin das Problem. Könnten Sie da noch etwas zu sagen?

Taylor

I'm sure that this is something that we do need to know much more about. My own group has made observations that relate to clinical medicine with prazosin. When the heart fails the pharmacokinetic profile of prazosin alters quite dramatically. I think this is the kind of information we really do need. I don't think we have that information yet on combined alpha-, and beta-blockade with labetalol. Naturally you are bringing forward topics which this symposium was meant to generate.

Silke

I wish to make a brief comment on the variability of plasma concentration in relationship to effect. It may be true that the standard deviation of plasma concentration is quite large. If one considers the variation in the response, that is the standard error around the reduction in blood pressure, this is showing a much smaller effect. In other words, you cannot show a linear relationship with the response in terms of blood pressure effect or heart rate effect, or the cardiac output effect. We cannot predict from labetalol plasma concentrations, what effect we will get. Some patients may become hypotensive with plasma concentrations of 100 or 200 ng/ml and other patients, for reasons we don't understand, for example following infarction, tolerate levels over 1000 ng/ml. There is always an element of the individual response which makes attempts to predict response in individual patients, based on a plasma concentration, of limited value.

Holti

I feel that the pharmacologists have not provided us with the information we really required. A drug acts at tissue level and not at blood level. Blood levels may be very high because drugs are bound so firmly to carrier proteins.

Woodcock

Labetalol is a drug with a high clearance where the clearance, as in the case of verapamil, probably depends on liver blood flow and therefore on cardiac output. The effect of cardiac output on drug metabolism and on liver blood flow, for all drugs, is only scantily investigated. Thus it is difficult to interprete serum levels and eliminations half-times when cardiac output is changing but this is important information. We know that with labetalol the serum concentrations that we obtain on chronic treatment are not the same as those predicted from single intravenous doses. There is a change in the elimination characteristics of labetalol on chronic application, and this is not only true for labetalol, but also for drugs like propranolol. In the future we need to obtain more pharmacokinetic information in chronic treatment and especially in patients with reduced cardiac outputs.

Taylor
It is time to bring the proceedings to a close and to summarize the main points. Dr. Corr's comments on the newly discovered pathogenic roll of alpha-receptors in ischemic myocardia might be a very important and rapidly expanding field, providing a new roll for alpha- and beta-blockers.

Dr. Jackson then reported preliminary findings in an open-study of alpha-beta-blockade in angina emphasizing three points. The first was this very small labetalol dose, compared to that for hypertension treatment, that he was using. He found it to be a drug with high tolerability as has been emphasized by Dr. Holti. He concluded by saying that many more studies are necessary in angina pectoris, and others have mentioned variant angina, and perhaps crescendo angina.

Dr. Chamberlain presented results of his studies with labetalol in normotensive patients. Although he did conclude that no further major studies are probably warranted in this field, I think that he also feels that we need more information.

Dr. Silke reviewed the potential of alpha-beta-blockade, particularly the acute effects on heamodynamics in patients with AMI and concomitant hypertension. This is an area where none of the other beta-blocking drugs have been found to be of use. He also compared his findings with those using nifedipine and could conclude that labetalol was at least and possibly, more effective than nifedipine, but this field of acute myocardial infarction has not been paid much attention in the past. I think therefore that the long-term circulatory, pharmacokinetics, and clinical benefits of combined alpha-beta-blockade in coronary heart disease have yet to be finally crystallized. All the evidence would seem at least to encourage clinical investigation to find the true role for such drugs in patients with coronary disease.

Woodcock (closing remarks)
In this 5th International Symposium on Methods in Clinical Pharmacology we have had the opportunity to exchange knowledge and opinions on this interesting theme alpha-, beta-blockade. The outcome is that we have experienced, without doubt, a most successful, stimulating, and enjoyable symposium. It is my first duty therefore in closing this symposium on behalf of everyone here, to extend our sincere thanks to Dr. Strauß and his collegues of the Cascan Company, Wiesbaden, for the sponsorship which they have generously given us. The speakers have done us an excellent service and we know that this does not happen from itself, but only comes from hard work. Symposium participants, whether addressing the podium, or listening, must invest energy and enthusiasm. Please allow me therefore to offer our thanks to both. Thank you also to our translators, audiovisuel technicians, and to the team at the registration bureau, who are part of us and have done a magnificant job. Professor Norbert Rietbrock and the symposium committee extend a sincere thank you to all, a safe journey and we look forward to meeting you once again soon.

Auf Wiedersehen!

Postskriptum

Wir danken unseren Freunden, Mitarbeitern und Kollegen, die das Symposium mit Rat, Tat und Einsatzbereitschaft unterstützt haben: Dr. R. Strauß, Eva-Maria Simmet-Bauer, Irmtrud Reben, Dr. H. Powilleit, U. Zickmann, Dr. W. Stehling, Helga Rebelein, Dr. W. Hotan, Beate Beutel, Elke Schrader, der Cascan GmbH & Co. KG Wiesbaden; Dr. S. H. Taylor vom University Department of Cardiovascular Studies, Leeds; Brigitte Käse, Prof. R. Kirsten von der Universitätsklinik, Frankfurt am Main.

Frankfurt am Main, im September 1984

Sachwortverzeichnis

für deutschsprachige Beiträge

Subject Index

for English contributions